You Don't Need a Hysterectomy

You Don't Need a Hysterectomy

2nd Edition

• • •

New and Effective Ways of Avoiding Major Surgery

Ivan K. Strausz, M.D.

Perseus Publishing
CAMBRIDGE, MASSACHUSETTS

2nd Edition Copyright 2001 © by Ivan K. Strausz, M.D.
ISBN: 0-7382-0449-8

Perseus Publishing is a member of the Perseus Books Group

Text design by Elizabeth Lahey
Set in Bembo 11 point

Printed in the United States of America.

Visit us on the World Wide Web at http://www.perseuspublishing.com

Perseus Publishing books are available at special discounts for bulk purchases in the U.S. by corporations, institutions, and other organizations. For more information, please contact the Special Markets Department at HarperCollins Publishers, 10 East 53rd Street, New York, NY 10022, or call 1–212–207–7528.

First printing, March 2001
1 2 3 4 5 6 7 8 9 10—03 02 01

• *Contents* •

• *List of Tables* •

• *List of Illustrations* •

• Foreword to the •
First Edition

Paula Brown Doress and Diana Laskin Siegal
Coauthors of *Ourselves, Growing Older*

The women's health movement that arose in the 1970s as part of the second wave of feminism brought new questions and insights about the ways that we as women view our bodies. We learned that our reproductive organs are not solely vehicles for childbearing, but like other body parts, have multiple functions. For example, the uterus and ovaries are involved in sexual response and secrete hormones both pre- and post-menopausally. Other reproductive organ functions may exist that are not yet fully understood. Thus, it is our opinion that the uterus is important to a woman's health and should not be removed unless absolutely necessary. Yet, for over a century in the United States, women's reproductive organs have been subject to medical abuse.

Consequently, more than one-third of all women in the United States today have had a hysterectomy by the age of sixty. It is estimated that 33 to 72 percent of hysterectomies are not medically necessary. Only 8 to 12 percent are performed to treat cancer or other life-threatening conditions. Though this information has been reported in the medical research literature and widely disseminated through feminist and consumer health publications, it has not always been clear how women can best make use of these facts when faced with a personal decision about hysterectomy.

It is therefore a great pleasure to recommend *You Don't Need a Hysterectomy*. In this book, Dr. Ivan Strausz challenges his colleagues' abuse of professional responsibility and trust. If you are struggling over whether your situation warrants surgery or whether other approaches, including simply waiting for menopause, would do just as well, this book will be helpful, clear, and informative for you.

Dr. Strausz presents a wealth of detailed information to help you understand your reproductive system and the processes that often lead physicians to recommend hysterectomy. Here, you will find uniquely helpful insights on endometriosis, fibroids, chronic pelvic pain, the heavy bleeding (or menorrhagia) characteristic of the pre-menopausal years, as well as cancers of the cervix, endometrium, and ovaries.

Women are less likely to be railroaded into surgery once they understand upsetting but ordinary occurrences such as erratic or heavy periods, the development of fibroids, small changes in cervical cells, and other fairly commonplace symptoms that precede unnecessary hysterectomies. Dr. Strausz explains these situations well and offers medical approaches for managing them. The reader who wants to try nonmedical approaches will have to look elsewhere.

Dr. Strausz is most critical of surgery and less critical of other medical approaches. For example, in our view, his chapter on menopause is more favorable to hormonal therapy for post-menopausal women than we are, though he does include some of the questions and controversies regarding such treatment.

Despite this difference in emphasis, we feel that Dr. Strausz presents the facts about hysterectomy forthrightly and factually in a helpfully designed format. He is open to learning from women, his editors, and the women's health literature, but most important, his patients. Unlike many physicians writing for the general reader, Dr. Strausz reports and discusses all sides of controversies within the medical community on the topic of hysterectomy. Some readers may find this approach confusing, but it is necessary if we are to make our own informed decisions. Dr. Strausz encourages such investigation and offers both information and opinions clearly stated so that the reader can draw her own conclusions.

• *Foreword to the* •
Second Edition

Much has changed since the early 1990s when the first edition of this book was written, but the story of unnecessary hysterectomies has continued largely unchanged. During most of the 1980s, hysterectomy numbers in the United States hovered around 650,000 a year. Between 1988 and 1994 there was a decrease to approximately 550,000 hysterectomies annually: an improvement, but not as much as might have been achieved. However, in 1995 and 1996, the numbers began to increase again. By 1997, there were slightly over 600,000 hysterectomies, and in 1998, there were 645,000 (these are the last two years for which statistics are currently available). In other words, after a transient drop, we are back where we started. It is clear that the business of performing hysterectomies has recovered nicely; it is a healthy and thriving undertaking again.

On the positive side, there has been a gratifying expansion of gynecological interest in and research into chronic pelvic pain, the reason for about 60,000 hysterectomies a year. Trying to understand this mysterious disease and publicizing what little was known about it during the 1980s led me to write the first edition of this book; this occurred at a time when I was acutely aware of the misery of many disappointed women whose problems with severe pelvic pain were not relieved by hysterectomy.

During the mid-1990s, a promising new treatment for chronic pelvic pain appeared: injections of medications that induce temporary menopause. This is not a treatment to be recommended lightly. However, many women with severe chronic pelvic pain (CPP) suffer so intensely from their many symptoms that any new and apparently successful treatment warrants careful consideration. Moreover, many of the unwanted side effects of these medications can now be controlled by hormonal means. Also, all the menopausal and other effects of these complex treatments are reversible. Should they prove difficult to accept, the injections can be discontinued, with the reasonably rapid disappearance of all unpleasant symptoms. This, of course, differs sharply from hysterectomy, which, if it does not relieve pain, is a major and irreversible setback for the woman who had pinned her hopes on surgery that would return her life to her.

During the last eight years, we have also learned that hysterectomy might help at least some women with chronic pelvic pain. These women, because their symptoms improved after hysterectomy, no longer crowd into gynecologists' offices. Gynecologists see "hysterectomy failures" much more often than they see "hysterectomy successes"; they remember these women well because of their many stubborn and continuing symptoms. The fate of these women colors the pessimistic view many gynecologists have of the operation. Hysterectomy for CPP remains such an exceptionally controversial subject among gynecologists and is so important to women considering such surgery that I have devoted an extensive section in Chapter 11 to discussing, in considerable detail, what is known about it.

Also, since the publication of the first edition of this book, a large number of new operations have come into use, potentially replacing hysterectomy as the gynecologist's first choice for most pelvic problems. Fibroids, bleeding problems, and endometriosis have been the main reasons for performing hysterectomies in recent decades; I am pleased to be able to report that the new medical and surgical treatments I'll describe offer considerable improvements over hysterectomy.

A discouraging development in the medical world has been the emergence of "health maintenance organizations" (or HMOs), currently prime providers of medical care for millions of women. HMOs have limited the costs of medical care. This is an important consideration for all of us as individuals, but also for labor unions and for corporations large and small intent on controlling costs. However, HMOs have also limited the time physicians are able to spend with their patients, an exceptionally troublesome development for all concerned. In addition, women may no longer have easy access to physicians who might be best suited to treat them or to the surgery that might help them. Wherever possible, I have paid attention to these difficult problems and have suggested solutions to help solve them.

I dedicate this edition to women with chronic pelvic pain, whose symptoms have often eluded an easy solution. I hope that with recent advances, their health will improve as much as the hysterectomy business has improved. I also hope that a close reading of this book will remedy at least some of their problems.

New York, September 2000

• *Acknowledgments* •

Much of whatever is valuable in this book is due to the untiring work of my agent, Ellen Levine, who organized my meager writing skills, provided much-needed editorial direction from the beginning to the end, and helped me in ways too numerous to mention.

I would also like to thank my editors, Nancy Miller, Meg Fry, and Carmen Wheatcroft. They understood complex biological ideas rapidly and frequently suggested ideas I should have had myself. They taught me to write sensitively for and about women and, most important, often gave my gynecological jargon a more professional finish.

Many others also helped to shape this book. The staff in the Medical Library at Metropolitan Hospital in New York City, for example, searched the medical literature for information from obscure sources with unfailing speed and courtesy. My colleague at New York Medical College and at Metropolitan Hospital, Dr. Elmer Agustin, read many chapters and offered ideas to expand and clarify my thinking. Harriette Johnson's comments on statistical concepts were invaluable. Dr. Richard Malen was helpful with suggestions on psychiatric matters. I am grateful to Drs. Robert S. Neuwirth at St. Luke's–Roosevelt Hospital Center, Hussein Amin of Albert Einstein College of Medicine, and Glenn Hofman of Mt. Sinai Medical Center, all in New York City, for their expertise. Dr. David Redwine of Bend, Oregon, gave me his thoughts on endometriosis; Drs. Andrea Rapkin from Los Angeles and Judith Lewis Herman from Somerville, Massachusetts, confirmed my ideas about chronic pelvic pain. In earlier years, much inspiration and education came from the Rape Intervention Program at St. Luke's–Roosevelt Hospital Center in New York City, particularly from Mary Anderson, Julie Blackman, Ellen Doherty, and Susan Xenarios. I could not have achieved much without help and encouragement from all the above.

• *Introduction* •

The United States leads the world in hysterectomy rates, an achievement that is hardly a reason for pride. American women are up to five or six times as likely to have a hysterectomy as are women from other medically sophisticated countries, a disparity difficult to justify. Gynecologists know that many hysterectomies are performed unnecessarily, because there are frank discussions of the subject in professional journals and textbooks. However, the prevailing attitude is that the unneeded operations are done elsewhere, by other gynecologists. Hospitals have rules that should prevent unnecessary surgery, but hysterectomy statistics show that these have had little impact.

The reasons for this unsatisfactory situation are, I believe, partly financial and partly a consequence of professional inertia: the tendency to continue to think tomorrow exactly as you thought yesterday. On the financial front, hospitals must watch their balance sheets as carefully as business executives do; empty sessions in operating rooms and hospital beds vacant for days on end are a much more immediate source of anxiety than a very remote abstraction: the fact that women have had surgery that could have been avoided. Also, routine hysterectomies provide a comfortable way of life for many physicians. However, in the medical universe, inertia may be as potent a force as gravity, just as strong as the pull of financial considerations. An excellent study published in February 2000 in *Obstetrics and Gynecology*, perhaps the most popular professional journal American gynecologists read, shows that hysterectomy is still often recommended without trying alternative treatments. The study also points out that official guidelines published by the American College of Obstetricians and Gynecologists and other prestigious organizations such as the Rand Corporation are routinely disregarded. This is old news; I mention the article because it contains a nugget of new information: Unnecessary hysterectomies are commonly performed by salaried gynecologists who do not profit directly from doing these operations. And, of course, there may be many other nonmedical reasons for some of the unnecessary hysterectomies. For instance, you may be interested in an exchange of letters published in the *British Medical Journal* in 1997. One of these was from John Bunker, a visiting American professor, who, in a sharp retort to his Italian colleagues, expressed his opinion that American and Swiss gynecologists may find it "often more efficient, and possibly less expensive, to operate than to take the time to educate a patient and to treat [her] medically."

This book teaches you how to identify a hysterectomy that is probably unnecessary. It also shows you how to avoid hysterectomy for diseases that prompt even responsible gynecologists to reach for the scalpel. Hysterectomies currently rank second only to cesarean sections on the list of operations commonly performed by obstetrician-gynecologists (OB/GYNs) in the United States. However, during the last twenty years, a large number of new diagnostic procedures, medications, and operations have become available. If gynecological care of high quality were available to all women, and if American women availed themselves of this care in good time (before, for instance, fibroids grew to unwieldy sizes), hysterectomy could be displaced from its current ranking, after cesarean sections, as the second most often performed obstetrics/gynecology (OB/GYN) operation.

Of course, there are exceptions, but with current technology, the only hysterectomies that are absolutely unavoidable are those performed for cancer or in response to a massive, life-threatening infection or hemorrhage. These problems account for an estimated 12 to 15 percent of American hysterectomies. The remainder are potentially avoidable or can be postponed for months (or even for years) with the new treatments. This delay may be an important advantage if you wish to, for example, finish your studies or take an important trip before undergoing surgery. Also, if you are close to your menopause, you may find that you can avoid surgery altogether by using medical treatments until its spontaneous onset. Most important, you may have emotional, philosophical, or simple practical reasons to avoid surgery, particularly if the need for the operation is less than clear-cut or if it can be postponed without jeopardizing your health and well-being.

Your success in avoiding hysterectomy will depend on your gynecological condition, on the medical community in which you live, and on your efforts in educating yourself about the choices open to you. However, neither patient advocacy nor patient welfare would be well served by recommendations based on ideological considerations against surgery without looking at medical factors. For the patient who truly needs one, hysterectomy is a good operation, one that may cure cancer, is virtually certain to relieve vaginal bleeding, and often helps pain. Unfortunately, many American gynecologists resort to hysterectomy carelessly and too often, a practice that almost amounts to systematic deception of women in favor of this operation. Too many hysterectomies are recommended by gynecologists whose ideas appear to date back to the end of the nineteenth century, when ovaries were removed simply because the operation was so much in vogue, and was in vogue for such absurd reasons, that women were flocking to surgeons asking for it. Sad to say, even today, when treatment alternatives are discussed, women often rely on incomplete or misleading information instead of an honest and full disclosure of well-established facts.

Your Diagnosis

Your diagnosis is not as fixed as you may think: it may warrant change after close scrutiny. Fibroids, growths of the uterus which are almost always noncancerous, may be confused with solid ovarian tumors, which are usually malignant. Heavy bleeding may be due to undetected polyps, which are fleshy and fingerlike benign growths of the lining layers of the womb, instead of fibroids. The list of possible errors is long, and not only because some diagnoses may be carelessly or imprecisely made. Diseases may mimic each other or offer only faint clues to their presence, eventually surprising even the most careful diagnostician. A brief look at some examples of diagnostic mistakes and difficulties follows:

•A businesswoman in her early thirties had suffered for years with abdominal pains. Her gynecologist performed a laparoscopy, an operation in which the surgeon inspects the organs in the pelvis and the abdominal cavity. He found no disease, but the pains continued. A year later, I repeated the laparoscopy and found subtle but definite signs of a disease called endometriosis. These signs might have appeared between the two operations, but more likely they went unnoticed at the time of the first laparoscopy. With the correct diagnosis, and with modern treatments, the woman's pains vanished. The chapters on endometriosis and chronic pelvic pain will explain how you can ensure that you will not encounter such a delay in treatment.

•Hysterectomy was scheduled for a woman who had an ovarian cyst. The presence of the cyst was confirmed by three ultrasound examinations, which use sound waves to outline internal organs. Heart disease and obesity put the patient at high risk. At surgery, no cyst was found. Afterward, the patient developed serious complications, including a pulmonary embolus, a clot of blood that lodges in the lungs, cutting off vital circulation.

The woman could have died of this, but she recovered after a two-week hospital stay, much of it in an intensive care unit. The error in her case was that the last vaginal examination and pelvic ultrasound (also called a sonogram, the terms are interchangeable) were performed five weeks before her operation. Contrary to common sense, neither was repeated the night before her surgery. Some ovarian cysts come and go; information that is five weeks old may not represent the current situation. The last chapter of this book, which deals with the ovaries and the menopause, discusses which ovarian cysts are harmless and should be left alone. It also explains which cysts should be investigated and treated aggressively, either because cancer is a possibility or because complications are likely.

•As a tragic but unavoidable event, I recall a pregnant woman whose sonograms showed, in addition to her pregnancy, shadows that were thought to be caused by three or four small fibroid tumors. Subsequent sonograms received similar interpretations. Much later, she needed a cesarean section, at which, to common astonishment, widespread ovarian cancer was found in addition to a few small fibroids. Careful reviews of her scans revealed no clues to the more important diagnosis; in fact, there was no practical way to make this diagnosis earlier. Shocking as that episode was, all that could be learned from it was that no investigation is invariably accurate. Such events may happen to patients in competent hands; your protection is that they happen very rarely. Fibroids and ovarian cancer, two important subjects, will be discussed in detail in corresponding Chapters 6 and 14.

•A woman we'll call Dea had used a copper loop intrauterine device (IUCD) for contraception for a number of years without problems. Her menstrual period, which was a week late, finally began while she was urinating. Dea felt a sharp cramp in her pelvis, so much worse than her usual cramps that she almost fainted. She fell sideways against the wall of the bathroom and hurt her shoulder. She went to a nearby emergency room, where she was examined; blood tests were taken, and her shoulder was x-rayed. Since none of the tests revealed any abnormalities, Dea received a pain medication and was sent home.

The shoulder pain worsened, and later the same day, Dea went to another emergency room. Her menstrual flow and cramps were also severe, but the staff paid no attention to this. The tests now showed a slight anemia, but the emergency room personnel were too busy to call the first hospital to compare the two blood counts. Her shoulder x-rays were again normal. Dea got another prescription for the same basic pain medication and was again sent home to rest.

The shoulder pains gradually got even more severe, and the next morning Dea went to a third hospital, where she was examined more carefully. Staff now noted that her stomach was slightly swollen, her pulse was fast, and her blood pressure was low—Dea was about to go into shock. Her blood count showed marked anemia. For the first time, a pregnancy test was ordered, and this came back positive. Now it was easy to understand what had happened. Dea had a large internal hemorrhage, caused by a tubal (ectopic) pregnancy that is not prevented by intrauterine devices. Ectopic pregnancies typically cause lower abdominal and shoulder pains accompanied by vaginal bleeding. Dea had all of these suggestive symptoms all along, but they were misunderstood in the first two emergency rooms. Within an hour, she had an operation and recovered rapidly.

I always teach medical students assigned to me for the OB/GYN course that any woman sexually active with a male partner is potentially pregnant and that they must not fail to think about this possibility. Chapter 6, which deals with fibroids, will also explain how you can check yourself for signs of a serious internal hemorrhage.

As you can see, it is not always easy to be sure that your diagnosis is correct. Diseases are unpredictable. Symptoms may be so subtle that no one realizes their significance until something unmistakable such as pain or bleeding focuses attention on them. Even if your gynecologist listens carefully to you and arranges all the investigations appropriate for your care, some unexpected development may drastically alter your situation. However, for most diseases discussed in this book, it is possible to be reasonably certain that your diagnosis is correct. Armed with the facts, you can also ensure that you will receive quality care. To help with these objectives, this book pays particular attention to questions you may have concerning your diagnosis. Careful reading of the materials dealing with your complaints will tell you if your diagnosis is probably correct, or perhaps incomplete, or downright incorrect. You will also find a detailed discussion of all your treatment options, from doing nothing to undergoing the latest medical and surgical treatments.

Your Gynecologist

The medical community that serves your area has much to do with your chances of successful diagnosis and treatment. If you live in a small town and the two gynecologists available both urge you to have a hysterectomy, it will require diplomacy of high order on your part to decline the surgery but continue to use either physician for your ongoing gynecological needs. A consultation with an expert at the nearest academic medical center should improve your ability to deal with the problem. In larger metropolitan areas, you ought to be able to find gynecologists with the requisite skills who are willing to help you avoid surgery. You are fortunate if you already have a gynecologist who is competent and whom you can trust. The difficulties of finding a good gynecologist are the same as the difficulties of finding any competent professional. The suggestions that follow should help you with your search.

As a minimum requirement, your gynecologist must be certified by passing two examinations—one written, one oral—conducted by the American Board of Obstetrics and Gynecology. Once certified, he or she is eligible to become a Fellow of the American College of Obstetricians and Gynecologists. No one is allowed to complete this examination until two years have passed following completion of training, so that his or her performance as a practicing gynecologist may be assessed as part of the examination. Having recently completed a training program would be one acceptable reason for a practitioner to not be board certified.

You can find out if a physician is board certified in any specialty by consulting a variety of publications that list the qualifications of American physicians. This information and more extensive biographical data are easily available from medical directories in public libraries. These will tell you when and from which medical school a physician graduated and where he or she was trained. This is good basic information to have, but it will not help you locate an excellent physician. The professionals most familiar with the capabilities of gynecologists in your community are the young residents who assist them. Operating room nurses are also shrewd judges of doctors' surgical skills: They see which surgeons get into trouble frequently, and they know who is called to rescue them. If you have any access to operating room nurses or OB/GYN residents, who may be the friends or relatives of people you know, consult with them.

You can also call, or better yet, visit the departmental administrator or executive secretary of the department of OB/GYN at a nearby medical school or large hospital. Explain that you need a referral, but first find out if gynecologists' names are handed out in rotation. (This system is fair, and is in common use). Explain what your problem is, and ask to be referred to an expert. This direct approach should net you the most qualified gynecologist, one with the intelligence and expertise you need, rather than one picked at random, or alphabetically. Even departments of OB/GYN in prestigious hospitals may have one or two gynecologists whose judgment and surgical skills are not as secure as they should be, and these may well be the same practitioners who will think that there is nothing wrong with performing a hysterectomy for inadequate reasons. A personal appeal for help will most likely steer you away from less competent gynecologists toward experts and specialists.

Asking another physician for a referral is not necessarily a wise idea. Your internist does not necessarily know which gynecologist is the best surgeon in town, or who is the most up-to-date with the use of hormones. He or she may give you the names of one or two excellent gynecologists, but you may also get a "reflex" recommendation to a physician with average abilities. If you trust your physician, whatever his or her specialty, preface your request by explaining that you need a carefully considered referral, one that will need to be researched through the chairperson of a reputable department of OB/GYN. Spell out the problem and emphasize your expectations; then proceed with the other approaches already outlined. If the same name crops up from different sources, you have probably found the best gynecologist for your problem.

Relying on the advice of family or friends should be left to the last, unless they are unusually critical persons who are sophisticated about medical care. These attributes are necessary to avoid a common error: mistaking confident airs and good bedside manners for clinical ability. Even successful care may not be proof of competence.

•A friend of mine, a professor at a prestigious university, was very impressed with the gynecologist who saved her daughter's life when her pregnancy lodged in a fallopian tube, rupturing it and causing a substantial intra-abdominal hemorrhage. However, the diagnosis and treatment were so obvious that a competent resident could have managed the emergency equally well, and perhaps better. In the course of the surgery, the gynecologist removed most of one of the young woman's ovaries, an outdated measure that should have been avoided. There may be adverse consequences for her fertility and future health should the remaining ovary eventually develop a disease that necessitates its removal.

This way of looking at medical care may be tough, but I think it is fair. Unfortunately, medical care of consistently high quality is often a Utopian—and therefore largely unobtainable—ideal. Few of us have constant access to caring and highly intelligent, humanitarian nurses and expert physicians. The introduction of computers into day-to-day clinical decisionmaking might at some future time improve the quality of care you receive; at present it is entirely up to you to find the best practitioners and hospitals available.

Taking Responsibility for Your Own Care

Even the most competent and conscientious gynecologist may not concentrate on you, your illness, and your treatment as thoroughly as needed. Also, too much medical care is delivered in a rushed setting, with an office full with other patients, telephone calls, and the odd emergency crowding the consultation that should be exclusively yours. Your success in avoiding hysterectomy will be proportional not only to the severity of your disease but to your determination in pursuing your goal. Just as the jailhouse lawyer pursues his freedom by learning the law, you must persevere with your aim of avoiding hysterectomy by learning gynecology. This book will assist you with a wealth of detail not usually found in medical self-help books. In some instances, after reading this book, you may be better informed about some aspect of gynecology than your gynecologist. This is, I think, the ideal situation, in which you have maximized your chances of receiving the best possible care.

A good friend of mine was repeatedly advised by her group of gynecologists to undergo hysterectomy: first for abnormal bleeding, then for abnormal Pap smears. This exceptionally intelligent and accomplished young woman called me each time surgery was recommended to discuss the situation. I usually sent her copies of relevant pages from textbooks and medical journals to read, and we always found ways of averting hysterectomy. Then, a few days after minor gynecological surgery, a sudden hemorrhage occurred. Her gynecologist did not heed either the bleeding she had or the telltale warning signs she told him about: the appearance of tiny rose-colored hemorrhagic spots all over her body.

In this emergency, she became my patient. It was unexpectedly difficult to operate on a close friend suffering from a life-threatening hemorrhage. She required complicated medical care, including abdominal surgery, but hysterectomy was again avoided. Now, twenty years later, she is past her menopause, but she still has her womb. It is not causing any symptoms, and I know that she is happy with the care she received from me. Her bleeding was not due to gynecological disease, and hysterectomy would not have helped. The bleeding was caused by a rare condition, the virtual disappearance from her blood of platelets, tiny cells essential in arresting bleeding by sealing the slow leakage that occurs gradually from normal blood vessels, and, in her case, from vessels bruised and cut during her recent gynecological surgery. The care she received from me and from the consultant specialists I brought in saved her life.

Financial Matters

Americans spend an astonishing amount of money on health care. According to a comparative analysis released in 1998 in Paris by the Organization for Economic Cooperation and Development, we spent approximately $4,000 per person for health care in 1997. The corresponding figure for Switzerland, the next most expensive country, was about $2,500 per person—a significant difference. If your insurance is good, it will pay all (or most) of your expenses. If you are uninsured or poorly insured, you are in a difficult situation, because the gynecological care outlined in this book is not inexpensive. There is only one way of getting expert medical or surgical care at a lower cost: by becoming a "clinic" or "service" patient in an academic hospital with an excellent reputation. This means that your care will be the responsibility of resident staff, who are supervised by older and more experienced personnel.

Clinic care has received poor press. Its quality may vary, but it may not be worse than what you may count on in private care. There will be discomforts such as long waits in full waiting rooms, and there may be a rotating staff of younger residents to look after you, but I have seen women receive better care at a good public facility than from certain practitioners in private practice. You may consider clinic care as a last resort only, but it is not necessarily a backward step. For instance, if you need laser surgery and cannot afford to get it through a private gynecologist, you may be better served as a clinic patient. If this is acceptable to you, the following steps should help you to obtain the best care for the least cost:

1. Pick the most prestigious and best hospital near your home that has a large OB/GYN clinic service.
2. Make an appointment to meet with the chief resident in charge of gynecological surgery.
3. Bring along all the documentation with a bearing on your disease: surgical reports, x-rays, copies of Pap smears, and pathology reports.
4. Explain what you would like to have done and ask if there is a senior gynecologist on the consulting staff of the hospital who might be able to help. If there is, the chief resident will know how to arrange the surgery. If you are in good health and there is no emergency, there may be a choice between being admitted to the hospital or using an ambulatory surgical facility (arriving in the morning and going home in the evening). If possible, choose the second option. Whoever pays the bills, hospital care is expensive. More important, mistakes are more likely to occur in the hospital than in your own home.
5. Never accept last-minute substitutions of either the surgeon or the procedure, unless some obvious emergency (such as a hemor-

rhage—your hemorrhage and not that of another patient) dictates this change. If need be, politely but firmly postpone the surgery until the previously agreed-upon plan can be carried out.

6. If the chief resident cannot help you, ask to be referred to another hospital that may be better staffed or equipped to serve your needs.

This book was written primarily to help women avert hysterectomy. However, since the book deals with frequent gynecological complaints, it should also help women who do not need surgery understand many of their symptoms. Doctors' explanations, I regret to say, are often incomplete and vague, and the current emphasis on "productivity"—taking care of more patients every working day—has made for even less time that can be spent on leisurely explanations or exchanges. Unless you help yourself by educating yourself, you may well receive inferior care. If you read about your symptoms as thoroughly as you can before your appointment, you will become an informed consumer. You will ask better questions and get better answers, assuring superior gynecological care.

··· I ···

Avoiding Hysterectomy

In October 1945, during festivities surrounding the fiftieth anniversary of the Chicago Lying-in Hospital, one of the speakers broke ranks with his celebrating colleagues. The dissenter was Norman Miller, an outspoken gynecologist from Ann Arbor, Michigan, who made the short trip to Chicago with a provocative address packed in his briefcase. Based on responses he received to a questionnaire he had sent to Midwestern gynecologists earlier the same year, the speech carried the pointed title, "Hysterectomy: Therapeutic Necessity or Surgical Racket?" Miller presented a terse condemnation of the common practice of performing hysterectomies for reasons that were dubious at best and nonexistent at worst.

The following year, Miller's paper was published in the *American Journal of Obstetrics and Gynecology*, the most prestigious and widely read OB/GYN journal of the day. Subsequent studies, all appearing in authoritative publications such as the *Journal of the American Medical Association* (in 1953), and the *New England Journal of Medicine* (in 1976), agreed with Norman Miller. Almost without exception, they showed that very likely at least 25 percent, and possibly as many as 43 percent, of hysterectomies performed in the United States were unnecessary. The scandal that began to brew was not confined to quarreling between idealistic reformers and mainstream practitioners but reached a subcommittee of the U.S. House of

Representatives in 1977. As a result, federal programs such as Medicare and Medicaid began to require a validating second opinion before hysterectomy and certain other operations were authorized.

Traditionally slow to change their ways and indifferent to the groundswell of criticism, American gynecologists responded resourcefully by finding reasons to perform, year after year, ever larger numbers of hysterectomies. The tide crested in 1975, when more than 740,000 American women underwent this major operation. After that year, hysterectomies continued to be performed at gradually decreasing, but still near record-breaking, levels. During the early 1980s, each year brought over 600,000 hysterectomies. In 1988, this number dropped to 571,000; in 1989, the number was reported at 533,000. Similar figures were reported annually until 1996, when nearly 600,000 hysterectomies were performed. In 1997 and 1998 (the last years for which such statistics are available), the figures were 603,000 and 645,000, respectively. These figures need certain qualifications—for instance, population growth might have been expected to cause modest increases in the numbers of hysterectomies, with newer operations causing a decrease—nevertheless, it seems to me that the hysterectomy business has recovered nicely and is healthy again. I am not writing this book to condemn all hysterectomies—many are performed with good reason, and these operations have good results. Unfortunately, too many others are done without a good reason; this book is dedicated to preventing the continued and indefensible deluge of unnecessary hysterectomies.

Hysterectomy statistics were first collected in 1965 by the National Center for Health Statistics (NCHS), a branch of the Department of Health and Human Services. According to the Center's figures, the hysterectomy business grew by an impressive 68 percent during the ten-year span from 1965 to 1975, a dramatic increase in striking contrast to the stable levels of most other surgical activities. During the 1960s and 1970s, hysterectomy was the most frequently performed surgery in the United States, even though only half the population could have it: women. Contemporary estimates showed that if the trend continued, at least a third, and possibly half, of all women would lose their wombs to surgery by the age of sixty-five.

Independent of hysterectomies, there was an even sharper upswing in the use of another major operation also performed by obstetrician-gynecologists. By 1981, cesarean sections overtook hysterectomy as the operation most often performed in the United States. However, women began to show increased vigilance and resistance to surgery that could be avoided. Books denouncing hysterectomy began to appear. These documented the continuing plague of unnecessary hysterectomies and discussed legitimate reasons for surgery such as large fibroids, severe endometriosis, and excessive bleeding. However, since there were not many alternatives, more space was devoted to hysterectomy and to ways of coping with this operation than to ways of avoiding it.

Until the 1970s, not much else could be done for most women who were told that they needed this operation. For instance, only a small number of hormones were available to control irregular and excessive bleeding, one of the most frequent causes of hysterectomy. Because their effectiveness was usually short-lived, gynecologists rarely persevered with hormones. Using available hormonal treatments, and despite curettages, the bleeding usually recurred. Not unreasonably, neither patients nor gynecologists had much enthusiasm for approaches that did not guarantee a cure. If the onset of menopause did not resolve the situation, surgery was the gynecologist's ace, the accepted way of restoring health and allowing the patient to resume her normal existence. Myomectomy, the piecemeal removal of fibroids, was practiced more by enthusiasts than by rank-and-file gynecologists. Fibroids could grow back after myomectomy, whereas hysterectomy offered a definite cure. Unnecessary hysterectomy could not be condoned, but the frequent recourse of American gynecologists to hysterectomy was understandable at least in part.

Of the approximately 600,000 women who still undergo this operation in the United States each year, about 500 will die as a direct consequence of the surgery. Others develop complications physicians call "morbidity." This word, derived from the Latin *morbus*, meaning disease, covers a wide range of adverse outcomes. Some are mere nuisances, such as transient fevers after surgery that vanish without treatment; others are serious complications. One of these, for example, is bowel obstruction, an abrupt and life-threatening emergency that must be corrected immediately by skilled surgery. In addition to surgical complications, some women feel psychologically traumatized by the loss of their uterus well after other women have recovered. Overall acceptance of the operation is good, particularly after symptoms such as pain and bleeding have been relieved. As discussed by Kristen H. Kjerulff and her associates in the March 2000 issue of *Obstetrics and Gynecology*, many women felt significantly improved after hysterectomy, with fewer symptoms, better psychologic functioning, and an improved quality of life. However, it is also true that a small percentage of women reacted very poorly, developing serious symptoms that were difficult to treat successfully after surgery.

Unfortunately for gynecologists, many of the ill effects of hysterectomy are immediate and easy to document. In addition to other drawbacks, the fate of the ovaries must be considered. The older a women is when she has a hysterectomy, the more likely it is that she will lose her ovaries. According to information published in 1997 by the Centers for Disease Control and Prevention (CDC), the large and prestigious governmental organization based in Atlanta, Georgia, 51 percent of all women who underwent hysterectomy between 1988 and 1993 were castrated in this fashion. The word *castration* has an ominous sound to it, partly because of the male fear of losing testicles, outward emblems of masculinity. Castration is the excision of gonads, testicles, or ovaries; its physiological consequences are more wide-ranging and damaging in women. And even if left behind, perfectly good ovaries may be inadvertently knocked out of action by an apparently uneventful hysterectomy.

Although expert opinion is far from unanimous, gynecologists are generally unaware of this possibility or are unconcerned with its results. Losing ovarian hormones has serious implications for women whose ovaries are erroneously thought to be intact and functioning: These women become menopausal within a year or two of the hysterectomy. If they do not get menopausal symptoms such as hot flashes, possibly neither the woman nor her gynecologist will understand the seriousness of the situation, and the estrogen these women have quietly lost may not be replaced. Veronica Ravnikar, a Boston gynecologist, also showed in 1989 that if a hormone prescription is given, the patient may not have it filled. Even if bought, the drugs may be discontinued within a few months without revisiting the prescriber for a discussion of the consequences. Because of the lack of estrogen, women may become prone to developing coronary artery disease and osteoporosis, the difficult-to-replace loss of bone tissue, which leads to fractures. These conditions are far easier to prevent than to treat. Hysterectomy with, or even without, the excision of the ovaries may be followed many years later by a heart attack or a fall that fractures a forearm or a hip.

Neither the woman's internist nor her orthopedic surgeon is likely to pay much attention to the patient's ancient gynecological history, even though her surgery may have been at least partly responsible for the heart attack or the fracture. This sequence is a travesty of intelligent and effective preventive care.

Of course, the benefits of hysterectomy are clear-cut when dealing with a serious hemorrhage. A woman may begin to bleed faster than her blood can be replaced with transfusions, and conventional measures may fail to stanch the hemorrhage. This can occur after normal childbirth or after a cesarean section; it may also happen to women who have large fibroids. In these cases, hysterectomy may be lifesaving because, particularly in an emergency, there are few other ways to save the woman's life. For other women who have cancer, hysterectomy may still be essential. But most hysterectomies are not performed to treat cancer or an uncontrollable hemorrhage. Nine out of ten of these operations are done electively, with the promise of eliminating troublesome symptoms and thereby improving the woman's quality of life. This may be true in some cases, but too often hysterectomy is performed with less benefit to the patient than commonly realized. Well before the scalpel is taken out of its sterile wrapper, a critical review could help avoid many operations. At long last, such strict reviews are beginning to be done not months or years following the surgery, but in time to prevent it.

In recent decades, the notion of avoiding hysterectomy has become a public issue of great importance. During these years, the panorama of medical care changed substantially. First came an almost fourfold increase in the use of cesarean sections, with benefits that almost all obstetricians and most patients appreciate, yet benefits that (due to statistical problems) remain elusively difficult to prove. At the same time, physicians began to face financial and consumer pressures to reduce their reliance on surgery. The financial pressures originated with those who paid most of the surgical bills: insurance companies, governmental agencies, and large corporations. Cutting medical costs became a national preoccupation, and within a few years, "second opinion" consultations and elaborate mechanisms for approving (or rejecting) surgery in advance became necessary for a whole range of operations. Executives, labor leaders, and physicians began to use a new language with punchy but complex phrases such as "outcome measurement," "evidence-based medicine," and "cost-effectiveness," concepts barely on the horizon twenty years earlier. Other pressures originated with consumer advocates and medical pioneers.

But change was slow in coming. It took decades before surgeons such as George Crile Jr. in Cleveland and Oliver Cope in Boston as well as consumer advocates like Rose Kushner finally convinced American surgeons of a single detail—that for early breast cancer, a partial mastectomy (popularly known as lumpectomy) was an acceptable treatment alternative to the more disfiguring, traditional radical mastectomy.

In the early 1980s, the AIDS epidemic arrived with an avalanche of news broadcasts—a situation that emerged day by day, but was always terrible. Soon it became known that transfusions of blood could cause AIDS, shown most dramatically by hemophiliacs who developed the disease after receiving transfusions. As a distant but unfailingly lethal specter began to loom closer and closer, large numbers of patients began to shy away from any elective surgery that might require transfusions. Women also became increasingly outspoken about their ideas and expectations from the medical establishment, and began to feel free to complain and criticize patterns in which they saw unfairness or misogyny. Not surprisingly, there were plenty of targets for their criticism. High American hysterectomy rates became not only one more focal point of public interest but also a concern of enormous significance to women who were advised to have the operation.

Fortunately, during the last two decades, the news began to improve, particularly for women who were suffering from diseases such as fibroids, endometriosis, and bleeding problems. These conditions have, in recent years, accounted for the majority of American hysterectomies. New ideas and treatments, previously only employed by a few gynecological pioneers in limited clinical trials, became available for more widespread use. Increasing numbers of myomectomies and other, newer operations began to be performed in preference to hysterectomy. Also, a burgeoning number of new medications appeared, competing with hysterectomy as well as the new surgical alternatives to it. A new and successful treatment also became available for women suffering from chronic pelvic pain—abdominal and pelvic pain often associated with other intractable symptoms. In short, effective new choices became available for a wide range of gynecological problems for which hysterectomy used to be recommended.

Some years ago in my private practice in New York City, I began to see patients refuse to accept hysterectomy in a passive way. One of my patients was Judith, an artist in her early forties, a smart and likeable woman. She had a number of small and medium-sized fibroids, which had recently begun to cause symptoms. Occasional heavy periods, unexpectedly severe menstrual cramps, and recurring bladder infections combined to spell the beginnings of trouble. She came to me for a second opinion and made a telltale comment, in dismissive tones, about her then-current gynecologist. He had recommended hysterectomy, and she wanted to find other means to deal with her problem. Judith noticed that the gynecologist (a man I knew as an average and reasonably competent practitioner, but not someone particularly attuned to intelligent and outspoken young women) was not interested in avoiding surgery.

Judith had three choices. She could have a hysterectomy or undergo myomectomy. Her uterus, normally the size and shape of a small pear, was now almost as large as a pineapple, and Judith's symptoms were beginning to be bothersome. By conventional gynecological teaching, these two factors, or "indications" as physicians call them, were adequate to justify either operation. If Judith decided to have surgery, she would have an approximately 2–3 percent chance of serious complications. But the fibroids were not all that large, and her symptoms were only recent. Myomectomy seemed a better operation for her, but there was no compelling reason to have this operation immediately. In fact, there was no urgency to the situation, and there was a third course open to her. This was the more conservative course of inaction: that is, waiting to see what would happen without surgery.

A rapid calculation showed that Judith's chances of running into serious trouble without an operation were much the same: about 2–3 percent. A sudden hemorrhage while she was at the wheel of her car, tied up in stalled traffic on a busy highway, was a dramatic but very unlikely possibility. Cancerous changes in the uterus or in the fibroids themselves were another possibility, but these happen to well under 1 percent of patients like Judith, and this risk was acceptable to her. My only concern was the possibility that this accomplished and personable woman might develop ovarian cancer while she was under observation. This occurs in about 1.0 or 1.5 percent of all women over their entire life span, whether they have fibroids or not. And whenever this happens, much soul-searching follows, with an inevitable questioning of the wisdom of not operating and removing the uterus with the ovaries. Clearly, I had to discuss this possibility with Judith, along with the fact that she would take much the same chance if she went

7

ahead with either hysterectomy or myomectomy but instructed me to leave her ovaries in place.

Judith was willing to accept the remote possibility of developing ovarian cancer, an intractable and often fatal condition discussed in Chapter 14. Since there was no need to make an immediate decision, I gave her written information about the advantages and disadvantages of removing the uterus with or without the ovaries and about myomectomy, asking her to return to see me when she was ready. When I saw her next, we spent a few more minutes on the difficulties of the timely diagnosis of ovarian and certain other cancers. Unfortunately, some of these have a bad outcome even if detected and treated early, which they rarely are.

When she left my office, Judith had decided against surgery. Instead, she had a prescription for iron tablets and an antiprostaglandin medication. These drugs, taken just before and during a period, are used to ameliorate menstrual cramps; they also tend to diminish the volume of menstrual flow. Similar drugs are now available over the counter, without a prescription. Judith agreed to talk to her regular gynecologist about scheduling ultrasound examinations once or twice a year. She also promised to remember standard gynecological maintenance recommendations: resuming taking iron tablets and getting occasional blood counts if the excessive bleeding continued, monthly breast self-examinations, with annual "check-up" examinations, including Pap smears, mammograms every two years until she was fifty, and annually afterward, and a few other tests.

This happened four or five years ago. Until recently, Judith still sent me, once every year or two, an invitation to the opening of an exhibition of her recent paintings. The message she generally whispers when the crowd thins out is good: "I'm doing fine," she says, or "All's well." She is clearly happy with the decision to avoid surgery and use simple measures instead. Her mother reached an easy menopause in her mid-forties, and if the daughter's luck holds, menopause will be safer and gentler than a surgical solution to her problem with fibroids. For this woman, a distinctly low-technology approach was successful in avoiding a procedure that someone more docile would have accepted without argument.

Patients have a legitimate need for detailed information. Unfortunately, scheduling patterns in busy physicians' offices often make it difficult for patients to receive this information. One of the most frequently voiced complaints about medical care in the United States is directed at the limited amount of time spent with the physician who is, or should be, the patient's mentor and her resource for health-care questions. Women almost unanimously complain that there are too many interruptions, that they have too little time to explain themselves, to voice concerns and feelings, and to have treatment options and other medical details discussed in depth. Of course, good gynecologists are usually successful, which means they are busy. Time becomes a precious commodity and, in most gynecological practices, not enough is spent on thorough discussions of treatment choices, complications, and alternatives. And instead of the logical alternative of making printed materials available for patients with various common problems, physicians too often take the easy way out: They distribute the glossy but simplistic handouts provided by the pharmaceutical industry.

Other systems of medical care are not necessarily any better at giving patients more time. On the contrary, general practitioners in Britain's much-vaunted National Health Service, recognized as a competent but far from luxurious system, usually give their patients well under ten minutes per visit. Having spent three years in that system, as well as over thirty years in New York, in practice and teaching OB/GYN, I am well aware of the shortcomings of both approaches to delivering health care of high quality. This book treats one of the shortcomings of the American system: the discouraging unwillingness to tackle decades of unnecessary surgery. There is much at stake in the struggle to eliminate unneeded surgery, and because there is no central authority or force to assure that the practice will not be tolerated, it continues unchecked.

Over the years, in my private practice, I gradually got into the habit of scheduling "double visits" of forty minutes for all potential surgical patients. Much as my patients appreciated this, it was unfair to women who did not need surgery. Other problems also need extra time. The teenager with excruciatingly painful periods, the young woman with her first pregnancy, and the woman who has premenstrual syndrome (PMS) or severe chronic fatigue all need and deserve more time. As the growth of medical knowledge expanded, somehow I had to find more time to spend with each patient. I found I could not double the time given to most patients: the practical, business side of medical care tends to interfere very sharply with Utopian ideals. This facet of modern medicine—and American medical practice in particular—has created serious problems for me; once in a while, I still wish I could have practiced obstetrics and gynecology in the tradition of one of those independently wealthy late nineteenth-century country squires who were physicians but who had no direct need to earn a living from practicing medicine. The issues connected with a possible hysterectomy are numerous and complex, and there is little prospect that any surgeon will find the time to discuss a large number of various concerns and cover them all consistently, thoroughly and evenhandedly in clearly comprehensible language. This book was written to do just that.

Originally the domain of the researcher and the superspecialist, the various treatments and operations outlined here as alternatives to hysterectomy are now widely available. Even so, too many patients tell me that they were advised to undergo hysterectomy when, on investigation, it appeared that the need for surgery was unconvincing. The gynecologist who recommended the operation obviously saw it as the best solution to the patient's gynecological problem, but the patient was skeptical enough to get other opinions. Even when hysterectomy was reasonable from a strictly medical point of view, the surgeon tended not to hear the patient's voice, which usually appealed for an alternative. And even when unavoidable or when successful in relieving symptoms, the operation was viewed by many women as a mutilating procedure.

Fortunately, with common sense and the judicious use of modern technology, today's informed woman can often avoid hysterectomy. The immediate problem is that many women (or, indeed, men) are not accustomed to accumulating impartial and complete information on their medical concerns and problems. Instead of reading a book or two, they are satisfied with brief but possibly incomplete or inaccurate explanations. However, if you refuse or postpone surgery, you need precise information about a range of gynecological possibilities. You and your doctor must now take the time and make the effort to consider the situation thoughtfully, developing an intelligent plan for the complex situation at hand. This book will help you to evolve such a plan and teach you how to achieve success by negotiating your plan with a surgically oriented and generally conservative gynecological establishment.

This book was not planned as an extremist condemnation of hysterectomy. Under some circumstances, hysterectomy is the best solution, and it would be misleading to pretend otherwise. Instead, I have tried to discuss all courses of action as impartially as possible. The ideas and methods described here are familiar to most responsible, up-to-date, mainstream gynecologists. At the book's conclusion, it will be evident that hysterectomy is no longer what it used to be: the automatic treatment for most pelvic illnesses, and the surgery most frequently proposed to prevent various gynecological problems.

My aim is to present a reexamination, a reappraisal of the reasons that lead to this operation, with a variety of modern ideas involving alternative treatments. Since many of the new managements are "high technology," you will find careful explanations of ideas and procedures in the pages that follow. You will also find an accurate account of treatment successes, advantages, disadvantages, complications, and failures. Armed with the relevant facts, you will be able to return to your gynecologist to discuss the situation and select the management best suited to your physical and emotional needs. If the ideas presented here cannot be discussed openly with your current gynecologist or if he or she cannot provide the treatments outlined in this book, you may have to find another specialist.

As you assess the advantages and disadvantages of various treatments, you must ask certain important questions. What exactly are you trying to avoid? How realistic is this avoidance? What are your alternatives? If you are trying to avoid surgery altogether, you may have to use drug treatments until you reach your natural menopause, and quite likely beyond. Medical treatments are acceptable to some women, but others may find it difficult to tolerate the drudgery of living with constant schedules of medications to be taken. One important treatment we'll discuss will make you menopausal as long as you are getting certain injections—clearly this is not a solution for minor symptoms. Also, you may be successful with medical treatments for years, but may later need surgery anyway.

The fear of blood transfusions is another factor to be considered. Should you need nonemergency surgery, you may make your own blood available for a possible transfusion two or three weeks later by banking two pints with the blood bank of the hospital where you plan to have your surgery. Research is also progressing toward making artificial blood available for transfusions instead of regular human blood donated by friends, family members, or strangers. Being transfused with your own blood would eliminate an event that is already extremely unlikely: the later development of transfusion-related illnesses, particularly AIDS. However, for the present, anytime you undergo surgery, you will be asked to give your consent to receive a transfusion of blood should an emergency develop. Remarkably, as discussed throughout this book, modern medical and surgical treatments can stop all but the heaviest hemorrhages, allowing effective treatment of the shock and the anemia that often follow heavy vaginal bleeding. Time is thus gained to consider the situation calmly and to arrive at a rational plan.

Our assumptions often turn out to be incorrect. William Osler, a Canadian who became one of the giants of American medicine at the turn of the century, summarized this well when he addressed a graduating class of young doctors. "Gentlemen," he said, "half of what we know is wrong." Osler paused and then continued: "Unfortunately, we do not know which half." We have progressed since Osler's days, but we must recognize a humbling fact, that on occasion we all accept ideas and facts that turn out to be wrong. Unfortunately, the drive toward an authoritative stance is very strong. It is reinforced by colleagues and patients who prefer confident, straightforward explanations, and not a meditative "Well, that's one more detail that's difficult to be sure about." Throughout the book, I have tried to differentiate between what we know with reasonable certainty and what remains uncertain.

The book's philosophy also explains the absence of references to counterculture treatments. Precise information about the effects of these is usually not available. Most appear innocuous enough but must be taken on faith; a few (such as potions that contain lead or mercury) are dangerous. Meanwhile, precious time is lost. A few of my patients have tried unorthodox diets or other experimental methods, but with no noticeable effect from any. I recall reacting strongly only once, with a patient whose cervix harbored a small but very abnormal-looking, granular region. Her **biopsies** (tiny pieces of tissue removed to be examined under a microscope) showed that the area would probably become malignant, most likely within six months or at most within a year. This woman needed treatment urgently, but she insisted on trying douches with a concentrated extract of garlic for at least six months first. It took careful diplomacy to convince her not to trust her life to a home remedy about which neither of us knew anything for certain, whose effects she could not investigate properly, and which I thought was very likely ineffective. But she held her ground, and I had to compromise.

In the end, we used the treatment I recommended as well as the one she insisted on. She used the garlic douches for a few days; then her cervix was treated by freezing it, which was the best medical treatment then available. She resumed the douches as soon as I thought it was safe to do so, and she recovered. In the end, both of us were satisfied that we played an important part in devising a unique, mutually respectful, individualized and successful treatment plan.

I don't mean to undercut or high-handedly dismiss other unconventional approaches, old or new. However, I cannot recommend them personally. The Romans, with their flair for concise statements, summarized this well 2,000 years ago. "*Caveat emptor,*" they said: "Let the buyer beware." This warning applies to any purchase, to any road taken or not taken, including surgery.

Academic medicine takes the question of genuine knowledge very seriously. Rigorous thinking and robust statistics are preferred to impressionistic opinions. It took physicians centuries before they began to understand that the effectiveness of various treatments was not an easy matter to be confident about. French mathematicians, with at least one eye on winning at gambling tables, had to understand the statistics of probability before they could begin to think about calculating the odds of assessing medical treatments. One of the first problems to be considered was the use of leeches for bloodletting, a time-honored treatment for a variety of ills. Studied in Paris in the middle of the nineteenth century, leeches were not found to help, and their use declined gradually.

Today even famous professors are apt to be questioned very closely about the exact reasoning behind their convictions. Personal opinions count for less and less—unless backed by carefully designed and statistically sophisticated studies. Unfortunately, these precise ways have not always filtered down into the busy marketplace of medical practice. Thus the ancient Roman injunction still applies: *Caveat emptor.*

Most readers may not want to read a whole book about problems that are not their own. They will be interested in reading all about their disease and ways of avoiding hysterectomy for that particular condition. The organization of the chapters provides easy access to the diseases and treatment choices discussed. However, there is much overlap in treatments. The potent menopause-inducing medications noted on page 164 became available to treat endometriosis over ten years ago. However, almost immediately, the same drugs, usually given as injections, came to be used to shrink fibroids and to check uterine bleeding. And, remarkably, during the

13

late 1990s, the shots have emerged as highly effective treatments for many women with chronic pelvic pain. **Laparoscopy**, an operation in which the contents of the abdomen and pelvis are carefully inspected, is commonly used in the diagnosis and treatment of many gynecological diseases, particularly endometriosis and chronic pelvic pain. To avoid repetition, many medical and surgical treatments have been grouped together in Chapters 8 and 9. The occasional repetition of information is based on my belief that few women will have reason to read this book from cover to cover. Essential items of information have been repeated as insurance against readers missing important facts.

I hope that this book will be useful as a source of accurate and honest information on many gynecological topics. The symptoms and diagnoses it addresses cover much of the gamut of gynecology. Fibroids and endometriosis are household words to a great many women, and the irregular and excessive bleeding that precedes menopause remains a common problem to others. Chronic pelvic pain (CPP) is said by some experts to affect over 9 million women in the United States, higher than the figure for PMS. Both conditions may be disruptive enough to interfere with personal and professional pursuits. Both are difficult to treat successfully; large numbers of gynecologists regard hysterectomy with the removal of both ovaries as an acceptable solution for stubborn cases of CPP. Women may be convinced that earlier surgery would have saved them years of unnecessary suffering; others blame hysterectomy for a variety of problems developing in its wake. This book contains complete and helpful information to help women assess these complex situations. It was written not only for women eager to avoid hysterectomy but also for women who need help with other gynecological problems. I also hope the book will prove useful with problems beyond those developing in the pelvis. Year after year, medical care grows not only increasingly sophisticated but also more rushed, complicated, and fragmented. In this setting women can empower themselves effectively only if they understand the full range of medical facts and practicalities outlined in these pages.

The Early Days of
Gynecological Surgery

Ovariotomy

The origins of the craft of surgery are lost in antiquity, but the start of modern gynecological surgery is well documented. The first successful operation took place on Christmas Day in 1809; to the disbelief and astonishment of medical experts, it was performed not in one of the hallowed and learned European universities, but in rural Kentucky. And, against all odds, the patient survived the operation. She was Mrs. Jane Todd Crawford, a woman of forty-six, who had a massively enlarged and painful tumor growing in her abdomen. Earlier, she thought that she was pregnant and was getting ready to deliver a child. Her pains increased greatly, but labor would not start. Two local physicians were baffled by her condition and requested a consultation from a surgeon, Ephraim McDowell of Danville, Kentucky, who traveled sixty miles over mountainous back roads to visit Mrs. Crawford. His diagnosis was entirely unexpected: Dr. McDowell thought it was not pregnancy that caused her complaints, but a large ovarian tumor. Even more shockingly, he recommended a drastic and unprecedented treatment: excising the tumor.

Ephraim McDowell learned the craft of surgery at the University of Edinburgh toward the end of the eighteenth century. By that time, the ancient capital of Scotland was also one of the most renowned medical centers in the world. The idea of removing a diseased ovary had occurred to McDowell's teachers in Edinburgh, but none of them had the courage to attempt it. Operating on limbs and even amputations were one thing; opening the abdominal cavity was quite another. From what little was known about abdominal surgery, prospects were good that no patient would survive such an operation.

Jane Crawford understood the experimental nature of the treatment offered to her and agreed to travel to Danville to undergo surgery. She rode there on horseback, probably taking the same mountain trails McDowell traveled over when he came to visit her. On the way, she supported the mass protruding from her abdomen against the saddle, the weight of the large tumor bruising her skin. She knew that she would be awake during the operation but could not know whether she would survive the ordeal.

Surgery had to be postponed a few days to allow the bruise to heal, after which it was scheduled for Christmas Day at the McDowell house in Danville. When the appointed day arrived, the patient's husband and family were there, milling around the house with a local crowd. The throng was not in a friendly mood; they were apparently ready to kill McDowell if his patient did not survive. Jane Todd Crawford may have swallowed a few drafts of a concoction that contained opium before the operation—we know that this was McDowell's practice for the relief of pain after surgery. However, there was no anesthesia as we know it today—almost fifty years would elapse before anesthetic gases came into use. Instead, the patient sang hymns and the Psalms to fortify herself against pain. The ovariotomy, as the operation was then called, lasted about twenty-five minutes. Jane Crawford recovered; McDowell was surprised to find her changing her bed the fifth day after the operation. Jane Crawford eventually outlived her surgeon, dying thirty-two years later at the age of seventy-eight. The era of abdominal surgery began with a gynecological procedure, but strangely enough, in the beginning no one believed that such an operation was accomplished with the patient remaining alive.

McDowell did two more ovariotomies with both patients surviving, an amazing achievement for those days. He then submitted his case reports for publication. The claim, particularly from an unknown surgeon in backward Kentucky, strained the imagination of all the experts. Ovariotomy was thought to be impossible. McDowell's paper was rejected by Philip Syng

Physick, the famous professor of surgery in faraway Philadelphia. Across the Atlantic, in London, James Johnson, editor of the prestigious *Medico-Chirurgical Review*, refused to publish McDowell's account for the same reason. It ultimately appeared in print in the United States eight years later, in 1817, in a Philadelphia journal called *Eclectic Repertory and Analytical Review*.

James Johnson did eventually publish McDowell's work. John Lizars, one of McDowell's Edinburgh classmates, reported four of his own ovariotomies in Johnson's *Medico-Chirurgical Review* in 1825. Only two of Lizars's patients were found to have ovarian tumors, but three of the four women died. With only one woman surviving, Lizars's experiences were typical of surgery in the early years of the nineteenth century. Not surprisingly, the paper was not well received. However, Lizars's report included a mention of McDowell's three successful operations. Ironically, Johnson had no quarrel accepting Lizars's disasters but was incredulous about McDowell's successes. To his credit, Johnson reversed himself the following year. The apology he published misspelled the surgeon's name, but Johnson openly asked for "God's and McDowel's pardon" for his uncharitable doubts about the operation.

McDowell, who never graduated from Edinburgh, must have been an unusually courageous and competent surgeon, performing about a dozen of these operations during the years that followed. At least eight of his patients survived, an achievement that would not be equaled till the closing decades of the century. Contemporary accounts also make it clear that the women undergoing ovariotomies without proper anesthesia deserve more than a casual mention. The excision of ovaries was excruciatingly painful, an ordeal that could only be compared to having an amputation without anesthesia.

By the mid-nineteenth century, general anesthesia became available, and surgeons began doing ovariotomies in England, Continental Europe, and the United States. Word soon spread that many women died, and patients began to dread these operations. In London, surgeons who undertook ovariotomy came to be known as "belly rippers." Some of the better hospitals simply forbade the operation, forcing surgeons to take their patients to other hospitals where ovariotomy was not outlawed. Reaction was even stronger at New York Hospital, where surgical records indicate that not one major gynecological procedure was undertaken between 1848 and 1851. However, not far away, in Lancaster, Pennsylvania, the Atlee brothers became successful physician-entrepreneurs, performing large numbers of ovariotomies for a variety of peculiar reasons including "ovarian madness," "hystero-epilepsy," and nymphomania, a term that probably described masturbation, or, equally likely, the parental suspicion of masturbation by a daughter. Washington Lee Atlee reportedly performed hundreds of these operations.

Further south, Robert Battey of Rome, Georgia, removed so many ovaries that the surgery became known as "Battey's operation" not only in the United States but also in England. Battey, who later became the chief surgeon of a number of hospitals in the Confederate Army, was an expert physician, and it may be instructive to see how he became a convinced ovariotomist who ultimately achieved international reputation. Battey performed his first successful ovariotomy in early 1865 when he excised a thirty-pound tumor from a colleague's wife. That same year, he was consulted by two young women with severe menstrual problems. He described the first as unusually charming, a young woman who suffered from "violent perturbations of her nervous and vascular system." She was twenty-one years old and had neither a uterus nor periods, but she also had an unspecified heart disease. It is impossible to know what caused her symptoms, but while Battey debated what he could do for her, she deteriorated and died of unknown causes. The memory of this disaster apparently haunted Battey for years.

The second young woman who also came to his care in 1865 was twenty-three years old and had even more severe complaints. Her periods caused convulsions and left her semicomatose; she developed gastric and rectal bleeding at regular intervals; and a pelvic abscess ruptured through her rectum. She reported that her sufferings were so extreme that there was no future for her in this life, and that death would be a relief. After consulting with prominent gynecologists and writing to Boston for advice, Battey operated on her seven years later, in 1872. He removed her ovaries, which were outwardly normal, and, like McDowell, watched her in his own house after the operation. She had a miraculous recovery, not only from the surgery but from all her symptoms.

These two women may have suffered from **endometriosis**, a condition in which the abnormal growth of endometrium, the tissue lining the womb, may cause a number of severe complications. They may have had other diseases, possibly including PMS. The important point is that the woman who did not have surgery died, whereas the other recovered after the operation. Battey was so impressed that he went on to perform hundreds of similar operations, ultimately admitting that many may have been unnecessary.

By the end of the nineteenth century, the wholesale removal of ovaries began to fall into disrepute, but the practice of castrating young women did not cease entirely. It continued well into the twentieth century, and by the time the practice began to diminish, some gynecologists were busy with another lucrative innovation: unnecessary hysterectomies.

It was no accident that abdominal surgery began with a gynecological operation. Other intra-abdominal organs are solidly anchored to each other and to various supporting structures, and are thus difficult to remove. In contrast, the ovaries are unique in that they are attached to the womb by means of two slender sheets of tissue, in effect with a single stem, almost resembling fruit hanging from a stalk. Once inside the abdomen, this stem is relatively easy to locate and to divide, allowing rapid (if exquisitely painful) surgery. Nevertheless, invading a body cavity to remove an organ was a radical step, almost like landing on the moon. Fears of the unknown and concerns about a fatal hemorrhage or overwhelming infection combined to prevent the unprecedented and dramatic innovation of operating on an internal organ.

These were unmistakably the Dark Ages of surgery. Ovarian cysts and tumors grew to massive sizes, sometimes exceeding 200 pounds, because few surgeons had the courage to attempt surgical removal. The reluctance to operate was easy to understand: The lack of anesthesia alone sufficed to explain why surgery was rarely undertaken. And whenever it was performed, the mortality of abdominal surgery usually exceeded 60 or 75 percent. In other words, you were more likely to die after surgery than you were to survive. These stark facts must be weighed against the equally desperate alternative of standing by and not operating. Women with tubal pregnancies; appendicitis; large, twisted ovarian cysts; ruptured abscesses; and gynecological cancer usually died—some rapidly, others more slowly. Diseases were poorly understood and often misdiagnosed. What was known was that these mysterious illnesses, consisting of severe abdominal pain and swelling, often ended with the patient's burial. Already in miserable pain, women were faced with a terrible quandary: With or without surgery, they were about to perish.

Something as simple today as appendectomy did not become relatively safe until the turn of the century. Before then, appendicitis was, for some reason, less common—but it was also, according to contemporary records, a disease that was almost uniformly fatal. Veterinary surgeons had successfully spayed livestock, removing the ovaries of farm animals, but military surgeons knew that if the abdominal wall was penetrated by a weapon such as a stiletto, even an apparently minimal wound was usually fatal. Some surgeons now embraced the new procedure of ovariotomy as an amazing breakthrough; others condemned it as lethal, because it often was. The introduction of anesthesia served to reduce the dread of surgery. Soon afterward, the use of antiseptics, designed to cleanse the surgeon's hands (as well as the patient's skin and the operating instruments), helped cut the toll of lethal postoperative infections. The stage was now set for the first modern hysterectomy.

Hysterectomy

The idea of removing the womb arose at least 2,000 years ago, as a consequence of a rare but catastrophic complication of delivering a baby, called **inversion of the uterus**. In this situation the uterus is inverted, turning inside out like a sock, as well as upside down. It rapidly becomes swollen and discolored and appears as a purple, gangrenous mass hanging outside the vagina. Unless the womb was rapidly replaced in the pelvis, a daringly skillful procedure, the woman was likely to go into shock and die within hours. If this did not happen, most likely she would become infected and die a few days later.

Uterine inversion may occur spontaneously after a normal birth. More often, though, it happens because unskilled attendants aggressively pull on the umbilical cord (called **navel-strings** in Elizabethan England) to speed up the delivery of the afterbirth. Skilled midwives and obstetricians have known for hundreds of years that this is dangerous, but in less competent hands, the practice prevailed well into the twentieth century. Injunctions appearing in textbooks to this day are outspoken about the dangers of pulling on the umbilical cord, citing the risk of uterine inversion. The renowned physician Soranus, who lived in the second century A.D., warned explicitly against pulling harshly on the umbilical cord, but William Smellie, the preeminent British obstetrician of the eighteenth century, did not discourage the practice in his book on midwifery called *Treatise on the Theory and Practice of Midwifery,* published in 1752.

Ancient midwives and other medical practitioners must have watched a number of these tortured deaths and realized that more aggressive treatment was necessary if the newly delivered mother were to be saved. Some, like Soranus, were reportedly skilled enough to cut away the gangrenous body parts safely. Soranus was born in Ephesus, a thriving port city in the Eastern Mediterranean, then under Greek control, and now in Turkey. He studied in Alexandria, practiced in Rome, and became one of the most respected of ancient physicians. In his book, *Gynecology,* he credits an earlier physician, Themison, with performing vaginal hysterectomies for inverted wombs. Similar skills were possibly also possessed by at least some Roman practitioners, women called *feminae medicae*, who provided medical and surgical care for women.

The Roman empire went into decline a century or two after Soranus's death. For the period of well over 1,000 years, there are only occasional glimpses of surgical advances, mostly from military surgeons who traveled with the great armies of the Renaissance. A few exceptionally skilled medieval midwives and physicians probably also knew how to remove the womb vaginally. We do not know how often this operation was undertaken, how much of the uterus was removed, how the bleeding and pain of the surgery were dealt with, or how many women survived the ordeal. Born of despair, these operations were in effect amputations of the inverted part of the womb hanging outside the vagina. Except for occasional reports of cesarean sections performed under desperate circumstances, abdominal surgery remained rare in this period.

With the advent of the Renaissance, Italian anatomists began to understand the functions of abdominal and pelvic organs and surgical progress began again. By the sixteenth century, outstanding military surgeons such as Ambroise Paré of France were busy practicing medicine, teaching and writing medical books. Paré knew that if gangrene appeared in a wounded arm or a leg, the limb had to be amputated without delay or the infection would cause a painful death. With only opium and hard liquor as (inefficient) anesthetics, surgeons had to move fast. Two centuries later, master surgeons such as Baron Joseph Lister of England (later Lord Lister) and Conrad van Langenbeck of Germany were apparently able to amputate limbs in half a minute, a speed neither necessary nor matched in modern practice.

Accounts of vaginal hysterectomy began to appear in sixteenth-century Germany, Italy, and Spain. As before, the operation was performed only as an emergency, in the management of the inverted uterus that could not be pushed up and thus replaced after a delivery. Professor Tulpius of Amsterdam, that magisterial presence in Rembrandt's *The Anatomy Lesson*, was reportedly able to perform this operation expertly. The speculum, the duck-billed instrument some women call "the clamp," was well known by this time in continental Europe. The British, with Victorian prudery, decried its use, particularly after a law that demanded regular speculum examinations of prostitutes was passed, but French surgeons took to them and used them freely, even though similar laws were passed in France. Checking women for venereal diseases was then the usual role for the speculum, but a variety of other abnormalities began to be recognized during speculum examinations.

Amputating a diseased cervix through the blades of a speculum gradually became a well-established practice. As surgeons became more courageous, they could excise fibroids and cancer growing from the cervix, and more and more of the uterus itself. Ultimately, surgeons began to wonder if the entire organ could be removed, particularly if it was beginning to "fall out." This condition was only too frequent at a time when it was not unusual for a woman to bear eight, or ten, or even a dozen children. Uterine prolapse was a common problem those days; if severe enough it was called *procidentia*, as shown on page 276.

Prolapse and procidentia develop in women who have had so many or such difficult deliveries that the ligaments anchoring the womb in its place are increasingly weakened and stretched. The uterus now begins to descend through the vaginal canal. It may finally prolapse completely, to hang outside the vagina, which itself has been, usually over the course of many years, turned inside out. However, considering the severity of other illnesses encountered in an age riddled by disease, this was a relatively harmless and usually pain-free abnormality, not warranting the dangers and pain of surgery. Instead, elaborate pieces of equipment had been available for centuries, often belts with metallic or bentwood contraptions shaped like the letter "J" attached to the belt, designed to reach up high into the vagina to hold the uterus in its place. However, on occasion this organ was not only prolapsed but also diseased. Most often, it was bleeding because of cancer or fibroids, and the loss of blood, if heavy enough, was an ominous threat to the patient's life. Because of this tendency for the uterus to prolapse and the similarity of the operation to amputations and other familiar operations done through the vagina, hysterectomy by the vaginal route began to be contemplated well before the first abdominal hysterectomy was.

Conrad von Langenbeck of Germany is usually credited with the first carefully planned vaginal hysterectomy. Performed in 1813 to eradicate cancer, his operation received the same total disbelief accorded to McDowell a few years previously. Langenbeck's assistant, an elderly surgeon suffering from gout, was reportedly not particularly helpful during the operation, and he died soon after. The uterus was lost. Langenbeck was ridiculed for years about the operation, whose other witness was dead. Twenty-six years later, the patient also died, and to settle the issue, an autopsy was performed. The uterus was entirely absent, and Langenbeck was vindicated.

In 1840, J. Z. Amussat, a French surgeon, performed the first vaginal removal of a fibroid tumor, an operation now called vaginal myomectomy. His patient probably died. Four years later, Washington L. Atlee performed the first successful abdominal myomectomy. The Atlee brothers, Washington L. and John Light, were mentioned earlier as busy and successful entrepreneurs and practitioners, conversant with ovariotomy and confident about performing abdominal surgery. The stage was now set for abdominal hysterectomy.

Langenbeck of Germany, along with A. M. Heath and Charles Clay, two surgeons from Manchester, England, were probably the first to perform this operation. All of their patients died, with Clay's surviving fifteen days until she was "dropped by a nurse," after which she also died. On June 26, 1853, Dr. Walter Burnham of Lowell, Massachusetts, performed the first operation with survival of the patient, although his was not exactly a planned procedure. Burnham thought his patient had an ovarian cyst, an abnormality familiar to surgeons by then. After Burnham started what he thought would be an ovariotomy, performing the operation without anesthesia, his patient suddenly began to vomit, and her spasms forced the tumor through the incision. To Burnham's shock, the tumor was not an ovarian cyst but a large fibroid uterus, one he could not replace back into the belly. Desperate to finish the operation, Burnham removed the uterus, leaving the cervix behind. The patient recovered.

Of Burnham's next fifteen patients, thirteen died, a proportion not at all unusual for those days. Gradually, surgical patients began to survive in larger numbers. Two developments facilitated this spectacular leap, from terrified patients in a barbaric scene to calmer and reasonably successful surgery. The first was the discovery of anesthesia, which must have gone far to reassure patients that their operations would be at least painless. Antisepsis, the other innovation, was aimed at preventing infections, which often killed patients a few days after surgery. Some prominent surgeons argued loudly against the notion that cleanliness was essential, but the more radical thinkers accepted it, buoyed by the fact that their patients began to survive.

Anesthesia was certainly nineteenth-century America's greatest contribution to medicine. In 1842, Crawford Long, a general practitioner from rural Georgia, was the first to put a patient to sleep using an inhaled anesthetic gas. This was ether, a new chemical imported from Germany, which began to be used in "ether frolics," in much the same way some teenagers began to sniff glue in the last century. Long did not publish his method until 1849. Meanwhile, in 1846, the dentist William Thomas Green Morton and his colleagues at Massachusetts General Hospital anesthetized a patient, thereby attracting widespread publicity.

In England, chloroform was mistakenly assumed to be safer and became better known than ether. Sir James Young Simpson of Edinburgh first used chloroform to anesthetize a woman in labor in 1847. This went against biblical principles and earned much immediate disapproval. Six years later and nearly 400 miles to the south, in London, chloroform was used to help Queen Victoria's pains when she was in labor. With evident success and royal approval, acceptance followed rapidly. Simpson became an instant celebrity throughout the Western world.

The more abstract concept of antisepsis took longer to gain acceptance. Bacteria surround us invisibly: They float in the air, they live on our skin and in the crevices of our bodies. Unaware of the existence of bacteria, surgeons had often moved casually back and forth, from autopsies and infected patients to operations and to deliveries, using their bare hands without using gloves or a disinfectant. Independently of each other, three physicians came to understand the development of infections after surgery or obstetric deliveries.

The first of the three was Ignaz Semmelweiss, a Hungarian physician who was practicing obstetrics in Vienna. By 1848, he began to suspect that obstetricians infected their patients by examining them with their bare hands soon after performing autopsies on the corpses of other women who had died of infections. His innovative solution, the careful scrubbing of obstetricians' hands with soap before vaginal examinations, was considered outrageous and revolutionary. Semmelweiss proved that his simple measure could help avoid infections and thus save the lives of women who had recently delivered a baby. (Had they stayed at home for the birth, they might have survived, and medical history would have gone on to a another giant: Joseph Lister of London.) However, a power struggle ensued, and Semmelweiss was forced to leave Vienna. Soon afterward, he suffered a nervous breakdown and endured a prolonged stay in a provincial asylum in Hungary. Semmelweiss died a few years later from an insect bite. Ironically, this was caused by a skin infection that led to fatal sepsis, a process not unlike the infections called *puerperal sepsis* that had killed the Viennese women.

Nearly twenty years later, carbolic acid was introduced as an effective antiseptic agent by Baron Joseph Lister in England. In the United States, Oliver Wendell Holmes, physician and writer, and father of the famous jurist, was advocating similar ideas at much the same time. Simultaneously, the relationship between bacteria and infections was discovered by Louis Pasteur in Paris, thereby giving antisepsis its modern scientific basis. Thomas Spencer Wells, a famous English surgeon, kept careful records of his 1,000 ovariotomies, all performed in the second half of the nineteenth century. Before antisepsis, about 25 percent of his patients died. Toward the end of the century, with anesthesia and carbolic acid as the antiseptic agent, this figure was reduced to 11 percent.

The first total abdominal hysterectomy in the United States, with the removal of the uterus as well as the cervix, was performed by Mary Amanda Dixon Jones in 1889. By now, the practice of abdominal surgery was established, barreling ahead like other contemporary innovations such as electricity or the steam engines that powered ships and locomotives. Unfortunately, while surgeons of genius developed the craft of surgery, practitioners with commercial ideas moved in, and found a defenseless and often lucrative target: women.

· · · 3 · · ·

Hysterectomy in the Twentieth Century

During the first half of the twentieth century, hysterectomy was the accepted treatment for relatively few diseases. Large families were the rule, and after many deliveries, as the ligaments supporting the womb grew lax, vaginal prolapse often developed and was a frequent reason for recommending hysterectomy. Heavy bleeding caused by fibroids was another common indication. Gynecological cancers were usually treated with hysterectomy, the major exception being cervical cancer, for which this operation produced inferior results. However, a more extensive, so-called radical, hysterectomy, which removed pelvic lymph nodes as well as more vaginal and ligamentous tissues than the standard hysterectomy, was found to be better treatment for early cases of cervical cancer. Since chemotherapy was then ineffective, radiation was the only other choice available. Radical hysterectomy and radiation saved the lives of many women whose cancer was detected before it had invaded deep into the cervix. Unfortunately, radiation always destroyed ovarian tissues, causing the immediate onset of menopause; it also damaged the vagina, leaving it too rigid and unyielding for intercourse. Thus, of the two available treatments, surgery and radiation, radical hysterectomy was actually kinder to women with early cervical cancer.

Hysterectomy was performed abdominally or vaginally, with a Continental preference for vaginal surgery, and an English and American preference for the abdominal route. However, this choice is not as important as understanding how, by the 1960s and 1970s, hysterectomies came to be performed with such abandon by American gynecologists.

Surgical principles were already well understood by the 1930s and 1940s. World War II and then the Korean War brought effective blood-transfusion services, a wide range of antibiotics began to be developed, and anesthesia was perfected. The successful surgery of acute wartime trauma cases with life-saving results in hospitals run by the armed services led to the expanded use of surgery in other fields, including gynecology. As surgery became safer, gynecologists began to resort to hysterectomy for purposes unheard of before. Precancerous changes in the cervix and endometrium began to be identified. Benign in the beginning, these abnormalities often turn malignant over the years; in the absence of other effective treatments, it seemed logical to remove diseased organs by means of hysterectomy.

Endometriosis began to be diagnosed more frequently, and the more severe forms began to be treated with hysterectomy. Illegal abortions, usually obtained under unsanitary circumstances, regularly started serious pelvic infections, and women and frightened teenagers often died from overwhelming sepsis caused by abortions. Other infections of the fallopian tubes, which connect the ovaries and the womb, were sexually acquired and usually caused by gonorrhea. Both varieties were a stubborn scourge, leading to surgery that was often excruciatingly difficult to perform. Often there was no choice: **Abscesses** (collections of pus) in the pelvis were common, and it was appreciated only too well that unless promptly treated by means of surgery, a ruptured abscess that suddenly spilled a large volume of pus into the abdominal cavity would kill the patient within a day or two. With or without surgery, there was a vast toll in suffering; infertility and chronic pelvic pain were then common outcomes. Hysterectomy was the most successful and best understood surgical management available in those days, and it began to be used freely.

Initially, the expansion in the use of hysterectomies was rational and useful, representing the more creditable side of gynecology. Unfortunately, these operations began to be performed in increasingly large numbers for a variety of other reasons. Sometimes the surgery was performed to provide birth control, with the suspicion that a husband's sexual inclinations or the couple's religious scruples could be circumvented with hysterectomy performed for reasons that were ostensibly medical. Reliable contraception was not as easily available as it is today: Diaphragms and condoms failed fairly often; birth control pills arrived during the early 1960s but took a while to become popular. Legal abortions were difficult to obtain, particularly for women who were poor or came from communities with strong religious objections to abortion. However, a slight prolapse of the womb was almost always present after two or three deliveries; hysterectomy for this condition, but perhaps more for birth control, was an acceptable way out of the contraceptive quandary for many women.

Gynecologists now began to perform the operation for diseases that did not warrant such an extreme solution. Chronic infections of the cervix are difficult to eradicate, but usually cause nothing worse than a persistent vaginal discharge. Nevertheless, hysterectomy was the treatment offered when **conization of the cervix**, the excision of a small, cone-shaped core of tissue from the cervix, could easily have been used instead. Even worse were the hysterectomies performed for backaches that were supposedly due to retroversion. This is a condition in which the womb is not inclined forward toward the pubic bones and the bladder, but "backward" toward the rectum. Sad to say, it took physicians hundreds of years to learn that this is usually a harmless condition and not a disease. Shades of ancient Greek notions about the wandering uterus, and the illnesses it could cause, persisted well into the twentieth century. Worst of all were the hysterectomies done on women who had small and harmless fibroids only, or women whose sole complaint was nervousness, or those who had no complaints and whose organs were normal. Nevertheless, without apparent reason, many of these women were subjected to hysterectomy.

The Useless Womb

By the mid-1960s, there was so little resistance to hysterectomies that the notion of removing a healthy but "unnecessary" womb was debated with great professional seriousness. The apotheosis of the elective hysterectomy movement found one of its most extreme expressions in 1971, set forth by Dr. Ralph C. Wright of New Britain, Connecticut, an affluent suburb of

Hartford. Dr. Wright, who died some years ago, was at the time chairman of the Department of Obstetrics and Gynecology at New Britain General Hospital. In an editorial he wrote for *Obstetrics and Gynecology,* then the most popular professional journal read by gynecologists, Dr. Wright expressed the opinion that elective hysterectomy was perfectly justifiable. Once a woman's family was completed, he wrote, eliminating cancer and nuisances such as bleeding and pain warranted surgery, and now the woman might as well have the operation: "The uterus has but one function: reproduction. After the last planned pregnancy, the uterus becomes a useless, bleeding, symptom-producing, potentially cancer-bearing organ and therefore should be removed."

These two sentences, the essence of his message, were italicized in Dr. Wright's editorial. This was an unabashedly partisan opinion, unencumbered by analysis, a weighing of pros and cons, or any recognition of the complexity of the issue. The morbidity and mortality of the surgery, recognized for a century, were apparently not worth mentioning. Feminists have looked at Dr. Wright's statement ever since with various degrees of anger, scorn, and hostility. Women discovered that his words showed how at least some of their trusted gynecologists viewed their mission. The more one looks at Dr. Wright's sentences, the more objectionable they appear. There is no decency here, nothing to suggest that a person is being discussed and not one of her organs, one she may regard with the pride men invariably bestow on theirs. The woman in question has lost her voice as well as her choice. If she has a hysterectomy, she may become one more uninformed victim of a potentially dangerous custom that benefits the medical establishment more than it helps her.

We could understand how such a notion might have gained popularity thirty years previously, prior to World War II. In those years, cancers of the cervix and endometrium usually went undetected until it was too late to effect a cure. Ovarian cancer was (and still is) another notorious killer of women, impossible to diagnose early and to treat successfully. About 1 woman in thirty or forty died, usually painfully, from one of these forms of cancer. But by 1971, the picture had brightened considerably. Thanks to Pap smears and biopsies, cervical cancers were largely preventable, and those not prevented but detected early could be treated with better chances of success. Endometrial cancers, which Pap smears could not screen for, were readily diagnosable with biopsies and with curettages, minor operations then almost always performed under general anesthesia. Only ovarian cancer remained a lurking threat, occurring in slightly over 1 percent of women, impossible to prevent or to treat effectively. But by 1971, it was obvious that for most women it did not make sense to remove normal organs to prevent cancer.

Dr. Wright, who may have seen himself as a crusader, did not pay attention to a simple fact: that the operation he was advocating would inadvertently kill about 1 woman for each 1,000 who underwent the operation. Moreover, those who died of surgical complications and anesthetic mishaps would die immediately, as young women, whereas those who developed a malignancy twenty or thirty years later might still be saved from dying of cancer. But Dr. Wright was not overly concerned about cancer. The elective hysterectomies he was advocating were to be done to improve the so-called quality of women's lives. His ideas were readily accepted in circles in which more attention was paid to rhetoric than to facts, circles in which the surgeon reigned supreme, almost a Godlike figure, whose ideas no one (and least of all his patients) disputed. Today, thirty years later, it would be difficult to disentangle his enthusiasm from quaint notions of performing useful surgery and from the very lucrative prospects of the undertaking he was proposing. Elective hysterectomy without a good indication may have disappeared from gynecological vocabularies, but hysterectomies that are unnecessary are still being performed by gynecologists in many hospitals.

Women did not argue at first, and the number of hysterectomies began to balloon year after year. We have already seen how this led to steep increases in the number of hysterectomies, which ultimately peaked at 740,000 in 1975. Elective hysterectomy never caught on in responsible hands and was the exception rather than the rule—at least in teaching hospitals in the Northeast. This view is supported by Mildred Agnes Morehead's 1962 study, which will be discussed in the next chapter.

And there was certainly no protest from gynecologists against unnecessary hysterectomies. Instead, surveys showed that elective hysterectomies were accepted wholeheartedly by gynecologists doubling as entrepreneurs, particularly in Southern states, where hysterectomy rates were always higher than elsewhere. When the American College of Obstetricians and Gynecologists (ACOG) debated elective hysterectomy at its annual meeting in 1971, an audiometer was used to gauge the preferences of American gynecologists. This instrument, which measures loudness, reportedly showed that when gynecologists were asked to show their opinion by clapping, those supporting the operation clapped louder and longer than their opponents. The excitement was, I think, an example of satisfaction with a lucrative commercial activity thinly disguised in humanitarian and pseudo-academic cloaks.

Breast cancer occurs in women much more often than does genital cancer, which strikes the cervix, the body of the uterus, and the ovaries. However, prophylactic removal of the breasts is thought justifiable exceedingly rarely. The reasons for this disparity may be the domain of the psychologist, the social theorist, or the feminist sociologist and can only be guessed at. Men's conspicuous fixation with women's breasts and women's consequent absorption with their breasts may well provide at least part of the answer.

Current figures from the American Cancer Society show that about one man in eleven will develop cancer of the prostate, a disease whose mortality is almost identical with that of breast cancer. The prostate is difficult to excise completely, although urologists can remove parts of it easily, by working through the urethra. The testicles are easier to remove, but most instances of the disease appear in young men, well before the age of forty. Testicles develop cancer slightly less than one-third as often as ovaries do, and the disease is far easier to treat successfully, with surgery and modern chemotherapy, than ovarian cancer. A male cultural distaste for excising organs held in high esteem may be the last decisive factor that explains why urologists do not suggest that the prostate (or the testicles) should be removed prophylactically.

We must also discuss the charge that the avalanche of hysterectomies had sexist origins: that is, because men were operating on women. There is some evidence that female gynecologists are less likely to resort to hysterectomy than are male gynecologists. Of course, women angry with gynecologists are much more likely to accept this line of reasoning than male gynecologists themselves. Physicians' wives have certainly had unusually high rates of hysterectomy, although Italian data show that female physicians themselves have fewer hysterectomies. One benevolent interpretation of these facts may be that, rightly or wrongly, male physicians genuinely believe in the advantages to be derived from hysterectomy. A less benevolent interpretation is that male physicians are deeply enmeshed in a system that undervalues women's internal sexual organs. Consequently, even male physicians' family members may undergo hysterectomy when a careful analysis of its advantages and disadvantages would argue against such surgery.

Hysterectomies may be compared to another kind of surgery performed more on men than on women, namely, **coronary artery bypass grafts** (CABG, usually called "cabbage surgery"), and performed in the treatment of severely diseased coronary arteries. The huge numbers of CABGs have elicited two conflicting responses. The first was that too many such operations were being performed with indications that were known to be less than adequate. The second response was yet another gender-based charge, that these operations were done mostly for men, much less often than for women, who also deserve the benefits to be reaped from CABGs. Another and more simple explanation for the increasing numbers of both hysterectomies and CABG surgery may be explained by an obvious fact. Surgeons operate to help their patients but also to earn a living, and it would be very naive to imagine that the warm glow of satisfaction with a successful and lucrative professional life was not part of the equation. It will be interesting to note whether women will get more equal cardiological treatment in the years to come, including cardiac surgery with doubtful benefits.

Reasons for Hysterectomy

Every few years an official professional body, or a textbook, or a prominent gynecologist publishes a list of valid "indications" as a guide to the profession. The list usually includes instances of gynecological cancer and severe hemorrhage—there is no argument about these indications. Fibroids, with certain qualifications, endometriosis and prolapse, again with certain qualifications, are usually listed next. These lists go on and on, usually with added justifications, qualifications, and explanations, to include a litany of possible indications. Nevertheless, even among experts there may be surprising variations about the necessity for hysterectomy. Certain cases, such as cancer or a major hemorrhage, receive unanimous agreement; others are much less clear-cut. Also, modern technology has repeatedly encroached and altered the terrain of indications. Vaginal bleeding is the prime example to consider here. Thirty years ago, hysterectomy may have been the most effective treatment for most women who were not close to the age of spontaneous menopause; today a variety of medical and surgical treatments, discussed in Chapters 8 and 9, can be tried as perfectly reasonable alternatives. And I must add that this is not merely my opinion: Other books have also argued against unnecessary hysterectomies. Further, in the April 15, 2000, issue of *Contemporary OB/GYN*, Richard Soderstrom, a well-known and highly respected gynecologist from Seattle with impeccable academic credentials, has estimated that one-third of American hysterectomies could be safely replaced with a less aggressive treatment, namely ablation of the endometrial surfaces of the womb.

While researching this book and hearing the stories of patients, friends, and family members, I have been regularly told of gynecologists with large practices that were heavily dependent on hysterectomy, more often in Southern and Western states, and usually well away from teaching hospitals. In 1990, a relative of mine who lived in Florida developed excessive vaginal bleeding. She was told almost immediately that she needed a hysterectomy because of her fibroids. This was unmistakably unnecessary since the bleeding was checked by me with minimal effort—a brief telephone conversation, to be exact—using a hormonal medication called Provera. She is still perfectly well now, over ten years later. Of course, one instance does not create a convincing argument. Rather, it is the overall pattern of unnecessary surgery, as reflected by its statistics, that needs to be recognized and stopped.

Careful reading of recent guidelines issued by the American College of Obstetricians and Gynecologists for their members makes it clear that the College currently recommends hysterectomy only when its benefits outweigh the costs, risks, and disadvantages of the surgery. For instance, hysterectomy for birth control purposes has been discouraged. Further, ACOG has very specific recommendations for performing hysterectomy as treatment for fibroids and for chronic pelvic pain. These are outlined in corresponding chapters; suffice it to say here that even fibroids enlarging the womb to the size of a pineapple are not automatically regarded as good reasons for undergoing surgery unless they cause symptoms such as persistent bleeding or pain. Similarly, chronic pelvic pain should not be treated by means of hysterectomy except after detailed assessment and counseling. This, I believe, is academic gynecology at its best. However, academic gynecology is not what most women receive, instead receiving what may be called street-level, this-is-the-way-we've-always-done-it gynecology, gynecology that is often more a commercial undertaking, marked by poorly in-dicated or unnecessary hysterectomies, than a healing and humanitarian activity. Lest you think that this is a harsh judgment, consider the details of a study mentioned in the Introduction, on page xvii. This recent study de-scribes in detail how practicing gynecologists routinely disregarded official (and sound) ACOG indications and recommendations for preoperative in-vestigations, instead proceeding posthaste to surgery.

In this context, you may be interested in an editorial article and the sub-sequent exchange of letters published in the *British Medical Journal* in 1997. I found the title of one letter particularly outrageous: "Performing Hys-terectomies in Low-Income Women May Be Easier Than Educating Them." Poor women, in the United States and elsewhere, are substantially more likely to undergo hysterectomy than their counterparts, whose bet-ter education and income protect them, if incompletely, against inferior medical care. As the editorial and the ensuing correspondence indicate, competent medical care may often be biased by the convenience of those who are supposed to provide it, a problem that may be encountered in health-care systems as dissimilar as the American and the Swiss.

Although this is rarely articulated, hysterectomy is radically different from other forms of surgery. Almost all other operations are performed to treat one major and clearly identifiable disease. Hysterectomy, on the other hand, is often chosen as the treatment for women who have two, three, or even more conditions, each possibly insufficient to warrant major surgery by itself. There is a "primary diagnosis"—the major reason for the surgery—but by gynecological tradition, the accumulation of lesser indica-tions may also be accepted as justification for the operation. One investi-gator, Dr. Brooks Ranney, a gynecologist in private practice in Yankton, South Dakota, has reported that fewer than one woman in twenty under-goes hysterectomy for a single diagnosis. The remainder had two to ten reasons to undergo hysterectomy, a state of affairs unknown in other branches of surgery.

There may be a hidden agenda as well: providing permanent birth con-trol. A thirty-year-old woman with three or four children, a few small fi-broids, and minimal prolapse, but few or no symptoms to worry about, might undergo hysterectomy with the ostensible indication of prolapse. She may also appear in the statistics as a woman who had a hysterectomy for fibroids. Nevertheless, the real reason for the surgery may have been that her husband was unwilling to undergo vasectomy, a relatively minor operation usually performed under local anesthesia in an outpatient setting, and our patient's desire for permanent and reliable contraception was the real deciding factor leading to hysterectomy.

Let us look at another hysterectomy, this one scheduled for a woman who has chronic pelvic pain and a mildly precancerous change in her cervix. She is admitted to the hospital with the diagnosis of chronic salpingitis, or recurring infections of the fallopian tubes, to which the pains are often attributed. The pathologist who examines the womb after its removal finds normal fallopian tubes. This is not an unusual development, as discussed in Chapter 13. The precancerous change, which was not severe enough to warrant hysterectomy, is identified. One or two slight areas of endometriosis, a disease discussed in Chapter 7, may also be noted. This disease may or may not have been responsible for the pain. This woman may leave the hospital with her records stating that the hysterectomy she had was her treatment for chronic salpingitis—the original reason for her hospital admission. Her operation could also appear under the rubric of endometriosis, a frequent diagnosis in recent years, or even in the uncomfortably large group labeled "miscellaneous," which includes women whose hysterectomies were done because of chronic pelvic pain. None of these diagnoses may be an honest description of the reasons for her hysterectomy, and possibly neither the woman nor her gynecologist may understand that the hysterectomy was not necessarily the best treatment available. If her pains disappear, no one will have reason to complain. However, if her chronic pains become worse or if she develops serious complications, both the patient and her gynecologist will regret that major surgery was undertaken as opposed to other, less aggressive approaches.

With these two examples, I am not arguing for or against hysterectomy for two imaginary patients. Real women who become candidates for hysterectomy must understand that the gynecological thinking that pushed them toward surgery may have been less precise than they knew.

Indications for Surgery

According to a statement issued in 1977 by the American College of Obstetricians and Gynecologists, gynecological surgery was to be ranked by necessity. Emergency surgery was defined as lifesaving: For instance, a major hemorrhage due to an ectopic pregnancy or a hemorrhage from a ruptured uterus warranted emergency surgery. Mandatory surgery was defined, for example, as surgery performed to treat cancer—not a situation in which, as a rule, there is much choice. The next three levels, seemingly distinct, blend into each other: "urgent," "advisable," and "elective" overlap each other significantly. These levels of necessity do not involve actual diagnoses. During recent years, as detailed in the last section of this chapter called "Statistics," you will find a breakdown of indications for hysterectomy. In brief, approximately 33.5 percent of these operations were performed because of fibroids, 19 percent were vaginal hysterectomies due to prolapse, 16 percent were for women with endometriosis, 10 percent were for cancer, 5.5 percent were for precancerous changes of the endometrial lining, and 16 percent were performed for miscellaneous other reasons.

Many hysterectomies are unnecessary by any criteria. Others are perfectly appropriate but could have been averted with reasonable safety. Yet others may have been avoidable, but only at the cost of certain inconveniences and risks that are well known and understood by doctors, but not always discussed with women. The remainder are, at least from a gynecological point of view, unavoidable, although some women may still refuse surgery. Finally, on rare occasions, a hysterectomy may be a lifesaving procedure. These distinctions, sometimes clear-cut but at times surprisingly subtle, are discussed throughout this book.

Much of the difficulty is linguistic. *Elective* is a word used with two related but distinct meanings in gynecology. It may mean surgery performed not to treat current disease but to avoid future gynecological disease or to prevent pregnancy. Elective is also used meaning that the operation is "indicated," meaning a disease is being treated but there is no emergency. At one end of the scale, much cosmetic surgery is elective. Reconstructing a large but otherwise normal nose or enlarging small breasts may be regarded as just as elective as buying or not buying an expensive handbag. However, in gynecology, tubal ligation is usually considered an elective procedure, even if it is desperately needed by someone who has problems with all contraceptives and keeps conceiving against her wishes and her interests. Instead of using a diaphragm for the next twenty years, accepting its advantages and disadvantages, including unwanted pregnancies, a woman may decide to have a so-called tubal ligation operation, accepting *its* advantages and disadvantages. Particularly if her husband (or the baby's father) disagrees with abortions, it seems to me that this tubal ligation is not elective. It is at least highly advisable, and perhaps urgent. "Elective," "advisable," and "indicated" surgery cannot be sharply defined and separated. The use of these words implies judgments more subjective than objective, reflecting regional thinking (more hysterectomies in the South than in the Northeast in the United States), a surgeon's training, reasoning, and habits, and the patient's desires and circumstances as well as the more scientific facts of the diagnosis and the patient's overall situation.

Over the years, with changes in surgical philosophy, better understanding of disease processes, and the appearance of new medications and surgical techniques, indications have often changed. For instance, in the 1960s, an abnormal Pap smear and cervical biopsy were often regarded as good reasons to perform an operation called conization of the cervix. The operation damaged a number of wombs, sometimes making conception or childbearing more complicated. On the other hand, cervical cancer was diagnosed and treated earlier with this operation, a tangible benefit. Ten years later, gynecologists began to use better diagnostic methods, particularly colposcopy, which allows a close look at the cervix with a microscope-like magnifier. Conization was largely replaced by procedures such as freezing the cervix, laser surgery and, even more recently and successfully, by electrosurgical methods of excising precancerous tissues.

Similarly, one of the most exciting innovations of the last two decades has been the introduction of a variety of operations that avoid hysterectomy by destroying endometrium. This has been done with electric current, laser technology, and heating or freezing endometrial tissues that cause excessive bleeding. There is a constant competition, an incessant tug-of-war between various medical and surgical treatments. Gynecologists compete with urologists in the treatment of involuntary losses of urine, and with so-called invasive radiologists in the treatment of fibroid tumors. The honest practitioner should favor the use of methods that are safe, effective, fast, and inexpensive, or at least have the best combination of these attributes. The diminished rate of conization and the widespread use of electrosurgery show that progress is possible. That hysterectomy rates have remained largely unchanged in spite of well-accepted and less aggressive alternatives tells us that (perhaps in common with the rest of the world) gynecologists have been too slow to improve, too slow to change their ways.

The Benefits of Hysterectomy

Hysterectomies intended to treat gynecological cancer or for emergency situations are usually very difficult (or impossible) to avoid. However, almost 90 percent are performed electively, and, as this book shows, it is possible to avoid many or most of these hysterectomies. Surgeons usually justify elective hysterectomy by citing a mixture of reasons, such as an improvement in the quality of life and, possibly, the prevention of cancer. The first must be for the woman to decide; the second is a complicated and oversold proposition.

Operating on healthy women to reduce their chances of cancer no longer makes sense, except for those with a strong family history of ovarian cancer. On rare occasions, such women have developed a form of cancer similar to ovarian cancer even though their ovaries had been removed. We'll return to this astounding (and discouraging) development later, in Chapter 14. However, ovarian cancer occurs relatively rarely, in about one woman in sixty or seventy. Most cases of cervical cancer, and many cases of endometrial cancer, may be prevented in time to avoid hysterectomy.

The cancer-preventing benefits of elective hysterectomy to healthy women who are forty years old can be calculated precisely, although you need a refined love of abstract calculations to appreciate such considerations. Overall, as a result of elective hysterectomies freely performed, women's average gain in their life expectancy is very little—about a month per woman. Since it takes about this long to recover from the operation, the actual gains are minuscule. This insignificant "gain" must be balanced against the fact that after elective hysterectomy a very small number of women die. This occurs following one of the occasional and unexpected disasters that happen during or immediately after surgery. Anesthesia-related deaths, fatal blockages of lung circulation by blood clots (pulmonary emboli), and sudden, overwhelming infections account for most of these deaths, which nullify the gains claimed for purely elective hysterectomies. In other words: You save a few lives from cancer with such operations, but you lose a few others due to unexpected disasters. On balance, too little is gained with this approach.

Proponents of elective hysterectomy have also claimed that improvements in patients' quality of life warrant this surgery. This proposal is difficult to prove either way, because subjective judgments are involved, and these do not fit statistical calculations. It should clearly be the woman's pre-rogative to decide whether she needs this operation to improve her life, and to have access to information that would facilitate this decision. Polls of women who have had a hysterectomy are discussed elsewhere in this book; most women are satisfied with their surgery, but about 8 percent consider themselves worse off than they were before surgery.

Calculations that compute the financial costs of elective hysterectomy usually show large expenses in return for very small benefits. The hospital costs of hysterectomies have been estimated at $3 billion in 1985; total costs (including hospitals and surgeons) had increased to $5 billion within the next ten years. An authoritative text on the subject, *Te Linde's Operative Gynecology*, edited by J. D. Thompson and J. A. Rock (Lippincott-Raven, 8th ed., 1997), shows that mainstream gynecologists now concede that elective or prophylactic hysterectomy is a very expensive proposition and cannot be accepted without argument.

Hysterectomy Procedures

Abdominal hysterectomy is almost always a total (or complete) hysterec-tomy, an operation in which the entire uterus, including the cervix, but not the ovaries, is removed. The older form of hysterectomy was usually de-scribed as subtotal (or supracervical), meaning that the uterus was excised, but the cervix, by far the most difficult part to remove, was left behind. In previous decades, many hysterectomies were performed by general sur-geons and general practitioners not well trained in gynecological surgery, who often left the cervix behind. Later, some women developed cervical cancer that was then particularly difficult to treat. For this reason, the over-whelming concern in those years was that the cervix, which had the strongest tendency to turn cancerous, must be removed.

Gynecologist Conrad Collins of New Orleans, by all accounts an unusu-ally stern disciplinarian, was apparently very anxious not to have any of his patients develop cervical cancer. As chairman at Charity Hospital in the 1940s through the mid-1950s, he insisted that every gynecologist excise the cervix with the uterus and reportedly threatened to fire surgeons who did not comply. Collins personally removed the cervix from women whose previous hysterectomies were done by surgeons who left the cervix behind and who complained of pain or a severe discharge, showing that 4.4 percent of these organs were cancerous. This was, at least to modern gynecologists, not an unexpected finding, since the hysterectomies were performed before annual gynecological examinations with Pap smears became a routine event. Collins and like-minded gynecologists gradually established the requirement that unless technical difficulties were overwhelming, all hysterectomies should be total. Today, with much better detection of early cervical cancer and increased concerns about surgical mishaps (and malpractice claims after surgical mishaps), the cervix is left behind more frequently. The standard hysterectomy today is still "total"—it includes the cervix.

The researches of Masters and Johnson (of *Human Sexuality* fame) and certain Scandinavian opinions argue against excising the cervix, but many post-hysterectomy surveys, detailed elsewhere in this book, suggest that the woman who was relaxed, orgasmic, and sexually happy before surgery will continue to be orgasmic and sexually satisfied afterward.

David Grimes, a professor of OB/GYN at the University of North Carolina School of Medicine reviewed this subject in the pages of *Clinical Obstetrics and Gynecology*, a quarterly journal, in December 1999. His conclusion was that "opinions (on this topic) have outstripped the evidence"—meaning that too many of the studies were seriously flawed and little was known with certainty. Nevertheless, I believe that for some women, a strong case may be made for not removing the cervix.

One of my patients, at the age of thirty-five, was exhausted with the gynecological care demanded by her severe endometriosis and large fibroids. She agreed to have a hysterectomy but was aggressive and smart enough to undertake a computer search of disadvantages. The results convinced her that her cervix should be left behind to improve the quality of her post-hysterectomy sexual life. A series of negative Pap smears, a normal colposcopy, and other investigations convinced me that cervical cancer was highly unlikely to develop at a later date in this woman.

I asked her to give me a signed note about our discussion of this decision, modified the surgical consent form, and did as requested. Now, more than ten years later, she's doing well and has not complained of any post-hysterectomy problems. However, leaving the cervix intact at the time of hysterectomy is not mainstream gynecology. The fear of cancer still pervades gynecological thinking, while the role the cervix plays in orgasm is open to debate.

If the ovaries and tubes are removed, the surgery is called a **salpingo-oophorectomy**, usually abbreviated to SO (*salpinges* is Latin for fallopian tubes; *oophorectomy* means excision of the ovaries). These additional procedures may be done on one side only, in which case the abbreviations LSO or RSO are used, or on both sides, in which case the surgery is abbreviated to BSO. These initials usually follow the initials TAH (for total abdominal hysterectomy) or VH (same, except done vaginally). LH stands for laparoscopic hysterectomy, LAVH for laparoscopically assisted vaginal hysterectomy. TAH/BSO is the most common abbreviation gynecologists use.

Hysterectomy may be performed by the vaginal or abdominal routes or laparoscopically. Since this book promises to help you avoid hysterectomy, an extended comparison of these procedures would be inappropriate. Briefly, the vaginal procedure requires more expert surgery, although if there is some prolapse, vaginal hysterectomy is easier. A fibroid uterus smaller than 10–12 cm in diameter, or the size of a three-months' pregnancy may be removed vaginally, but as the uterus grows larger, it is increasingly difficult to do this. Hormonal medications may be used to shrink the uterus before scheduling surgery. If the surgeon needs to take an unobstructed look at all abdominal and pelvic organs, an essential task during cancer surgery, the abdominal route is preferable. However, some experts can perform even wide-ranging cancer surgery laparoscopically.

Laparoscopic surgery caught on in the United States during the 1970s but was initially performed mostly as a diagnostic procedure—to help provide accurate gynecological diagnoses through the careful inspection of internal organs. I usually summarize this for my medical students by stating, "Feeling (the manual examination) is guessing, looking is knowing." Soon instruments were designed to operate on fallopian tubes: first to interrupt them, as a contraceptive measure; then to repair the damage caused by pregnancies that lodged within fallopian tubes or to repair tubes damaged by infections. It was only during the early 1990s that the instruments and skills required to perform hysterectomy through a laparoscope became available. This innovation needs complex equipment as well as considerable surgical expertise and dexterity. Laparoscopy may also be a helpful adjunct during vaginal hysterectomy—called laparoscopically assisted vaginal hysterectomy, or LAVH. If a long abdominal incision is avoided, there will be less pain after the surgery is completed, fewer adhesions (shown in Figure

10.1) will develop, and the patient will enjoy an earlier return to normal activities. Laparoscopic surgery is discussed in Chapter 11.

Statistics

Looking at the total numbers of hysterectomies performed annually in the United States between 1980 and 1993, tabulated from hospital discharge summaries and compiled by the Centers for Disease Control and Prevention, it is apparent that there has been a modest decrease over the fourteen-year period reported in 1997, the latest detailed report available. Between 1980 and 1987, approximately 650,000 hysterectomies were performed annually; between 1988 and 1993, this decreased to about 560,000 a year. However, the most recent numbers, obtained directly from CDC, unfortunately show a gradual upswing to previous levels:

1994:   556,000
1995:   583,000
1996:   591,000
1997:   603,000
1998:   645,000

The United States certainly leads the world in hysterectomies. However, in spite of the availability of good alternatives, the recent and discouraging increases detailed above indicate that it will continue to do so. However, these large numbers are clearly a consequence of the large number of adult women in this country; obviously, a smaller country will have fewer hysterectomies. This statistical difficulty is corrected by using a measurement called the **hysterectomy rate**, which indicates the number of hysterectomies per 1,000 adult women. American data show a peak of 8.8 hysterectomies per 1,000 women over the age of fifteen in 1975, with a distinct diminution afterward. During the 1980s, hysterectomy rates fluctuated between a high of 7.2 in 1981 and a low of 6.5 in 1986. In 1987, the National Hospital Discharge Survey was redesigned; rates obtained after 1987 are in the 5.3 to 5.7 range, but these figures are no longer comparable to previous rates. European hysterectomy rates, as we'll see, are always lower and sometimes substantially lower.

43

A subtle flaw in the use of hysterectomy rates is that it makes no allowances for those women who have already had the operation. A number of years with very high hysterectomy rates will substantially deplete the pool of candidates who are available to undergo this operation. Hysterectomy rates would plummet—not because of different gynecological practices but because a large proportion of each group of 1,000 women had already undergone the operation and were no longer candidates for it. This difficulty is corrected by a sophisticated recalculation of the original data. This time, the proportion of women with a womb still in place who underwent hysterectomy is measured and divided by the number of hysterectomies performed. These figures are available for certain years only. Again, there was a peak in 1975, with 10.4 hysterectomies per 1,000 women with an intact uterus in their pelvis. This number decreased to 8.7 in 1980, and there was a much smaller decrease to 8.6 in 1984, the last year for which these figures are currently available. These decreases are not particularly reassuring: The rate in 1984, at 8.6, was still higher than it was in 1965 or 1970, when hysterectomies were already being performed too freely.

Let us now look at the reasons ("indications") for performing hysterectomies in recent years. According to data collected by the Centers for Disease Control and Prevention, and excluding radical surgery for cervical cancer, there were about 8,600,000 hysterectomies performed in the United States during the fourteen years between 1980 and 1993. More detailed information is available for more recent years: Between 1988 and 1993, there were about 3,350,000 hysterectomies; the primary diagnoses given by the hospitals reporting the latter operations have been the following:

Experts believe that pelvic pain is responsible for 10–12 percent of hysterectomies. The list of diagnoses presented in Table 3.1 does not include chronic pelvic pain; surgery for such pains is included under miscellaneous hysterectomies. If operations for CPP were subtracted from the line labeled "Miscellaneous" and were given a line of their own, the proportion of hysterectomies performed for these undefined reasons would be reduced to about 5 percent, giving us a more precise breakdown of the causes of American hysterectomies during recent years.

Table 3.1 shows the causes of hysterectomies during the years 1988 through 1993, but new options have recently become available that could reduce a proportion of these operations performed in most of the diag-

TABLE 3.1   Hysterectomies in the United States, 1988–1993

Diagnosis	Number of Hysterectomies[a]	Percentage of Total
Fibroids	1,118,000	33.4
Endometriosis	632,000	18.9
Prolapse	549,000	16.4
Cancer	340,000	10.1
Endometrial hyperplasia	179,000	5.3
Miscellaneous other	533,000	15.9
Total	3,351,000	100.0

[a] Figures are rounded to the nearest 1,000

nostic groups listed above. Reliable and safe treatments are now available for fibroids, endometriosis, prolapse, and chronic pelvic pain, and even for precancerous (premalignant) conditions of the cervix that reasonably justified hysterectomy in previous decades. The new treatments may be medical, surgical, or combinations of these, and they are outlined throughout this book.

American hysterectomy rates are much higher than European rates. As reported by Oxford epidemiologists Angela Coulter, Klim McPherson, and Martin Vessey in a 1988 article entitled, "Do British Women Undergo Too Many or Too Few Hysterectomies?" in *Social Science and Medicine,* a British journal, women in the National Health Service (NHS) had a hysterectomy rate of only 2.8 per 1,000 in 1985. This figure excludes hysterectomies performed outside the NHS. About 10 percent of Britons, mostly the affluent, have left the NHS; women enrolled with non-NHS insurance apparently had a higher, but unquoted, hysterectomy rate. This mirrors another uncomfortable fact that has emerged as a pattern. Patients enrolled with insurers that pay physicians high fees tend to undergo more investigations and operations than patients with poor insurance.

An argument may be made that the NHS is underfinanced and understaffed. British expenditures on health care are remarkably low for a major European power. While overall satisfaction with the NHS is high, dissatisfaction with waiting lists and cancellations of nonemergency cases (including elective hysterectomies) has also been voiced. The shortcomings and problems of the NHS are a recurring staple of British press coverage; "Grandmother Dies After Surgery Cancelled Eight Times" is one headline

I recall from many years ago. Political charges and countercharges about the sorry state of the NHS boil up with great regularity. In comparing the NHS to the American system, we are comparing a severely stressed service to one that rewards action very handsomely and is therefore exceptionally activist. There is no evidence that women in the NHS are suffering ill health because they cannot obtain indicated hysterectomies. One expert, Professor Lilford from Manchester, has calmly blamed women, writing in an editorial in the *British Medical Journal* in 1997 that "much of the variation in hysterectomy rates is . . . attributable to the psychosocial factors that influence demand." One of Lilford's major arguments was that the heavy bleeding women complained of was, when measured, not so heavy after all; I'd have expected gynecologists to understand this and explain it to their patients, before resorting to surgery. It may be concluded that a lower hysterectomy rate is perfectly compatible with good gynecological health.

Coulter, McPherson, and Vessey refer to rates of other countries. Canada, in 1979, was slightly below U.S. rates, at 6.2 per 1,000 women over fifteen. In the middle of the pack were the Netherlands (1981), Australia (1976), and Denmark (1981), with rates of 3.9, 3.8, and 3.6 hysterectomies respectively per 1,000 women. The lowest figures came from Sweden, where the 1977 figure was 1.3, and Norway (1977) at 1.1 per 1,000 women. A search of the standard medical database Medline reveals that recent corresponding figures are available mostly for Scandinavian countries. As before, Norwegian rates are the lowest: fewer than 2 hysterectomies per 1,000 women over the age of fifteen between 1988 and 1990, and Finnish rates were still well under 4 per 1,000 during the late 1980s.

The markedly different hysterectomy rates among various countries cannot be explained by thinking that American women are more sick or that European women need hysterectomies but cannot get them in their state-funded or "socialized" health-care systems. One minor exception may be noted: African-American women are more likely to need surgery because they grow more, and larger, fibroid tumors. However, this difference is insufficient to explain the differences between Scandinavian and American hysterectomy rates. The likeliest explanation for high American hysterectomy rates is simply the strong preference of American gynecologists for this operation, a theme that emerges repeatedly whenever scholars attempt to explain the fact that published American hysterectomy rates appear to be the highest in the world by far.

• • • 4 • • •

Voices Against Hysterectomy

Unnecessary Hysterectomy

Edward Shorter, a Canadian historian, has written detailed accounts of the physical and medical misfortunes of women in the Western world during the last three centuries. His book *A History of Women's Bodies* (Basic Books, 1982; Pelican Books, 1984) details a numbing sequence of insults and injustices suffered by women. Some were caused by disease, others were at the hands of husbands, yet others were by various medical practitioners with their often primitive or misguided efforts to heal. Shorter's argument is that owing to constant physical labor, difficulties with pregnancies and physical illnesses, poor medical care, and men who were often brutish and oppressive, women were in no shape to fight back against abuse and discrimination. With better contraception and medical care, along with improved standards of living, educational opportunities became feasible, and many of the burdens were lifted. These changes enabled women to begin their fight for equality.

The dour misogyny of the nineteenth century is easy to discern in the early development of gynecological surgery. In those days, hysterectomy was too difficult an operation to be undertaken casually. However, with the widespread acceptance of anesthesia, the removal of ovaries became fairly safe and not particularly difficult. As mentioned earlier, surgeons such as the Atlee brothers of Pennsylvania and Robert Battey of Georgia earned renown for removing the ovaries of hundreds of women for reasons that struck even some of their colleagues as ridiculous. **Nymphomania** and **hystero-neurosis** were two such "reasons" for operating on women. According to historians such as Ben Barker-Benham, Wendy Mitchinson, and Edward Shorter, the contemporary meaning of nymphomania was the male suspicion that the women—some of them inmates in mental hospitals, but others the wives or daughters of middle-class citizens—were masturbating excessively. Hystero-neurosis, a diagnosis often made in an age not given to diagnostic precision, was a catch-all phase, meaning hysterical fits, headaches, lethargy, and insomnia, which were then prevalent among women. These symptoms have been thoughtfully analyzed by Elaine Showalter in her books *The Female Malady* (Pantheon Books, 1985) and *Hystories* (Columbia University Press, 1998) and also by Edward Shorter in his book *From Paralysis to Fatigue* (The Free Press, 1992). And while the nineteenth century was rife with diagnoses and treatments for patients of either sex that appear preposterous today, it must be noted that it was rare for men to undergo mutilating surgery on their genitals to cure illness. True, boys were castrated, at the behest of their parents, to preserve their high-pitched soprano and alto voices, and rapists and other sexual offenders may occasionally have been punished by castration. The French monk Abelard was castrated early in the twelfth century for having an affair with his noble-born pupil Heloise; the horrifying severity of the punishment reverberating down the centuries, but there was no large-scale excision of male gonads to change undesirable patterns of behavior.

The first woman to become a physician in America was Elizabeth Blackwell, who graduated from a now-defunct medical school in Geneva, New York, in 1849. Blackwell was among those appalled by the wholesale excision of ovaries, but their protests were drowned by the chorus of contemporary opinions supporting such surgery. By contemporary accounts, this virtual stampede was encouraged by many physicians regardless of their gender and accepted by women in search of a solution for a variety of problems. There were testimonials to the amazingly curative effects of removing the ovaries of young women as well as a few scathing dismissals of the practice, but it took almost 100 years before gynecologists began to challenge the widespread practice of unnecessary surgery.

In a 1945 study of 246 hysterectomies in ten hospitals in three Midwestern states, gynecologist Norman Miller of Ann Arbor, Michigan, was startled to discover a peculiar practice of his colleagues. Miller found that, based on information he received from gynecologists performing the operations, far too often the hysterectomies were unnecessary. In one-third, there was no apparent reason to perform the operation, since all the tissues that were removed were normal. Nearly 17 percent of the women had no symptoms, no suspected disease on pelvic examination, and no microscopic evidence of disease in the organs removed. Many had complained of headaches, fatigue, irritability, or nervousness, symptoms that hysterectomy could not help and symptoms that could be made worse if the ovaries are also removed. Miller's respondents probably thought they were not doing anything unusual in performing the hysterectomies; quite likely it was simply business as usual. An impartial and thoughtful analysis of their own activities was apparently not to be had from these professionals.

In describing these operations, Norman Miller's language was accurate and colorful in a way no longer found in medical journals. He referred to them as "acute remunerative or hip-pocket hysterectomies" and described the scene he surveyed as "stunning" and "astonishing." To Miller, it was a "bewildering discovery" that hysterectomy specimens were free of pathology or, even worse, that the disease ultimately identified was an unsuspected pregnancy. Miller concluded, "If what we have observed in this look behind the scenes is confirmed by further studies, then we may be sure when the curtain rises we shall witness a tragedy painful and far-reaching in its implications."

Seven years later, in 1953, a much larger study of over 6,000 hysterectomies revealed findings that were disturbingly similar. This time, the critic was gynecologist James C. Doyle of Beverly Hills. The previous year Doyle had published an article in the *Journal of the American Medical Association,* reporting the unnecessary removal of 704 ovaries from 546 women. In the same journal, Doyle showed that 39 percent of the hysterectomies he reviewed were unnecessary. His article makes it plain that apart from unnecessary surgery, the quality of care received by these women was often appallingly poor. There were 65 women whose uterine cancers were not diagnosed until after the hysterectomy because standard investigations such as Pap smears and biopsies or curettages were not carried out. At a time when pregnancy tests were in widespread use and reasonably accurate, undiagnosed pregnancies were a frequent reason for unnecessary hysterectomies. For instance, the operation was often performed to control bleeding due to a miscarriage. Curettage, a much easier and well-established procedure, would have sufficed to stop the bleeding. It is difficult to imagine why hysterectomy was performed; I am embarrassed to state that plain incompetence is one possibility.

Doyle also pointed out that some hospitals were particularly responsible for excessive rates of unnecessary surgery. In looking at 35 privately administered California hospitals, he found that in 4 hospitals with the best overall record, 76 to 95 percent of the hysterectomies were warranted. You may think that 76 percent is not an admirable percentage, but this figure looks good in comparison to unnecessary surgery at the 4 worst hospitals Doyle found. By his reasonable criteria, the hysterectomies performed in these 4 hospitals were necessary in only 16, 19, 31, and 33 percent of cases, respectively.

Doyle singled out one hospital, identified only by the code letter "W," for particular attention. In addition to the exceptionally high proportion (84 percent) of unnecessary hysterectomies, in this hospital 33 percent of the organs removed showed no disease whatever. Much worse, the preoperative diagnosis was found to be correct in only 46 percent of cases, and in 3 percent, hysterectomy was actually contraindicated. This is an emphatically strong word, used when, due to medical circumstances, experts condemn the use of an operation. Miller and Doyle were twenty or thirty years ahead of their colleagues in drawing attention to incompetent and unnecessary surgery. In those days, there was no public outcry against medical care that was dangerous as well as worthless.

Subsequent studies began to trickle in, confirming that many hysterectomies were preventable. Whenever expert gynecologists checked the work of their colleagues, they found that 10–40 percent of hysterectomies they scrutinized were undertaken for questionable reasons. Open surveillance and publicity were often all that were required to produce drastic reductions in the abuse that became known as unnecessary hysterectomy.

A 1962 study of the medical care received by Teamster families in the New York area revealed that over 30 percent of hysterectomies were unnecessary. Nine years later, Mildred A. Morehead, M.D., one of the senior authors of that study, collaborated in writing a similar paper, in which expert reviewers concluded that 43 percent were unjustified. This article addressed the evaluation of the quality of care given by physicians and found that "the teaching hospital is clearly superior overall." This statement is important. Most segments of the medical establishment run into difficulties (and disasters) on occasion, so perhaps the best move is to stay out of hospitals as long as you can. However, if you need gynecological surgery or other medical care that needs a hospital stay, I believe that you are likely to obtain the best quality in hospitals run by, or affiliated with, medical schools.

Experts from Saskatchewan, Canada, undertook a study of hysterectomy because the use of the operation increased by 72 percent from 1964 to 1971, with an increase of only 7.6 percent in the number of women over the age of fifteen. A list of indications was compiled; those operations not meeting the criteria drawn up by experts were classified as unnecessary. Overall, during the years of surveillance, the proportion of unjustified hysterectomies in Saskatchewan dropped from 23.7 percent to 7.8 percent. Even more to the point, in two hospitals with the worst records, the percentages dropped more steeply, from 59 percent to 16 percent, and from 45 percent to 13 percent.

Writing for *Scientific American* in 1982, John Wennberg and Alan Gittelson drew attention to inexplicably wide variations in hysterectomy rates in Maine. In one unnamed city, the rate was so high that if it persisted, 70 percent of the women would have undergone hysterectomy by the age of seventy-five. In another similar Maine city, less than twenty miles away, the hysterectomy rate was substantially lower. If its hysterectomy rate persisted, only 25 percent of the women there stood to lose their wombs from surgery. There were no striking differences in the health of women between the two cities. Looking for a reason, Wennberg and Gittelson came up with one answer only: In the first city, surgeons were "enthusiastic about hysterectomy"; in the second, they were "more skeptical of its value."

In 1982, a review of the indications for hysterectomy in the quarterly publication *Clinical Obstetrics and Gynecology* published by J. B. Lippincott Company conceded that 10–40 percent of all American hysterectomies were probably unnecessary.

A 1991 survey, carried out by Blue Cross/Blue Shield of Minnesota, indicated that nearly 17 percent of 495 hysterectomies reviewed were thought to be medically inappropriate.

One of the most recent articles to address this topic appeared in *Obstetrics and Gynecology* in February 2000. Called "The Appropriateness of Recommendations for Hysterectomy," the paper was written by members of the staff at a variety of prestigious organizations such as the Department of Obstetrics and Gynecology at the University of California at Los Angeles (UCLA), the Rand Corporation of Los Angeles, and the University of Michigan in Ann Arbor. Using Rand Corporation standards as well as their own criteria and established and well-known ACOG recommendations, this study reported that fully 70 percent of the nearly 500 hysterectomies they surveyed from August 1993 through July 1995 were inappropriately recommended. The most common failures reported were "lack of adequate diagnostic evaluation" and "failure to try alternative treatments" before surgery. Further, there were 71 women to whom one of three specific ACOG criteria for hysterectomy applied; but the problems of 76 percent of these women did not meet official ACOG criteria for hysterectomy. What made this study even more remarkable was that the reviews were all performed in so-called capitated medical groups: In other words, the surgeons were salaried and did not gain financially from performing the operations—rather, they worked very hard at jobs they could easily have avoided! This finding diminishes the particularly sharp charge that surgery was undertaken for financial gain, a painful point to contemplate, but it supports the equally serious accusation that unnecessary hysterectomies were simply an accepted and satisfactory way of life for the ninety-seven gynecologists whose work was evaluated.

And, of course, these conclusions were derived from yesterday's hysterectomies, performed on yesterday's patients. Today, as long as cancer and severe hemorrhage are excluded, many hysterectomies, even those previously regarded as necessary, are potentially avoidable. Further, it is discouraging to note that while various alternatives have been available for decades and others have arrived more recently, the new procedures have largely failed to influence hysterectomy rates.

Systematic injustice is not limited to North America. Writing in 1945, Miller cited the 1939 opinion of the prominent Irish obstetrician Bethel Solomons, who was clearly unhappy with his colleagues' surgical habits. Solomons wrote, "I would say a gynecologist is not a gynecologist until he ceases to perform unnecessary hysterectomies, for this operation has become nearly as overdone as the operations for tonsillectomy, appendectomy and curettage."

In Switzerland, the canton of Ticino saw a steep increase of 65 percent in the hysterectomy rate, from 860 hysterectomies per 100,000 women between the ages of 39 and 49 in 1977, to 1,422 operations in 1982. A publicity and information campaign was consequently undertaken from February through October 1984. This resulted in decreasing the number of hysterectomies by one-third. In the neighboring canton of Bern, with no publicity, the hysterectomy rate remained stable, with only moderate fluctuations between 1977 and 1985. A careful look at the data shows that throughout the years of the study, hysterectomies were performed about 50 percent more often in Bern, with Ticino gynecologists almost catching up with the high rates of their Bern colleagues and then falling back again. The likeliest explanation of these facts is that hysterectomy has more to do with gynecological ambitions, habits, and customs than with the health needs of the women whom the gynecologists were supposed to serve.

There was only one study in which the majority of hysterectomies were found to be appropriate. This study was performed under the aegis of the New York County Medical Society, composed of licensed and expert physicians practicing in Manhattan. In 1972, these physicians concluded that less than 1 percent of the 1,901 hysterectomies reviewed were unnecessary. However, all other reviews, all performed by competent physicians, found that an unacceptably high proportion of hysterectomies were unnecessary. In scientific matters, the views of the majority of experts are usually considered to be correct; there is no reason to believe that unnecessary hysterectomies are an exception to this rule.

Arguing against too easy acceptance of the idea that large numbers of hysterectomies may be unnecessary, medical apologists may stress that necessity is too vague and undefinable a concept to apply to surgical procedures. This philosophical argument need not detain us much. The most respected American textbook of gynecological surgery, *Te Linde's Operative Gynecology* (Lippincott-Raven Publishers, 8th ed., 1997), devotes many pages to topics such as inappropriate indications for hysterectomy and unnecessary hysterectomy.

Responsible gynecologists have no trouble identifying unnecessary hysterectomies, which have given the profession a sour reputation in many quarters. This book will show, disease by disease, how it might be possible to avoid even those hysterectomies that today's gynecologists consider either necessary or at least perfectly acceptable. Since your gynecologist may plan to remove your ovaries along with your womb, you will find a chapter devoted to discussing the advantages and disadvantages of excising these organs. The statistical information presented in the previous chapter and the hysterectomy reviews in this one make it clear that too many gynecologists have a very flawed idea of the correct use of this operation.

Unnecessary hysterectomies are not performed in a scientific or humanitarian fashion, in response to women's medical needs or complaints. Instead, they appear to depend entirely on the gynecologist's ideas about the appropriateness of the operation.

A few years ago, a woman physician in a major metropolitan medical center told me of her near-hysterectomy experience with her gynecologist, who was a respected and socially prominent physician, whom I knew. She had been his patient for many years when her periods began to turn heavier. He found a small fibroid uterus, and subsequent examinations revealed a pattern of steady growth. Contrary to current practice, not a single sonogram was ordered. Six months later, with the womb now reportedly "larger than a grapefruit," hysterectomy was recommended and was about to be scheduled. The woman, who had never before questioned any of her gynecologist's recommendations, decided to get a second opinion. The gynecologist she chose was surprised because he felt barely any enlargement. An ultrasound scan was finally ordered and confirmed the second gynecologist's estimate. The woman, who had gradually become a senior figure at another hospital, felt angry about the deception, but not angry enough to lodge a complaint. As many women do, she chalked it up to experience and simply changed gynecologists. Years later, when she told me her story, I heard that training for a marathon made her lose quite a few pounds of weight. I suspect that this interfered with the rhythmic pattern of her ovulatory cycles, causing irregular periods—but this is merely a guess. Most likely, she did not need surgery; she needed information and reassurance. But the chicanery involving his overestimates of uterine size and of not ordering any sonograms still rankles. I was saddened to come across rank duplicity from a practitioner I knew fairly well. It was also brazen on his part to inflict a self-serving and unmistakably dishonest recommendation on a prominent colleague.

Your situation will be different if you do not have a private gynecologist but are a "service" or "clinic" patient, in the hands of resident staff, learners who are under constant supervision, particularly during surgery. The information you receive may be less than what you would get from a private practitioner, so that you must educate yourself thoroughly about your treatment options. The quality of the care you will receive will, as always,

depend on the humanistic and medical attributes of the nurses and gynecologists providing your care. It is easy to cite examples of excellent or
poor quality care in either private or "service" settings. Resident staff are
less experienced, but they are also less likely to rely overmuch on obsolete
and abandoned ideas. As already stated, teaching hospitals are preferable, although no place is without physicians (and nurses) who may be euphemis-
tically described as suboptimal.

There is an additional important feature about being a "service" patient
in a teaching hospital. The economic incentives to perform surgery are
usually less important than they are in private practice but are replaced by
a system that seeks surgical cases for different reasons. The more a resident
gynecologist operates, the more skillful he or she becomes. Vaginal hysterectomy in particular is a skill difficult to acquire without first assisting at
many cases and then going on to do more cases. A surgical training program that does not provide sufficient surgical experience would be in
trouble within a year or two, unless the numbers of operations were increased. One solution is to send young doctors-in-training (residents) from
large teaching hospitals to smaller, rural hospitals. Indications for surgery
are less stringently scrutinized in these hospitals, and uterine prolapse is
more frequent, because rural women usually have more children. Consequently, much surgical experience is gained, but at the expense of women
who live somewhere else. Another solution is to relax standard surgical criteria and pump up the number of operations at the medical center by performing hysterectomies that are not as well indicated as they should be.
Either system encourages surgery that may be avoidable.

Apart from the income to be made, are there other reasons for unnecessary hysterectomies? The most benign explanation, that "surgical enthusiasm" is a way of life in gynecology, may well be true, but what exactly does
such a statement mean? The thrill and prestige of being a gynecologist
with a busy surgical schedule is probably a major factor. Surgical work
boosts the ego: It is precise and demanding, a source of satisfaction when
successful, excruciating when difficulties pile up. Female physicians and the
wives of physicians have exceptionally high rates of hysterectomy, although
female gynecologists, as noted, are less likely to perform hysterectomies
than some of their male colleagues. I believe that unquestioning acceptance of unnecessary surgery and the prospect of economic gains combine
to dictate many hysterectomies.

If you are a clinic patient, you have a right to discuss your care with the gynecologist in charge of your care. This person must be someone who has finished a residency program. If you are told that your case is unusual, you can insist that a senior gynecologist or the chief of the service be consulted. This may not work if your case appears to be a common condition, frequently handled by the resident staff. If you cannot afford a private consultation, you may be able to get a low-cost or free consultation from another clinic, at another hospital. However, these consultations become more difficult to arrange if you are already in a hospital, bleeding and hooked up to intravenous infusion sets. As always, it is essential to plan ahead judiciously.

From the consumer's point of view, the safeguards against unnecessary surgery consist of eternal vigilance with as much information about your gynecological diagnosis as you can obtain. The gynecologist who proposes that hysterectomy is the best solution of your problem must be able to answer the following questions:

1. Is this operation really necessary? This question is answered in those sections of the book that deal with the diseases the surgery is supposed to help. If you are looking forward to the surgery, this is usually because there is much bleeding or pain. Make sure you ask the surgeon if you are likely to derive the benefit you expect from the operation. If you are anxious to avoid the surgery at all costs, this book shows you how this may be achieved.

2. What is the disease that appears to necessitate hysterectomy? Be cautious if the operation is being recommended for a number of separate problems: Each may be manageable with measures other than a major operation, and each must be discussed individually. This is time-consuming, and your gynecologist may not have the patience to go through every option available to you. This book contains an enormous amount of information, questions that must be answered, and even the possible consequences of your decisions in the years to come. Support groups, listed in the Resources section at the end of the book, are also a good way of gathering information. If you are careful and consider all the guidelines listed, you will be prepared and make the best use of the time that becomes available for discussing your problems. You

may even find that you can decide some questions directly for yourself.

3. What would be the consequences of not doing a hysterectomy? Vague references to preventing trouble or cancer are not acceptable. Unless your symptoms have worsened, you have time to research the situation.

4. What other ways are there to treat your condition? This book outlines all the treatment options available for various gynecological diseases. Do not accept hysterectomy as a solution too quickly.

5. How certain is it that hysterectomy will improve your most troublesome gynecological symptoms? Some complaints are relatively easy to correct: For instance, hysterectomy will invariably put an end to abnormal vaginal bleeding. Other complaints (for instance, pain or the involuntary loss of urine on coughing or sneezing) may or may not respond to hysterectomy. The gynecologist who assures you that all your symptoms will disappear may be correct but may also be a superior salesperson with a well-practiced routine. You should have a clear idea *before* surgery of how likely it is that your gynecological symptoms will improve and what the next step is if they do not.

Do not be embarrassed or reticent about asking for a second, or even a third, session to discuss any proposed surgery. You are discussing a major step in your life. Your gynecologist must be willing to concentrate on you and your problem for a reasonable amount of time. A second opinion is essential. Unless you are exceptionally well organized and have an excellent memory for details, take notes. In theory, tape-recording a conversation is fine, but such an approach may make the doctor being interviewed excessively cautious, defensive, and long-winded. More important is your selection of the gynecologist who will provide the second opinion. He or she should never be a friend or partner of the gynecologist who recommended hysterectomy in the first place.

If you have no choice because your insurance directs you to a certain physician for a second opinion, at least find out if the two work at the same hospital. Ideally, they should not know each other. In larger cities, there should be no difficulty in finding a gynecologist to provide a second opinion acceptable to you as well as your insurance company. If you live in a smaller town and have only one or two gynecologists to turn to in an emergency, inevitably your choices are reduced. However, a consultation with a reliable gynecologist in another city should not be to difficult to arrange and should give you an independent opinion of your exact needs for surgery.

The selection of physicians has been discussed in the Introduction to this book. For the purposes of a second opinion consultation, as much information as possible should be available to save you the trouble (and possibly the expense) of a second visit. Ask for copies of reports and keep the following:

- Blood tests: blood counts, pregnancy tests, and so on
- Pathology reports: Pap smears, biopsies, surgical reports
- X-rays, ultrasounds, scans: the reports as well as the x-ray plates and scans, if this is possible
- Mammogram reports if you are over thirty-five years old or at high risk of breast cancer
- Operative reports

You may prefer to have as your future gynecologist someone who has provided a second opinion for you and whose manners and opinions you prefer. From an ethical point of view, this physician should not accept you as a patient. This rule derives partly from old-fashioned notions of chivalry, according to which you and your original gynecologist have a prior claim to each other. In addition, the value of the second opinion is not meant to be tainted by financial considerations such as the income to be derived from a new patient, who may sooner or later need surgery. However, the rule is sometimes breached, and sometimes for good reason.

Any patient, and particularly women who may need surgery, must understand that money is part of the exchange between doctors and patients. Unless you belong to an HMO or have signed an elaborate agreement with your insurance company that prohibits switching doctors, you are a free agent whose main concern must be to obtain the best care available. If your original gynecologist recommended hysterectomy and the "second opinion" gynecologist advised against surgery, you should consider obtaining a third opinion. After three opinions, if you would prefer to continue with the second (or third) gynecologist, you must discuss your decision with your insurance company. This is time-consuming, almost legal work, but it is a prudent way to ensure the continuity of your care and of your insurance coverage.

Do not confuse a wonderful bedside manner with competence. One of my most outstanding teachers, a professor of medicine in Cape Town, South Africa, could not make a living from private practice, and ultimately abandoned the effort. His memory was photographic, his judgments unfailingly excellent—but he was too impatient and brusque to be a congenial, well-loved physician. A physician with a ready smile and an open, engaging personality is preferable; but more to the point, you should ask precise questions and receive precise answers. Most questions you will ask will be related to disease you are thought to have. The questions you must ask will be listed, disease by disease and chapter by chapter, throughout this book.

It may be comforting to know that there are certain invisible safeguards working on your behalf, although they are difficult for outsiders to evaluate. In good hospitals, a so-called tissue committee examines the outcome of every operation performed. The surgeon who cuts out normal organs instead of the diseased tissues the pathologist expects to receive may be contacted by the hospital's tissue committee and asked to explain the background and purpose of the surgery. Some tissue committees are aggressive and powerful; others have no real authority and may not criticize anyone. Surgical work may not be scrutinized closely until a number of operations result in bad outcomes. Of course, an uneventful recovery does not mean that surgery was necessary. Since such information is not easily available, your only safeguard consists of choosing a reputable hospital when surgical care is unavoidable. If needed, you can still ask the hospital's OB/GYN department to recommend a gynecologist for another opinion.

Hysterectomy is not the only surgery with a tainted history. Tonsillectomies, gallbladder surgery, hemorrhoidectomies, coronary artery bypass surgery, and even appendectomies have been shown to be open to questionable use or flagrant abuse. During my residency in St. Louis several decades ago, I knew of one American hospital in which patients thought they underwent cholecystectomies (excisions of the gallbladder), after which the recovery was miraculously free of pain and complications. Some time later, symptoms would recur, and further tests would show that the gallbladder had not been removed. Quite likely, the skin had been incised and sutured, a sham that did not require abdominal drainage tubes, catheters, and intravenous fluids. The hospital in question closed its doors many years ago, and such open abuses are no longer feasible, but operations that benefit surgeons more than patients have endured.

Reflecting on the history of ovariotomy and unnecessary hysterectomies, it is evident that poorly indicated gynecological surgery has been with us almost as long as gynecological surgery itself. However, you do not have to go to medical school to distinguish necessary from unnecessary surgery. What you need is a level-headed appraisal of the medical facts of your condition:

1. Be as certain of your diagnosis as possible. Understand that only rarely is surgery necessary to find out exactly what is happening in your body, but occasionally laparoscopy (or even laparotomy) may become essential to find out if a tumor is cancerous.

2. Line up all the available managements, including doing nothing; taking pain medications, antibiotics, or hormonal treatments; or resorting to surgery. Additional consultations, telephone hot lines, support groups, even an hour or two spent in a bookstore with medical self-help books and textbooks may point you in new and helpful directions. Medical information available in a variety of Web sites is another possibility, but with one cautionary note: Anyone can post any information with little fear of contradiction.

3. Try to examine each participant's motives for preferring one mode of treatment over another, particularly when it comes to advocating surgery. You must make every effort to evaluate carefully all the opinions you get, bearing in mind that every person you turn to may have an agenda that includes not only your interests but quite possibly theirs as well. The holistic practitioner who recommends acupuncture for your fibroid tumors is, as far as I am concerned, a charlatan, but it may not be politically correct to stress this.

The Disadvantages of Surgery

Over thirty years ago, when I was a young resident in gynecology in St. Louis, Missouri, a socially prominent woman in her forties was admitted to my hospital late one afternoon. She had developed a sudden illness consisting of vomiting with abdominal pain and swelling. A series of x-rays confirmed our suspicions: She had acutely blocked bowels, known as intestinal obstruction, and she required emergency surgery. When we operated on her at 4 A.M., my colleagues and I found a thick ring of firm, rubbery tissue, almost like a napkin ring, encircling a short length of her colon. Above this ring, the colon was bulging; below, it was collapsed and empty. To our shock, the diagnosis seemed to be obvious: cancer of the colon. The surgical team I was assisting relieved the obstruction by cutting out the thickened tissue and a margin of normal-looking colon. But judging by the distinctly swollen lymph nodes in the area, the suspected cancer had spread well beyond what could be removed, and we had no illusions that the surgery saved her life. We removed one of the swollen lymph nodes to check the cause of the enlargement and completed some additional surgery, and finished by 7 A.M.

Other surprises awaited us. The next afternoon, the hospital pathologist called to tell us that the microscopic exam did not show cancer. Instead, he found endometriosis, a complex disease discussed in Chapter 7. The woman's glands were enlarged because they were bursting with endometriosis. Today, using a technique called "frozen sections," the pathologist may be able to give the correct diagnosis within fifteen minutes of getting a small sample of tissue, but we had no such help in the middle of the night in the 1960s.

Since endometriosis of the bowel consistently mimics other diseases, our error was not particularly embarrassing. However, the patient was not improving. Her abdomen, which was less gas filled immediately after surgery, was getting distended again. Further x-rays explained why: The surgeon (or one of his assistants, perhaps me) had inadvertently left behind a pair of scissors in the woman's abdomen, between loops of her bowel. Red-faced, we reopened her to retrieve the scissors, and she recovered quickly. The episode stayed with me because in looking after one woman, we experienced two awful shocks and one joyous surprise in a day and a half. Medicine is never boring, and surprises are far from exceptional.

The oft-repeated charge that 25–50 percent of all hysterectomies cause complications is true, but the statement is misleading all the same. Many so-called complications are inconsequential. For instance, a transient low-grade fever must, by definition, be counted as a complication, but it is not worrisome. On the positive side, some hospitals have reported thousands of consecutive hysterectomies without a single death. Of course, operating on healthy young women who may not need surgery in the first place is an excellent way to ensure few complications. This chapter is not concerned with the need for surgery, but with its adverse effects.

While operating poses risks, not operating may not be safe for some. If appendicitis or an ectopic pregnancy is suspected, for example, avoiding surgery is dangerous. A proportion of appendices will be removed unnecessarily, just to make sure that no case of appendicitis is misdiagnosed. The situation is the same if a potentially lethal condition such as tubal (ectopic) pregnancy is suspected. The risks and benefits of surgery must always be compared to the risk and benefits of not operating. Fortunately, it is rare that postponing elective hysterectomy causes serious trouble later.

The complications of hysterectomy that concern gynecologists, either because the complication is frequent or because it is serious, are discussed next. The list is far from complete, since a detailed discussion of the complications of hysterectomy is beyond the scope of this book. In Table 4.1, "Complications of Hysterectomy," I have tried to indicate the likelihood of some of the complications by using simple descriptions such as "frequent" and "rare." Whenever feasible, percentages are given.

The most frequent complications are postoperative infections, due to wound (incisional) infections (these occur in 5–10 percent of all patients), infections at the top of the vagina (where it is closed after hysterectomy, which occur in 2–5 percent), and urinary tract infections (which probably occur in 20–30 percent). All these are usually easy to treat successfully.

The **mortality** related to hysterectomy (a woman's chances of dying because of the surgery) has been studied carefully so that accurate information is available to women. Overall, in recent large studies, 12–15 women died for every 10,000 hysterectomies performed, or a rate slightly above 0.1 percent. The risks are higher in certain groups:

- Pregnancy-related hysterectomy (ruptured uterus, hemorrhage): 29.2 per 10,000
- Cancer-related hysterectomy: 37.8 per 10,000
- Mortality in women over 75 years of age: 173.3 per 10,000

Women who have medical diseases such as diabetes and hypertension are more likely to develop complications, including death, after surgery. Con-

TABLE 4.1   Complications of Hysterectomy

Anesthesia-related complications	Unsuccessful spinal anesthesia: rare
	Cardiac arrest: very rare, but possibly lethal
	Vomiting under anesthesia: rare, but potentially serious, leading to pneumonia
Complications during surgery	Hemorrhage: rare, under 1 percent
	Erroneous diagnoses: frequency difficult to estimate
	Damage to surrounding organs: bowel, bladder, uterus; about 1–2 percent
	Need for additional, unintended surgery: rare
	Transfusion reactions: about 1 percent
Postoperative complications	Infections: mostly skin, bladder, vagina, lungs: frequent, 15–35 percent, but rarely serious
	Venous clotting: frequent, but major complications rare
	Delayed return of bowel function, urinary tract function: frequent, but usually of little consquence
	Incision does not heal, breaks open: 1 percent
	Thrombo-embolic disease: under 1 percent, but potentially fatal
Delayed complications	Readmission to hospital: rare
	Incisional hernias: rare
	Intestinal obstruction from adhesions: very rare
	Ovarian cysts: probably about 3–5 percent
	Ovarian cancer: if ovaries left behind, about 1 percent
Hormonal changes (see Chapter 14)	Heart disease
	Bone loss (osteoporosis): delayed, but frequent if ovaries removed and estrogen not replaced
	Premature ovarian failure (premature menopause): frequency difficult to estimate
Emotional consequences	Depression and anxiety: frequent, but transient
	Sexual difficulties: discussed later in this chapter
Surgical mortality	Dying during or within a month of surgery: Slightly above 0.1 percent overall, less for younger women (see information above)

versely, among healthy young women who undergo hysterectomy electively, fewer than 1 per 1,000 die of the operation.

The extensive list of rare complications creates concerns about a balanced discussion with patients. The surgeon has moral and legal obligations to describe the complications of the surgery being planned with the patient. In some states, including California and New York, the law demands that an additional hysterectomy consent must be signed. Alternatives may have to be discussed, including the fact that the patient understands that after hysterectomy she will no longer be able to conceive. This consent must be signed, even if the woman is well past her menopause at the time of the operation.

In addition to complications, before any surgery, you and your physician must also discuss alternative managements, pre- and postoperative care, and a host of other matters. At this point, you may encounter the fact that surgeons usually have no interest in a complete discussion of risks. Such discussions take a long time and risk frightening the patient away from surgery. Patients, often under stress, may not be able to absorb all the information provided.

One of my reasons for writing this book has been the realization that a full and impartial discussion between surgeon and patient is probably an ideal that can be met only rarely. Often, I have been able to discuss all the relevant facts only after setting aside an hour without interruptions of any kind, something not easy to arrange in a busy OB/GYN practice. Unfortunately, most of us probably spend more time on finding the right house or the best car for the money than on investigating major surgery we are about to undergo.

To be fully informed, women can draw on the following sources:

- The medical professionals involved in their care
- Support groups, listed in the Resources section at the end of this book
- Books and other informational materials, obtainable from libraries, bookshops, or computer databases and networks
- The Internet—with cautions discussed on page 323.

Preventing Complications

The rise in malpractice litigation has forced most surgeons to be extremely cautious in taking measures to guard against all foreseeable complications. For instance, antibiotics are usually started before surgery to prevent infections after surgery. Heparin, an agent that slows down the coagulation of blood (or "thins the blood," as some describe it), may also be used in an effort to prevent the formation of clots in leg and pelvic veins during surgery. Without drug therapy, such clots may break away and be carried to the lungs, where they may obstruct large vessels. This results in thromboembolic disease and may prove fatal.

Other complications are caused by diseases coexisting with the disease that led to the need for surgery. Obesity, diabetes, asthma, high blood pressure, and heart disease may all lead to complications that are difficult to prevent. Complex surgical problems, such as operating on women who have multiple large abscesses, make for unavoidably long and difficult surgery, after which the surgeon cannot guarantee good results—for instance, fertility may be lost irretrievably.

What can women do to minimize their chances of developing complications? Scrupulous care before surgery by following these steps may result in less trouble afterward:

1. Obtain the services of the best professionals and hospital available. This, by far the most important precaution, is discussed in the Introduction and throughout the book.
2. Stop smoking for at least several weeks before surgery. As most women are aware, smoking is bad for your health in various ways, but many cannot do without cigarettes. If you are completely addicted, you may consider the new nicotine-containing patches to satisfy your cravings for nicotine. They are expensive, but they will give your lungs a break at a time when they should be in the best shape for surgery.
3. If you are overweight and need elective surgery, try to lose the excess weight.
4. Be sure your surgeon knows the medications you are taking currently and have taken recently. Birth control pills should be stopped at least four weeks before surgery, something that is not feasible for emergencies. Medications for high blood pressure, asthma, and even aspirin may, combined with other drugs, cause serious complications. You may regard counterculture medications, including herbs, as perfectly safe; on occasion, this assumption has caused major problems.
5. Careful preoperative cleansing of the skin and vaginal tissues is important. A thorough shower and a douche with an agent such

as Betadyne are often used by hospitals the night before elective surgery.

6. Some of the most preventable complications are the emotional aftereffects of hysterectomy. Good rapport with the surgeon is critical. A thorough understanding of the purpose and effects of any operation are so essential that much of the next section is devoted to these topics.

7. Be sure your surgeon knows what other illnesses you have or may have. If you have other medical problems, such as, for instance, hypertension or diabetes, make sure that all your specialists contact your gynecologist before surgery. This may appear obvious and simple, yet only too often these professionals do not connect with each other carefully enough to ensure quality care.

8. After the operation, within a few hours of waking up from the anesthetic (or recovering from spinal anesthesia), you should cough up any secretions accumulating in your lungs. This is particularly important in women who are heavy smokers or who have lung problems such as chronic bronchitis and emphysema. Not lying motionless in one position for hours and hours is also extremely important. Roll over from side to side as early as you can, and move your legs about as much and as often as you can. As soon as the surgeon asks you to, try to get up and begin to take a few steps and sit in an armchair. These measures may prevent postoperative pneumonia. Even more important, they will help prevent thrombophlebitis (the postoperative formation of clots in your leg or pelvic veins) and thromboembolic disease (the obstruction of lung circulation by clots that have become detached from their origins and been carried to the lungs), a major cause of complications, including sudden death.

The Physical Effects of Hysterectomy on Sexuality

According to some women, and supported by at least some research, the surgical removal of the uterus and cervix may diminish sexual response. Virginia Masters and William Johnson have shown that the intact womb, including the cervix, plays a role during sexual arousal. Also, women may believe that uterine contractions are an important part of orgasm. Finnish research indicates that the cervix has a rich supply of nerves; these are interrupted when the cervix is excised. Fortunately, removal of the cervix in not nearly as essential today as it was fifty years ago. This remains an open question, but (as we shall see) surveys have found that sexual satisfaction may not be dependent on the presence of either the uterus or the cervix. The relief of painful symptoms and effective contraception are two good reasons why most women are sexually intact following hysterectomy.

Hysterectomy may shorten the vagina, and scar tissue may cause pain on intercourse. In my experience, women who were orgasmic and sexually fulfilled before surgery usually resumed their sexual activities successfully within 4–6 weeks after hysterectomy. Vaginal hysterectomy may be combined with another vaginal operation, in which lax tissues, usually the consequence of many deliveries, are tightened. This is called "anterior and posterior repair" (A&P repair), because the loosened front and rear walls of the vagina are tightened by the surgery. The A&P repair may cause more vaginal scarring than an abdominal hysterectomy. If the surgeon is not careful, he may tighten the vagina so much that intercourse becomes difficult. As men age and lose their youthful erections, a thoroughly tightened vagina makes intercourse difficult. If this happens, careful dilatation of the vagina with graduated dilators (or fingers) usually solves the problem within a month or two. This needs no gynecological intervention—it is something the woman (or her lover) can do. It is rarely necessary to reoperate to undo some of the repair and to loosen excessively tightened vaginal tissues.

Masters and Johnson have shown that during emotionally satisfying intercourse, the vagina distends. This ensures that any disparity in size between a large penis and a small vagina rarely causes sexual difficulties. Also, a few women are born without a vagina or have a rudimentary vagina only. In one method of artificially creating one, a small pouch is made where the vagina is normally located, after which the regular use of dilators (possibly including a penis) gradually builds an increasingly capacious vagina. These facts make me somewhat cautious about uncritically accepting claims of sexual problems due to reduced vaginal length.

During hysterectomy, as a rule, little vaginal length is lost, but during a radical hysterectomy, performed to deal with cancer, one-third or as much as half the vagina may be removed. Radiation may also be administered. In such instances, the vagina may be significantly shortened, and radiation usually causes a distinct hardening of the vaginal walls. It also destroys ovarian function, causing the onset of menopause. The sexual rehabilitation of these women is often difficult, but it must be remembered that the vagina is not the only sexual organ. The clitoris continues to function, and orgasm has been known to continue unchanged after the above treatment.

The sexual partners of women who have undergone radiation are generally older. Their sexual drives are now diminished, either due to age or possibly due to worries about being in intimate contact with two feared specters: cancer and radiation. The good news is that if these women and their partners are properly counseled, they may resume intercourse without too much trouble. In some hospitals, particularly larger or cancer-oriented hospitals, staff are available to help with sexual problems after extensive surgery.

The Emotional Complications of Hysterectomy

A century ago, the great German psychologist Richard von Krafft-Ebing, whose professional life was devoted to the study of sexual matters, noted that hysterectomy was more likely to cause mental illness than other operations. Difficulties after hysterectomy may be caused by physical and hormonal consequences of the operation, intertwined with the woman's emotional response to the loss of her womb. Gloria A. Bachmann, M.D., of the Department of OB/GYN at the University of Medicine and Dentistry of New Jersey–Robert Wood Johnson Medical School is an expert who has written extensively on hysterectomy. She emphasizes that the womb has enormous symbolic significance as a life-giving organ, a source of strength and vitality as well as one connected with sexual pleasure and female competence. The uterus is the source of menstruation and, with the ovaries, is also an organ that is perceived as a preserver of youth and attractiveness.

Commenting on elective hysterectomy in the *New England Journal of Medicine* in 1976, Malkah T. Notman, M.D., from the Department of Psychiatry of Cambridge Hospital in Massachusetts, another expert on hysterectomy, summarized these ideas. Her statement that "femininity has been linked with reproductive wholeness" catches the essence of women's feelings. Small wonder, then, that hysterectomy is at least potentially surgery with a negative effect on women's psyche and their sense of bodily integrity, surgery that may be followed by emotional upheavals. This is a difficult area for male gynecologists anxious to support women's feelings. While the loss of reproductive abilities should perhaps not be viewed as a loss of femininity, at the same time, this is a perfectly reasonable way to react to such surgery.

Although the uterus may have been diseased and the cause of much trouble, after hysterectomy its loss may understandably be mourned. The absence of menstruation is particularly disturbing to some women, many of whom wish to know about the effects of retaining in the body all the so-called bad blood that used to seep out with menstruation. In fact, if the endometrial lining is removed, all bleeding from that surface ceases. Furthermore, menstrual blood is normal blood, which begins to decompose on its way out of the vagina, and is not "bad" in any way. Not menstruating because the endometrium has been removed has no deleterious consequences, does not build up toxins in the body, and to many women constitutes a therapeutic success.

Unless carefully counseled, many women feel that they are sexually less attractive, incomplete, or somehow diminished by hysterectomy. And there is nothing unexpected or wrong with such feelings. Men's attachment to their genital organs runs at least as deep as women's attachment to theirs. This may derive from the obvious external presence of the male apparatus, compared to the largely hidden female organs. The loss of the penis or the testicles is an enormous blow to most men, who are horrified by, and resistant to, losing *their* sexual organs. One indication of this concern is a common experience of gynecologists who are asked to perform tubal ligations on women. This is a more extensive operation, often chosen in preference to vasectomy because husbands habitually shy away from surgery on their genital organs. Vasectomy, an operation that divides the small ducts that carry sperm from the testicles to the penis, can be done rapidly and easily and requires only local anesthesia.

An unsympathetic husband (or gynecologist, or hospital personnel) can undermine hours of reassurance. Fear of pain and the loss of control and depersonalization of a bad hospital experience also tend to make hysterectomy a potentially troubling experience. The mythology of femininity seems violated by hysterectomy. The notion of a post-hysterectomy syndrome, a group of complaints noted specifically after hysterectomy, was not new but was popularized during the 1970s by the English general practitioner D. H. Richards. The syndrome consists of symptoms such as depression, diminished sexual drive, a variety of sexual dysfunctions, menopausal symptoms (whether the ovaries were removed or not), and an increased need for psychiatric help following hysterectomy. In his first paper, Richards claimed that 38 percent of all such patients suffered from post-hysterectomy sexual dysfunction. In a subsequent study, Richards found that 70 percent of women developed depression within three years of surgery, but only 30 percent developed depression after other operations. Numerous other studies in recent decades have found that 10–37 percent of women were similarly affected by hysterectomy. Richard's figures were somewhat higher but were consistent with the findings of some researchers.

There are many confusing aspects of the syndrome. For instance, most physicians writing on the subject did not distinguish between women undergoing hysterectomy only and women undergoing hysterectomy with removal of the ovaries. Among women who had their ovaries removed, we do not know how many received estrogen replacement therapy immediately after surgery. Removing the ovaries during premenopausal years causes the immediate loss of most of the essential hormone estrogen. The younger the woman whose ovaries are removed, the more she will feel the effects of this loss.

Working in London, an Anglo-American team composed of Drs. Siddle, Sarrel, and Whitehead found that even if the ovaries are not removed, ovarian function in at least some women is diminished by hysterectomy. These women become menopausal sooner after hysterectomy than women who reach a natural menopause. Interference with ovarian blood supply, caused by the surgery, is usually held responsible for this change. It is also possible that the uterus makes hormones or other substances that may influence the ovaries and possibly other bodily functions. There is good evidence that this occurs in mammals, although the evidence is less clear in women. Uterine prostaglandins, for instance, may have a role in maintaining ovarian health, although they may not be secreted for long after menopause. More research is needed in this direction. Meanwhile, gynecologists must pay more attention to the need for estrogen after hysterectomy, since at least some of the adverse effects of the operation may be mitigated by the proper replacement of estrogen.

More recently, other investigators have shown that the frequency of such symptoms as depression and sexual dysfunction, which make up the post-hysterectomy syndrome, was also high in women before hysterectomy. For instance, the British psychiatrist Gath showed, in two important papers published in 1982 in the *British Journal of Psychiatry,* that the likelihood of depression developing was not increased by hysterectomy. One modern view is that the woman who was well adjusted before hysterectomy, who had good reason to have the operation, and who was thoroughly informed in advance will not be depressed or otherwise affected afterward.

John Kincey, a psychologist, and T. McFarlane, a gynecologist, give an evenhanded review of the psychological aspects of hysterectomy in *Psychology and Gynaecological Problems* (Tavislock Publishers, London and New York, 1984). They conclude that hysterectomy is not a major causal factor in post-hysterectomy problems. This 1984 volume was edited by Annabel Broome and Louise Wallace in the United Kingdom; their contributors included more women than men. The tone of the collection, academic and feminist, makes it likely that this is not an account promoted by gynecologists and colored by male prejudice.

In a presentation organized by the Department of OB/GYN of the Albert Einstein College of Medicine in New York City in 1991, Gloria Bachmann repeated a similar view. With proper care, women should have no trouble dealing with the aftereffects of hysterectomy. Of course, this is emphatically not an endorsement of hysterectomy. It is a reminder that adverse psychological aftereffects are often recognizable in advance, may be preventable, and are usually far from unmanageable.

Showing that depression occurs after hysterectomy may be compared to proving that much grief follows a first visit to a divorce lawyer. The statement is unmistakably true, yet misleading all the same: It does not take into account all the events that culminated in the legal encounter. In a way, of course, blaming preexisting troubles may be an example of that well-known phenomenon of blaming the victim. The woman who is acutely depressed because of her recent hysterectomy will not be particularly impressed (or helped) by such statements. The accent must be on making sure that every hysterectomy performed is actually needed and on identifying women who, for any reason, are likely to develop severe symptoms afterward. Women who underwent an emergency hysterectomy or who have had depressive episodes in the past but whose surgery was not preceded by

71

any discussion of possible aftereffects are particularly likely to develop the syndrome that now bears Richards's name. Other tipoffs to the post-hysterectomy syndrome are listed below:

- Previous difficulties in dealing with major stress
- Multiple physical complaints, particularly abdominal or pelvic pain, headaches, and lethargy
- Numerous hospital admissions and operations
- Expectations of sexual or emotional difficulties after surgery
- The absence of a satisfying career
- A desire to have children, particularly if there are none
- Lack of an obvious support system
- An unusually strong belief in the significance of the womb

Gloria Bachmann's views, although backed by much research, may be constructed by some as the view of the mostly male, mainstream American College of Obstetricians and Gynecologists. Another view is that of Nora Coffey, whose reaction to her hysterectomy was so disastrously bad that she founded HERS, the Hysterectomy Educational Resources and Services Foundation. HERS is located in Bala Cynwyd, Pennsylvania, and may be reached at (610) 667-7757. In addition to a twenty-four-hour hot line, the group has counseling sessions, a newsletter, and various informational services with access to the latest information, all at a moderate cost or no cost at all. However, HERS appears to believe that hysterectomy is immensely damaging to most women, a view contradicted by surveys that show excellent recovery by most women.

The issue of serious problems after hysterectomy is very important. One survey of long-term outcomes of hysterectomy was published in late 1991, in the *British Journal of Obstetrics and Gynecology*. The author was Margot J. Schofield, a research fellow in the Faculty of Medicine at the University of Newcastle in Australia, in its Discipline of Behavioural Science in Relation to Medicine. Dr. Schofield is a social scientist, not a gynecologist; her opinions about hysterectomy were, we hope, unbiased. The study was based on telephone interviews and questionnaires completed by 175 women, 51 percent of whom had a hysterectomy only, 13 percent of whom had removal of the womb and one ovary, and 36 percent of whom lost both ovaries. Schofield's findings were not unexpected:

- Women accepted hysterectomy because they were "fed up with symptoms" such as bleeding and pain. Most women found that they improved after hysterectomy.
- More than half the women surveyed developed symptoms they attributed to the hysterectomy. Menopausal complaints were reported the most frequently.
- A high percentage, 96 percent, of the women were satisfied that they received good treatment, but 4 percent thought that their condition deteriorated because of the surgery.
- Before hysterectomy, 23 percent had painful intercourse; of these women, 85 percent improved in this regard. Before surgery, 36 percent felt a low interest in sex. Fifty-six percent of these women improved, 40 percent stayed the same, and 5 percent were made worse (percentages rounded).

The most recent such survey, called "Sexuality After Hysterectomy," was published by Scott Farrell and Katharina Kieser from Dalhousie University of Halifax, Nova Scotia, in Canada. Appearing in the June 2000 issue of *Obstetrics and Gynecology,* the article found that while most studies were poorly designed, "the available evidence shows that the quality of life is improved for most women who had hysterectomy, and that hysterectomy did not adversely affect sexuality." However, the authors found that 8 percent of these operations were followed by serious problems.

There is a profound contradiction between views according to which hysterectomy does not cause depression or interferes with sexual happiness and views such as those espoused by HERS. However, we know that approximately 600,000 hysterectomies are performed year after year. If just 2 percent of these women have an exceptionally poor physical or psychological outcome, for any possible reason, within ten years there may be 120,000 women who are furious about the surgery they had. This is a sizable and vocal constituency, one whose existence I recall being discussed only once—by Gloria Bachmann. Through my pelvic pain clinic, I met about six women who were similarly convinced that hysterectomy ruined their lives. My argument is not against all hysterectomies; it is against unnecessary hysterectomies and against any elective surgery for which the patient is not properly prepared.

Psychological Support for
Hysterectomy Patients

Women contemplating gynecological surgery will usually find that most surgeons are not particularly adept at giving psychological support to their patients. As Ann B. Barnes and Caroline B. Tinkham of Harvard Medical School state:

> Surgeons tend to be activists rather than empathetic listeners and many of them need to distance themselves from the patient's feeling and fears as a kind of protective insulation. Some do not hear the patient and instead relate to a uterus or a breast or an appendix, and not a human being in distress.

This is not merely a matter of style. The absence of psychological support can have a profound effect on the entire surgical experience. The enormous popularity of childbirth movements such as the Lamaze method (and others) derives from the fact that a well-informed and well-supported woman goes through labor in a shorter time and with less pain than an unprepared woman does. The woman who has been well prepared for hysterectomy (or indeed any major surgery or stress) responds better and recovers faster than her unprepared sister. As already noted, emergency hysterectomies, while lifesaving, may carry an unusually high emotional toll.

For a variety of reasons, today's obstetrician-gynecologist is overcommitted. Even if the original intention was to provide all the information and support needed by a woman facing a complex situation, chances are that pressures from the full waiting room, the telephone, paperwork to be completed, and the emergencies of other patients cut short the leisurely and thoughtful discussion most patients would like to have. This is a typically American activity, called running a successful business. It is an activity that I do not expect to change, even though such change would inevitably result in better care. In my experience, physicians with a radically strong commitment to humanitarian causes do not go into surgical specialties. In consequence, surgeons are rarely empathetic listeners. Marian S. Neefus and Mary E. Taylor, two health educators from North Carolina, found that well over 90 percent of patients about to undergo hysterectomy were anxious for information about the physical and sexual effects of the surgery they were about to undergo. However, this information was rarely made available to them.

Sad to say, women who are often so giving with emotional support are not helped by medicine. Instead, when hysterectomy is contemplated, they must turn to other support systems, more often than not organized and staffed by women. If you need more information than you find in this book, refer to the Resources section at the back of this book for a list of organizations available for information and comfort. When facing possible hysterectomy, women must ask the gynecologist recommending surgery a number of important questions. Some of these were noted earlier in this chapter. Others follow:

1. How will I react to this operation? Think through in advance how upset you'll be after the surgery. If you have trouble even thinking about this or if any aspect of the surgery you are about to undergo bothers you intensely, you should first discuss your fears with your surgeon. However, you may do better with professional help. This may come from any qualified source such as social workers, psychologists, the clergy, psychiatrists, or psychotherapists. You may wish to speak to more than one person before selecting someone you will trust. Women assume that when it comes to hysterectomy, another woman will be a better source of advice than a man, and this assumption may well be true.

2. How much support can I expect from my husband, lover, friends, or others in the weeks and months after the operation? I will never forget two women, whose husbands left them, totally unexpectedly, at the worst possible time. One was beginning to go into labor when she learned that her husband of ten years had abandoned her for a younger woman. The other heard much the same story three days after her hysterectomy. It took an unusual amount of attention and care to get these two women back to their previous selves. Of course, outright abandonment is only the most flagrant and unforgivable act. Many women will have to deal with lesser offenses: poor emotional support, the inability of men to voice and discuss concerns, or their inability to understand that a dozen red roses in the hospital room, while a pleasant surprise, is not sufficient evidence of caring.

... 5 ...

How Your Body Works

To understand this book, you need to know how your body is built—this is anatomy, and how it functions—the medical name for this is physiology. This chapter covers these essentials; it also describes common medical and gynecological tests and procedures.

Anatomy

In healthy young women, the **uterus** (or womb) is a pear-sized and pear-shaped organ, kept in place at the top of the vagina by stout ligaments. Near the top, on either side, the ovaries and fallopian tubes are attached (Figure 5.1). The uterus is composed of interlaced bundles of muscle fibers. Tough, inelastic fibrous tissues keep the **cervix,** a firm barrel of tissue, closed for nine months during each pregnancy. As the fetus matures, the cervix becomes softer and more pliable. Toward the end of the ninth month, the interwoven layers of muscle the uterus is composed of begin their regular and forceful contractions, gradually opening the cervix and expelling the newborn.

All the tissues just mentioned surround and protect a narrow space called the **uterine cavity.** This space is lined by specialized layers of cells,

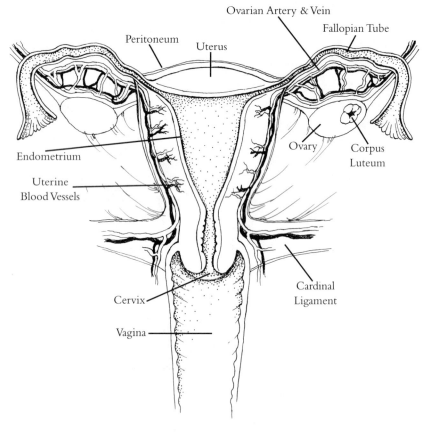

FIGURE 5.1   Cross-Section View of Normal Anatomy

usually less than one-fourth of an inch thick, called the **endometrium.**
Most bleeding from the womb originates from this layer, and much of this
book is concerned with this vital area of your body.

The womb is fixed in its place, supported by unyielding ligaments
spreading out from the cervix. This is an ingenious arrangement that allows
the upper, muscular part of the uterus to expand freely and greatly during
pregnancy, leaving the fibrous anchoring and supporting structures in the
region of the cervix undisturbed. The most important ligaments are called
the sacro-uterine and cardinal ligaments. If these ligaments are weakened
by pregnancies or difficult deliveries, the uterus begins to descend down
the vagina. This is called **prolapse,** a frequently cited reason for hysterec-

tomy by the vaginal route. If the uterus "falls out" completely, emerging outside the vaginal lips, the condition is called **procidentia**; this is shown in Figure 13.1. It was previously assumed that prolapse and procidentia would be most effectively treated by surgery that included hysterectomy, but we now know that this is untrue. If you have prolapse or procidentia, surgery may be difficult to avoid unless you are willing to keep **pessaries,** doughnut-shaped rubber or plastic rings, or other devices in your vagina forever, removing them periodically to be cleaned. If you cannot use one of the many available devices, you may have to accept the dryness, irritation and discomfort of the prolapse, and the fact that over the years it is likely to get worse gradually. Surgery is the only remaining alternative. Hysterectomy is not essential, but it is one choice; as the prolapse worsens, other operations may become difficult to avoid.

The outside of the uterus is covered by a pearly white, glistening, thin layer called the **peritoneum.** This sheet of tissue encloses and protects all the supporting structures, blood vessels, nerves, and lymphatic channels[1] needed to keep the uterus functioning.

The peritoneum covers every organ in the abdominal cavities of women as well as men. **Peritonitis,** often caused by bacteria acquired during intercourse with an infected partner, is a serious infection of an important space called the **peritoneal cavity.** The lowermost portion of this space is often referred to as the **pelvic cavity.** If peritonitis is not treated aggressively, usually with antibiotics, and possibly by means of surgery, or a combination of both, peritonitis may prove fatal. With modern treatments, this is extremely rare.

The **bladder** is closely attached to the front of the lower portion of the uterus just above the cervix. When empty, the bladder is undetectable on physical examination and almost invisible on ultrasound examination. When full, the base remains attached to the uterus, but the dome expands and billows over the top of the uterus, pushing it backward, toward the rectum. The uterus is now temporarily retroverted, or, as my patients usually say, "tipped backward"—if anything, a better description. It returns to

---

[1]The lymphatic system, probably familiar from its importance in breast cancer surgery, is a slowly moving circulation of body fluids from almost all the tissues in the body (except the brain) into tiny lymphatic channels, then on to a series of lymph glands, and finally back into the bloodstream. Lymphatics are also an essential part of your immune system.

a more forward position as soon as the bladder is emptied. A full bladder misleads the examiner's fingers and should therefore be emptied before any vaginal examination, unless an abdominal ultrasound scan is about to be performed—this examination needs a full bladder.

Retroversion, or backward tipping, of the uterus is usually a harmless condition. It would be unnecessary to dwell on this were it not for the fact that retroversion has been held responsible for backaches, pelvic pain, constipation, infertility, and a variety of other ills. My personal opinion is that retroversion is very unlikely to cause any of the symptoms listed. Severe retroversion, sometimes called retroflexion, may cause a sharp, stabbing pain felt with each thrust during intercourse, although such sensations may have other causes, and it would take a detailed gynecological consultation to decide whether the retroversion was indeed responsible for the pain. Various suspension operations, designed to correct retroversion, have been a popular gynecological pursuit for decades; it is doubtful whether more than a fraction of these operations ever helped a patient. About a dozen of these operations were in vogue until the sixties, then all but disappearing from American hospitals—an indication of the low esteem in which they came to be held. Hysterectomy, as we shall see, is another, very complex story, with a different outcome.

The pelvic cavity is protected on all sides by the bones of the pelvis: the pubic bones in front, the sacrum behind, and the hip bones to the sides. All the organs and tissues discussed here are located deep in the pelvic cavity, which is the lowermost extension of the peritoneal cavity. Above the womb, in the peritoneal cavity, the small bowels and the colon lie in coils: the small bowel in the center, the large bowel peripherally. The **omentum**, a fatty mass of protective tissue, slides over and around these organs. Below the womb, in the depths of the pelvis, is the **vagina**, attached to the lower segment of the womb in the vicinity of the cervix. The vagina is not only the delicate structure described in reverent terms by advertisers of hygienic products. It is a sensitive but exceedingly tough structure, a skinlike layer that almost never ruptures during intercourse, childbirth, or even wrenching trauma, such as may occur in a severe car accident.

The uterus is remarkable for several reasons. For instance, despite decades of study, we do not know precisely why it goes into labor after nine months of pregnancy, why sometimes it goes into labor prematurely or three weeks late, well after the expected date of delivery. The endometrium is also unusual in its exquisite sensitivity to hormonal influences, infinitely more than any other tissue in the body. Estrogen excites the endometrium to grow at an explosive rate, particularly during the first half of the menstrual cycle. It has been estimated that if the endometrial lining were to maintain this furious pace of growth for a year, it would, by the end of the year, weigh almost a ton. Of course, this does not happen. Toward the end of each menstrual cycle, unless pregnancy occurs, there is an abrupt withdrawal of the ovarian hormones estrogen and progesterone. This causes acute spasms of the tiny arteries that supply blood to this layer. Rapidly, vessels deep in the endometrium now begin to rupture and bleed, and the surface layer peels away in the familiar process of menstruation.

We owe our knowledge of these microscopic events during menstruation to the researches of the famous American physiologist Joseph Eldridge Markee. Working during the 1930s, Markee painstakingly transplanted tiny pieces of an anesthetized monkey's endometrium into the eye of the same animal, to a site in which changes of transplanted tissues could be watched with an **ophthalmoscope,** the instrument opticians and ophthalmologists use to peer into their patients' eyes. Markee's ingenious procedure expanded our knowledge of menstruation considerably.

With menstruation come uterine contractions, which force most of the blood, containing microscopic clumps of living endometrial cells, out through the cervix. A much smaller volume may be forced to flow backward, through the fallopian tubes, into the pelvis. The retrograde flow of endometrial tissue was first described during the 1920s by the American surgeon John Albertson Sampson. This process occurs in most menstruating women, but in some it may cause endometriosis, a prominent cause of hysterectomy.

Ovulation

The key physiologic event from early teenage years to menopause is ovulation, an event caused by a cascade of carefully modulated hormonal events. **Hormones** are messenger chemicals, made in one area of the body, usually in a gland. Released into the bloodstream (or other fluids) to travel to other areas of the body and to other tissues, hormones have profound effects. The response of the endometrium to fluctuating levels of estrogen and progesterone is an example of developments initiated and maintained by hormones. As we shall see, the endometrium undergoes repeated cycles of flowering, menstruation, and hibernation in response to these hormones.

The first signal that leads to ovulation is the release of a substance called **gonadotropin releasing hormone** (GnRH) from groups of nerve cells in the brain. These cells are in the **hypothalamus,** an area about three inches behind the eyeballs and just above the **pituitary gland,** which is located roughly above the soft palate in the back of your throat. GnRH begins to be made by the fetus and continues to be secreted later, during infancy and childhood. In preteen girls, it is released continuously, like a slowly and regularly dripping tap, but this pattern of secretion changes with puberty. The same hormone is now released in spurts, usually about an hour apart, with very little secretion between spurts. The change in the pattern is probably due to the maturation of **hypothalamic nerve cells** sensitive to estrogens; another important influence is the volume of fatty tissues developing in the bodies of young women. Various tissues, but particularly fat cells, can convert other hormones into estrogen, a process known as **peripheral conversion.** The hormone that first directs the hypothalamus to start the cycles of young girls is the estrogen made in fat cells.

GnRH from the hypothalamus flows directly to the pituitary gland. This so-called master gland orchestrates the activities of many other glands in the body: the thyroid, the adrenals, the ovaries in women and the testicles in men. The arrival of GnRH in the pituitary results in the secretion of two hormones. These are called **follicle stimulating hormone** (abbreviated to FSH) and **luteinizing hormone** (abbreviated to LH). If your periods occur in regular twenty-eight-day cycles, this happens because FSH and LH are released from the pituitary in a cyclic pattern, with an average cycle length of a lunar month, or twenty-eight days. If your periods are less regular, you may be interested in learning that regardless of the length of your cycles, ovulation usually commences about two weeks before the menstrual period it leads to.

Under the influence of FSH and LH, ovarian cells and tissues begin to make certain other hormones. Just after menstruation, the ovary secretes estrogen only. There are three basic estrogens, **estrone, estradiol,** and **estriol**. Estrone is produced mostly by fat cells all over the body. The main estrogen during years of sexual maturity is estradiol; this hormone is also the most potent of the three. Estriol is secreted almost exclusively during pregnancy, when it is produced in large amounts in the placenta. All of these hormones are converted and broken down into other hormonal compounds, most of which continue to function as weaker (less potent, less effective) estrogens.

Before ovulation, estrogen is produced mostly by groups of cells that surround developing egg cells. One of these egg cells is selected to mature fully, to become the single ovum to be readied for possible fertilization. All other cells wither away to enable this one cell to flower, unless twins (or triplets, and so on) are due to be conceived. Estrogen stimulates the endometrium to start multiplying and thickening. The first phase of the cycle and the appearance of the endometrium under the influence of estrogen are both called **proliferative**.

Ovulation occurs next, an event essential for both conception and menstruation. Its regular presence signifies sexual maturity; its permanent cessation signifies the onset of menopause. With ovulation, there is a miniature (and usually pain free) explosion in the ovary as the ovum is expelled. A yellow nodule called the *corpus luteum* (Latin for "yellow body") forms from cells that used to surround the ovum. The *corpus luteum* now begins to produce two hormones. Estrogens appear in ever-larger amounts, and progesterone begins to be made as well. These two hormones stimulate the endometrium, which responds by becoming thicker, with the endometrial glands ultimately beginning to secrete mucus. This layer is now described as **secretory**, and, under a microscope, is composed of tiny glandular structures not unlike closely packed sheets of sweat glands. The endometrium is now ready for one of two events: to start shedding (menstruation) or to receive and nourish a pregnancy. If pregnancy occurs, hormonal signals are sent to the *corpus luteum* to keep functioning and to continue producing its hormones. In the absence of this signal, the *corpus luteum* shrinks, and with rapidly falling hormone levels, the superficial layer of endometrium begins to break away from its moorings. As these tissues are flushed out, cramps begin to be felt and menstruation begins. Menstrual cells and fluids are mostly expelled through the cervix and the vagina, but, as discussed in Chapter 7, a smaller proportion may be flushed out "backward," through the fallopian tubes, into the peritoneal cavity.

After menstruation, the ovaries begin to secrete a fresh supply of estrogen, and the endometrium begins to regenerate. Estrogen next restarts the hypothalamus, and another cycle begins. As estrogen levels increase, endometrial growth resumes, and after three or four weeks, a new layer again covers the inside of the uterine cavity, ready for pregnancy or for menstruation.

The delicacy and precision of this process have no counterpart in men, whose sexual functions are simple in comparison. This explains women's frequent need for gynecologists, so different from men's typically lesser needs for urologists. The only organ to cause frequent problems in men is the prostate, but these do not usually start till men reach their mid-forties and fifties. For unknown reasons, prostate cancer has lately been diagnosed increasingly often in younger men, paralleling increases in breast cancer rates in younger women—but that story is not our focus in this book.

The processes leading to ovulation are easily disrupted. Thyroid disease or diabetes may interfere with ovulation. Travel or emotional shocks may cause a late or skipped menstrual period. Too much or too little estrogen may interfere with ovulation. Much estrogen appears in the tissues of obese women because their fat cells are busy producing estrone. This last process is often a feature of menopausal years, discussed in Chapter 14. Too little estrogen may be encountered in anorexic women or those who exercise strenuously, a fact well known to ballet dancers and marathon runners, who tend to have fewer fat cells in their bodies. With the loss of estrogen, the carefully balanced ebb and flow of hormones ceases, and ovulation (and menstruation) disappear.

Serious effects may follow if there is either too much or too little estrogen in your body year after year. Cancer of the endometrium is found more often in women who are significantly overweight and do not ovulate regularly. **Osteoporosis**, the loss of bone tissue, is a particular risk to women who are thin and **anovulatory** (that is, lack ovulation). Osteoporosis may be halted as weight is gained, but is very difficult to reverse. Ultimately, it may cause fractures of the spine, the upper thighbone (generally called hip fractures), and the bones of your wrist—any bone thinned by osteoporosis may fracture when stressed.

A fuller account of these changes is not necessary here, but they may be found in a number of sources. For example, *Our Bodies, Ourselves for the New Century: A Book by and for Women Written by the Boston Women's Health*

Book Collective (Touchstone Books/Simon and Schuster, 1998) gives an excellent outline of basic physiology and is easily available from bookstores and libraries.

The Gynecological Examination

The standard gynecological examination consists of measuring the blood pressure; examining the breasts and the armpits, the abdomen, and the lymph glands in the groin; looking at and examining the vaginal lips, the perineal area, and the clitoris, then the vagina through a speculum. Finally, the bimanual (using both hands) examination: checking the vagina and the contents of the pelvis—the uterus, the ovaries, and certain other structures. The pelvic examination is incomplete without a rectal examination.

The abdominal examination may reveal large masses, such as a pregnancy, or massive fibroids, or ovarian tumors. A collection of fluid (which may mimic a large ovarian cyst) is an ominous sign in women. In the United States, it often indicates that widespread ovarian cancer may be found; less often it may be due to alcoholic liver damage. Elsewhere in the world, it may be due to infections such as tuberculous peritonitis or to tropical diseases. Infections and a host of gynecological and other diseases may all cause abdominal tenderness. Unfortunately, so many conditions cause tenderness that this sensation serves mostly as a warning that something serious may be developing—although more often no disease is ever found.

The speculum examination reveals the vaginal walls and the cervix. Vaginal infections, the need for a Papanicolaou (Pap) smear, and tests for various cervical diseases are the usual reasons for doing a speculum examination. Cultures for gonorrhea and other infections such as chlamydia may be obtained through the blades of the speculum. Special examinations for cancer and surgical procedures to be described later may also be performed using a speculum.

The bimanual vaginal examination is performed with two fingers in the vagina and the other hand over the lower abdomen. In a thin patient who is not too upset by the examination and who does not have a permanently retroverted uterus, enlargements or other changes of the uterus, tubes, or ovaries are palpable with great confidence. Retroversion is no longer regarded as a serious condition. It may be a simple anatomical variant: as normal, and as significant, as, for example, large nostrils. At other times, retroversion may be age-related (it is more frequent in older women) or, rarely, a sign of disease: Endometriosis and repeated tubal infections may be responsible for the retroversion.

A competent pelvic examination may detect fibroid tumors smaller than one inch in diameter. This is an unimpressive fact until you realize that, for instance, tumors in the kidneys or the liver cannot be felt until they are much larger. A tumor in the liver may not be palpable even if it measured over two inches in diameter; in some sites a fibroid just 0.5 inches across can be felt with ease and confidence. An early pregnancy may be suspected (or diagnosed), or an ectopic pregnancy, or an ovarian cyst. If the uterus is retroverted, it is less accessible to the gynecologist's fingers, and the examination may be uninformative. If the examination is too rough, an involuntary contraction of abdominal and vaginal muscles will follow, also interfering with a thorough examination. An **ultrasound examination** (also called a **sonogram**) is now the best way to determine the size and location of the internal organs.

I include ultrasound as a method of examination because there is an increasing tendency, certainly among younger gynecologists, to perform ultrasound examinations routinely with gynecological office visits. An abdominal ultrasound examination, for which a full bladder is essential, is invaluable for giving information about larger pelvic masses. Vaginal sonography does not require a full bladder and is exceptionally useful with smaller masses deep in the pelvis. Ovarian cancer screening may be feasible through routine ultrasound examinations, a subject that will be discussed in Chapter 14. Women who have been advised to have hysterectomy, whether for fibroids or for ovarian cysts, generally receive a large number of ultrasound examinations. For this reason, a level of expertise with ultrasound-related matters is essential; you will find this information detailed in the next section.

Last, the rectal examination. Not a dignified experience for anyone to go through, it is nevertheless an essential part of the gynecological checkup. If the uterus is retroverted, the rectal examination allows the gynecologist to examine the underside of the womb and to appreciate its size—neither may be feasible during the vaginal examination. A negative examination virtually "rules out" rectal cancer. Specimens may be obtained to check on bleeding higher up in the alimentary tract, a clue to cancer and other diseases.

Gynecological Investigations

Several types of tests are used in gynecology:

1. Pregnancy tests. The use of any contraceptive, previous tubal ligation, even a conviction of infertility do not guarantee that you will not get pregnant, because all contraceptives (and all operations ever designed to prevent pregnancy) have failed occasionally. Very rarely, pregnancy may even occur without intercourse: seminal fluid, containing sperm, has been known to leak out during sexual play without actual intercourse, and before male orgasm is ever reached, to penetrate the vagina and ascend toward the fallopian tubes. Thus, it is possible to conceive while technically remaining a virgin. Exceptionally rarely, a normal pregnancy has been found after vaginal hysterectomy or during the first few months after you thought—with good reason—that you had reached your menopause.

Today's urine and blood tests rarely make mistakes. The blood tests are slightly more reliable, becoming positive well before a period is missed. Modern urine tests should be positive within about a week of the missed period. Home pregnancy kits are convenient and cheap, but their accuracy has been questioned. They are probably correct 85–95 percent of the time, which is not accurate enough. If you cannot get an appointment with a physician within a day or two, a rapid test may be done in a hospital GYN clinic or in an abortion clinic, easily located through the Yellow Pages and listed under "Clinics." Pregnancy tests may be done free of charge, or for a small fee. The results of the urine test should be ready within minutes; blood test results are usually available within six hours, certainly within a day.

2. Pap smears. These are inexpensive and efficient tests that assess the cervix for precancerous and cancerous changes. However, they are useful only with the detection of cervical cancer and certain vaginal infections; they give no information about cancer anywhere else in the pelvis.

The development of cervical cancer was an unobserved, secret process that killed countless women until a New York pathologist called Papanicolaou, a recent immigrant from Greece, began to study cells shed from the cervix. His studies, performed during the late 1920s, showed that cervical cancer may be diagnosed well before abnormalities are visible to the naked eye, if the cervical cells are collected on a glass slide, stained (colored with dyes), and examined under a microscope. At first Papanicolaou was regarded as a foreign-born crackpot, and it took about twenty years for his lifesaving ideas to be accepted. However, by the end of World War II, or soon after, Pap smears, as they came to be known, were a reasonably well-established screening test in the United States. Today, with rare exceptions, the women who develop cancer of the cervix are women who have not obtained regular Pap smears. The tragedy is that women who develop cervical cancer are often easy to pick out as likely victims. They are indigent women, occasionally HIV positive, or involved in prostitution, or trading drugs for sex—in short, women at the bottom of the socioeconomic ladder, women who fell through the safety net provided by basic gynecological care. Others I have encountered with cervical cancer were recent immigrants to the United States from areas without basic health care; still other women were probably infected with the human papillomavirus as teenagers and developed cervical cancer years later, after they had abandoned annual Pap smears.

Pap smears are far from foolproof: an unexpectedly high proportion of women with cervical cancer, at least 10–15 percent, have reassuring but misleadingly negative test results. However, the solution of this problem is relatively easy and is outlined below. Meanwhile, regular Pap smears at intervals not exceeding one year and investigating women with certain abnormal smears rapidly have almost eliminated tissue abnormalities that might later lead to cancer. Consequently, Pap smears have drastically reduced women's chances of developing cervical cancer; you will find this topic further discussed in Chapter 12.

There have been a few attempts to eliminate the gynecologist by enabling women to take their own Pap smears. Obtaining samples of cervical cells with specially designed tampons and douches has been tried, but these methods have not proved accurate enough to replace Pap smears obtained by nurses or by gynecologists. Cells from within the cervical canal are the most likely to be missing from samples obtained by means of tampons and douches, limiting the use of this potentially inexpensive innovation.

Standard Pap smears are "read" (inspected and reported) by technicians. Vaginal infections, bleeding, and technician fatigue (or overwork) tend to produce so-called false-negative reports. If the area turning cancerous is high in the cervical canal, fewer cells might be picked up when the smear is being taken—another source of error. As the term indicates, such reports are apt to cause a tragedy: Because the report is negative, the diagnosis of cervical cancer may not be made, or may be made much later than it might have been. Another possible error is the false-positive report: In this case, the report reads as if a cancerous (or precancerous) change were detected, although no such disease is found. Such reports cause unnecessary anxiety and lead to unnecessary investigations. Newer tests such as Thin-Prep and others might give more accurate results—fewer false-positive and false-negative reports—but at a higher cost. If the contents of this paragraph make you nervous, the easiest and most economical solution is to have two (or even three) Pap smears at intervals of a few months. Women good at math will understand the method rapidly: If the error-rate is 15 percent, after three negative smears your chances of getting erroneous information have been reduced to 15 percent of 15 percent of 15 percent—a probability small enough to be regarded as very close to zero.

3. Cervical biopsies. In these tests, small pieces of cervical skin are pinched off with a forceps, an instrument with sharp, scissorlike edges. Biopsies are taken if Pap smears are abnormal or if the cervix looks abnormal. This procedure is painless or slightly painful. If they are anxious about possible pain, I generally ask my patients to take a medication (for instance, Motrin or a similar antiprostaglandin drug or Tylenol with 1/4 or 1/2 grains of codeine) just before they arrive for the procedure. Even more important is my offer to stop the procedure immediately should it prove too painful. In my experience, it happens about once a year in a practice of average size that a biopsy cannot be obtained with relative ease.

4. Endocervical curettage is a way of obtaining cells and tissue from the cervical canal; it is usually performed during colposcopy.

5. Endometrial biopsies. These biopsies obtain small samples of the uterine lining. These are important when investigating abnormal vaginal bleeding. For instance, the easiest and cheapest way of looking for endometrial cancer is to examine small pieces of the tissue under the microscope. This sample may be obtained through the cervix with a thin plastic suction tube or with a tiny steel curette, an instrument that is slightly larger, but much harder, and therefore more painful to use. **Curettage** (a **D&C**) does the same, but with a still-larger curette, in a more elaborate and expensive, but at least totally painless way—except for the discomforts of full anesthesia.

The pain caused by endometrial biopsies is difficult to predict. Women whose cervix was previously dilated by a delivery or two feel less pain. Conversely, the patient with a tightly closed cervix (for instance, the woman without children) or one who is post-menopausal may feel more pain. Local anesthesia, called a **paracervical block**, may help but is itself painful to administer; this is rarely done. Some gynecologists have recommended the use of 20-percent xylocaine gel in the cervical canal to diminish the pain of taking a biopsy. When I tried this method, it helped less than I hoped it would.

6. **Colposcopy** consists of looking at the cervix through an instrument, the **colposcope**, that magnifies it about tenfold. The colposcope is a combined telescope and microscope. It is most often used when investigating an abnormal Pap smear, although a few gynecologists do it routinely. Cervical and endocervical biopsies, described above, are routinely—or almost routinely—taken during colposcopy.

7. **Hysteroscopy** is the modern way of inspecting the endometrial surfaces. Ideally performed as an outpatient procedure ("office hysteroscopy"), it is the best way of evaluating any abnormal bleeding not severe enough to be called a hemorrhage. The operation is described under gynecological operations in Chapter 9. Hysteroscopy may be combined with tissue sampling by means of a small curette, or with full curettage, or various forms of surgery. The more extensive the surgery, the less likely it is that it will be performed in a doctor's office as opposed to an ambulatory surgery unit or in a standard hospital operating room.

Scans

Internal organs may be looked at without an operation by means of a number of noninvasive (i.e., nonsurgical) investigations called **scans**. Scans use high-frequency sound waves, or x-rays, or magnetic waves, generally giving reliable information about internal organs and thereby making for more accurate diagnoses. Unfortunately, it is also true that on occasion scans have given misleading information, causing anxiety, the need for more tests, or even surgery that turns out to be unnecessary. This is the reverse of a silver lining: Great advances almost always bring exceptions and complications to be dealt with.

Some years ago, I did a routine checkup on a woman of about sixty, who had no symptoms at all. Her blood pressure and breasts were normal, but the pelvic examination was difficult and I could not make out any of the structures I can usually feel. In addition to Pap smears, mammograms, and a few other tests, I recommended that she should have a sonogram of her pelvis. The report showed an unusually thick endometrial layer instead of the thin sheet of tissue usually seen in post-menopausal women. I took a biopsy, which verified the sonographer's suspicion of endometrial cancer. A few years have elapsed since the hysterectomy, but the patient has remained perfectly well. Her disease was diagnosed months before it advanced enough to spread or to cause bleeding, mostly because the sonographer was alert enough to notice the thickened lining. The same week, a colleague's patient got into trouble because of another sonogram. This showed, in a patient about the same age, an ovarian cyst between one and two inches across. When this cyst did not go away, laparoscopy was scheduled. The laparoscopy was difficult, and the surgeon inadvertently tore a small hole into the patient's colon. It took a major operation to repair this hole, but the patient recovered. The ovarian cyst, which caused the operation, was small and perfectly harmless. These two instances show the two faces of sonography: the exceptionally helpful and the misleading. As discussed a few pages ago, "false-positive" and "false-negative" results are common; it is part of the gynecologist's job to be aware of these possibilities in almost every encounter with patients.

1. **Sonograms**, also called ultrasound scans, are in extensive, daily use in modern gynecology. Sonar was developed during World War II to detect submerged enemy submarines. Equipment aboard naval vessels would direct beams of sound waves into surrounding waters and detect echoes bouncing back from submarine hulls. The Scottish gynecologist Ian Donald was familiar with sonar from his days in the Royal Navy, and after the end of World War II, he became the best known of many researchers who helped develop sonography. Ultrasound scans are now accurate enough to count an unborn baby's fingers in the womb. Except for the discomfort of a full bladder required for much abdominal sonography, the method is pain free. Also, sound waves are entirely harmless, an opinion backed by careful research. We have already discussed the use of abdominal and vaginal scans in gynecology. Sonography has drastically changed obstetrical practices. However revolutionary these improvements may have been, they are not our focus in this book.

Do not be overly concerned if a sonographer casually mentions ovarian cysts or fibroids. First find out exactly how large the structures they identified were; if under an inch in size, they are probably harmless. Tell the sonographer that you know exact sizes are important and to be sure that this information is included in the report to be sent out. Read the corresponding sections of this book, and you will then be ready to discuss the sonographic findings with your gynecologist.

2. **X-rays** are excellent for showing bones, because the calcium in them shows clearly on x-ray screens and on photographic plates. The softer tissues that gynecologists are concerned with, such as the ovaries or the muscles that make up most of the womb, do not show up in simple x-rays. More specialized x-rays are available, for instance, to outline the shapes of cavities within organs filled with liquids that are easy to identify on an x-ray plate. Only one of these, called a **hysterogram**, is used with any frequency in women who may need hysterectomy, although it is done routinely, particularly in the course of infertility-related investigations. Hysterograms consist of filling the uterine cavity with a liquid containing barium, an element that, like calcium, shows up precisely on x-ray plates. The hysterogram that is now taken outlines the internal shape of the uterine cavity and may show fibroids or polyps projecting into that cavity. Hysteroscopy and sonograms have virtually replaced hysterograms in gynecology but are still used often enough to be mentioned. Another innovation is a **sonohysterogram**, a sonogram taken with a watery solution in the uterus.

X-rays are potentially injurious to tissue. Damage becomes probable only after heavy exposure, when a large number of pictures have been taken (for instance, five or six plates each of your gallbladder and your kidneys). The cumulative effects of smaller doses are difficult to be sure about but cannot be good for you. If there is any chance you may be pregnant, you must avoid exposure to x-rays. Radiation physicists and physicians suspect that x-rays may surreptitiously damage the cells in your ovaries, regardless of pregnancy. This unlikely but possible scenario involves radiation-induced damage to ova, the female egg cells. If a slightly damaged ovum is fertilized some years later, it may be aborted or congenital anomalies may appear in the newborn.

3. **Hysterosalpingography** consists of getting an x-ray picture of the uterine cavity with the fallopian tubes. Its use diminished with the advent

of hysteroscopy and laparoscopy, and, as has been noted, is currently used mostly in the course of infertility investigations.

4. **Computerized axial tomography** (**CT** or **CAT**) **scans** take detailed x-ray pictures of sections (thin slices) of regions such as the pelvis, one slice at a time. Substantially more expensive than sonograms, this method is used increasingly often in gynecology. CT scans give more precise information than sonograms, although often the increased precision is not essential. Its main use is in identifying cancerous growths deep in the body. Despite the cost, the use of these scans is increasing rapidly.

5. **Magnetic resonance imaging** (**MRI**) **scans** used to be called NMR scans (nuclear magnetic resonance), but the word "nuclear" was thought worrisome and inappropriate. X-rays are not used with these scans. Instead, a powerful magnet is trained on living tissues, after which the behavior of certain subatomic particles is measured by scanners linked to computers. MRI scans are safe technical marvels that give us a little more (and different) information than CT or ultrasound scans, but again at a substantially increased cost.

6. **Mammography** is not related to avoiding hysterectomy, but it is such an essential gynecological investigation that it deserves mention. It simply won't do to look after a woman, carefully preserve her pelvic organs, prevent the development of gynecological complications, and all the time not use a basic screening technique that may detect early breast cancer. Mammograms should be a routine in the care of women after the age of thirty-five, particularly if there is a family history of breast cancer or if the woman has never delivered a child (pregnancy is thought to have a protective effect against breast cancer).

Breast cancer grows very slowly, and the specialized soft-tissue x-rays used in mammography are excellent at picking up areas that may be cancerous (or merely suspicious) well before they can be felt with your fingers or those of a physician. Studies show that cancers discovered through mammography are smaller and need less extensive surgery, thus avoiding more disfiguring operations.

Current American Cancer Society guidelines for the early detection of cancer are the following:

- Women 40 years old and older should have an annual mammogram and an annual clinical breast examination (CBE) conducted by a health-care professional and should perform monthly breast self-examination. The CBE should be scheduled close to the annual mammogram.

- Women ages 20–39 should have a clinical breast examination conducted by a health-care professional every three years and should perform monthly breast self-examination.

More cancers are discovered by women examining themselves than by their doctors, although fewer women would die of breast and other cancers if the self-examiners would also have regular gynecological examinations and mammograms. The exceedingly small doses of x-ray radiation used in mammography are thought to be of little significance compared to the benefits of the procedure.

··· 6 ···

Fibroids

Fibroids are by far the most common tumor in the human body. By the time women reach their late forties or early fifties, as many as 20–50 percent have at least a few of these potentially troublesome tumors hidden deep in their womb; modern investigations have yielded even higher figures. However, most of these women have two, or three, or five small fibroids only, each nodule measuring well under half an inch in diameter and perhaps even smaller in size. These fibroids are as a rule entirely harmless, a disease by definition only, and not in any need of surgery. But the enormous frequency just noted, combined with the tendency to grow and cause symptoms, make fibroids the culprit of endless numbers of visits to gynecologists, general practitioners, gynecological clinics, emergency departments, and finally to operating rooms.

Fibroids are rubbery-hard tumors; they are almost always benign and are usually located deep within the body of the uterus. They are responsible for an enormous volume of investigations and treatments: Abnormal bleeding alone leads to over a million GYN office visits a year. Countless biopsies, curettages, and about 175,000 hysterectomies a year are performed because of fibroids. This chapter is devoted to fibroid tumors in general; medical treatments will be discussed in Chapter 8, and surgical treatments such as hysterectomies and myomectomies (the piecemeal removal of individual fibroids) as well as certain more recently developed procedures will be considered in Chapter 9.

After causing few difficulties for years, symptoms may flare up, and sooner or later, your gynecologist may tell you that hysterectomy is the best solution. Such an ultimatum should be avoidable with modern treatments, but you and your gynecologist will have to keep these potentially troublesome growths under careful surveillance. If not treated expertly before they get too large or numerous, hysterectomy may become the most logical operation to recommend.

Description and Causes

The word fibroid is a misnomer, but it is in everyday use, too solidly entrenched to be replaced even though it is inaccurate. Correct medical terms for fibroids are *leiomyoma, fibromyoma, leiomyofibroma,* or simply *myoma.* Fibroids are not derived from fibrous tissue, the tough, white, sinewy material typically found in ligaments and tendons; they develop from muscle cells, with the Greek root *myo* denoting the origins of these tumors from muscle tissues. Accurate or not, the simple word "fibroid" (or "fireball," as one of my patients once called them) is preferred by women and gynecologists alike.

Fibroid nodules are pink, gray, or ivory-yellow in color, with a potato-like diversity in shape. If you cut across a fibroid, you will see a jumbled and whorled pattern, a cross between the concentric layers of a halved onion and the grainy cut surface of a raw potato. Starting from a single cell and gradually growing into tumors as small as grains of rice, fibroids continue to increase in size fitfully and very slowly. Their growth begins to accelerate with the onset of menstruation. In a few years, any one of these tumors can grow into a much larger mass, although more often there will be four to six to ten, or even dozens, of tumors of varying size, mostly located within the muscular layers of the womb. Individual tumors may wind up as large as a walnut, a lemon, a grapefruit, or a football, and a few grow even larger.

Huge fibroids, usually seen in women who have steadfastly refused surgery, may be as large as watermelons. The largest fibroid ever removed weighed 143 pounds; the patient died soon after surgery in 1888. More recently, in a case reported from Texas in 1973, a 100-pound tumor was successfully removed from a fifty-eight-year-old woman, whose fibroid took twenty years to reach its gargantuan size. Ultimately, she went to see a gynecologist, reportedly because a voice spoke to her, saying, "Child, the time has come and I am going to deliver you." As reported by a British gynecologist, also in 1973, at least fifty-three fibroid-filled wombs have grown to weigh over 50 pounds. Tumors of this size must have immobilized these unfortunate women, but remarkably enough, ovarian cysts have been known to grow substantially larger than fibroids.

Each fibroid arose years (or decades) previously from a single cell. This ancestral cell was originally cradled somewhere deep within the layers of the uterus, where it slowly began to multiply among other muscle cells. The initial growth of a fibroid may be at a snail's pace, but in the end, huge tumors may be evident. Fortunately, fibroids do not always grow. Some stay the same size for years; others begin to grow after years of inactivity, and a few shrink spontaneously even before the onset of menopause, when most fibroids begin to diminish in size.

As they grow, fibroids usually remain deep within the layers of muscles comprising the uterus. Others bulge inward, into the uterine cavity, or outward, toward the intestines or bladder. A few are forced out altogether, possibly by contractions, but remain attached to the body of the uterus by a **pedicle**, a stalk that may be thick and short, or a slender band an inch or two long. Now they are called **pedunculated**: they hang loose, tethered in the abdomen or within the cavity of the womb.

Rarely, fibroids do very peculiar things. They may attach themselves to other organs such as the bowel, or grow, as long grapelike chains of fibroids, into pelvic veins, ultimately reaching the heart. Others may be found growing within an ovary, or in other abdominal organs, or in the breast, and even in your lungs. These variants are very rare; most often fibroids remain in the uterus, remaining the same size or increasing in size slowly and intermittently. Over the years, other fibroids may appear, also gradually growing and slowly distorting the shape of the uterus. Sudden and unaccountable spurts of growth are not unknown and must be investigated—we'll return to this topic shortly.

As already stated, it is only at menopause that this pattern of growth is reversed. Fibroids are highly dependent on estrogen, a hormone they absorb, make, and store. After menopause, as estrogen levels decline, fibroids commonly begin to shrink. If the estrogen lost with menopause is replaced (for instance, in an effort to control hot flashes), the fibroids may begin to swell again, at least slightly. The hormonal dependence of fibroids has been exploited by new treatments that control these tumors by medical (that is, nonsurgical) means.

The development of fibroids exclusively after the onset of menstrual periods and, decades later, their menopausal shrinkage all imply a hormonal connection, mostly involving the hormone estrogen. Chromosomal abnormalities have also been noted in cells comprising fibroids. Some experts believe that these genetic defects, influenced by estrogen, result in the appearance of abnormal cells; as these begin to multiply, fibroids are ultimately noted.

Much more is known about what causes fibroids, but this knowledge is largely obscure and inconclusive. Exceptionally large doses of estrogen are needed to stimulate the growth of fibroids in animals, and when the hormone is stopped, the fibroids vanish entirely. Subtle hormonal changes have also been described in the pituitary glands of women with fibroids. For instance, when their blood sugar drops to low levels, these women secrete large amounts of growth hormone—but no one has ever suggested that avoiding low levels of sugar in the blood might stave off fibroids.

There are two areas of great interest to women worried about fibroids: preventing the appearance of these tumors, and treating them with simple methods. Regrettably, the information available on these subjects is neither reliable nor useful. There are occasional reports in the popular press describing the shrinkage of fibroids attributed to herbal teas, to vegetable oils such as evening primrose oil, or to tinctures prepared from the American white ash tree. Such reports are anecdotal, which is a diplomatic way of saying that these reports are hearsay, difficult to take seriously. As already noted, we know that occasionally fibroids shrink without any treatment. For instance, large fibroids may degenerate spontaneously; as they degenerate, they shrink in size. Women have told me that acupuncture has been recommended to them as treatment for fibroids; exercise and stress avoidance, relaxation, vitamins, herbal medications, zinc and other trace minerals all seem to have adherents. Eliminating coffee as well as meats and cholesterol-containing foods is another staple advice. These measures are healthy and safe enough, but it is doubtful that they have any effect on fibroids. Gynecologists regard fibroids as autonomous: They are not influ-

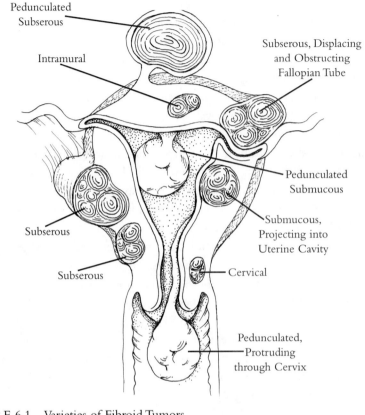

Pedunculated
Subserous

Intramural

Subserous, Displacing
and Obstructing
Fallopian Tube

Pedunculated
Submucous

Submucous,
Projecting into
Uterine Cavity

Subserous

Cervical

Subserous

Pedunculated,
Protruding
through Cervix

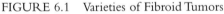

FIGURE 6.1   Varieties of Fibroid Tumors

enced by anything except their steady supply of blood, bringing oxygen, nutrients, and hormones, particularly estrogen.

Writing in a well-known feminist magazine some years ago, one counterculture practitioner startled me by blaming women themselves for their fibroids. His claim was that anxiety made women tie themselves up in fibrous knots, and to treat these, the anxiety had to be dealt with first! Publishing such articles is trendy but misinformed, and a serious disservice to readers who may not be able to assess biological issues for themselves.

Of course, your acceptance of medical ideas depends on your need for reliable documentation of effects. As my patients have occasionally reported to me, herbalists and natural healers always offered them optimistic promises: a sound enough practice-builder, but a far cry from effective help. In my experience, counterculture approaches have not helped women with fibroids. However, I recognize that to many women, neither medical science nor mainstream gynecology may have the last word. For a genuinely scientific investigation, a large number of patients with fibroids would be needed, gynecologists and ultrasound experts to track the growth of the tumors over many years as well as biochemists, statisticians, and computers, and the approval of reviewing organizations. I am not confident that such a study will ever be undertaken. Potential profits from expensive drugs for fibroids have financed such investigations, and the results of these studies are detailed elsewhere in this book. However, because of its economic structure, Western medicine may never find out if there are cheap, simple, and effective agents to prevent fibroids or to shrink them before they begin to cause symptoms.

At this time, only a few useful facts stand out. The shrinkage observed after menopause has been noted already. We also know that fibroids often run in families, affecting the mothers, grandmothers, sisters, and daughters of women with these tumors. Obesity and infertility are risk factors; pregnancies and birth control pills (BCPs) offer some protection. Fibroids rarely cause trouble before the age of twenty, usually appearing when women are in their late twenties or thirties. For reasons that are probably genetic, fibroids are more numerous, larger, and appear at a younger age among African-American women.

Gynecologists generally describe the size of a fibroid uterus in terms of pregnancies: for example, an "eight-weeker," which is as large as a womb at eight weeks of pregnancy—this is small and usually harmless. One that has grown to three months' size, by which time symptoms usually begin to appear, is moderately enlarged. These days, a fibroid uterus whose overall size (the womb plus the fibroids within its layers) is similar to a five- or six-month pregnancy is considered very large. Avoiding a hysterectomy in a uterus with such large fibroids is still feasible (but not easy) with modern methods, but these fibroids should have been treated much earlier.

Fibroids are almost always benign. According to most experts, cancerous changes occur in about one woman in 200. These tumors are called **sarcomatous,** sarcomas being aggressive, rapidly growing cancers. Since there is no agreed-upon definition of exactly what rate of growth is required to raise this concern, "rapid growth" is a subjective assessment. Once pregnancy has been ruled out, a myomatous (fibroid-containing) uterus that was 4 inches across three months ago, but is now 6–7 inches in diameter is growing suspiciously fast. Even among such rapidly growing tumors, at least in pre-menopausal women, most fibroids are not malignant. However, *after menopause, an increase in size or the appearance of new symptoms, and particularly bleeding, are unusual and must be investigated promptly.* Since even today's most sophisticated scans cannot unfailingly tell a benign fibroid from a sarcomatous growth or a solid ovarian tumor, diagnostic surgery (often hysterectomy) may be required—but this is a rare event. Sonograms are notorious for erroneous interpretations, CT and MRI scans usually receive more accurate readings.

Symptoms

Small fibroids usually cause no problems at all, and even those deep within uterine walls and those growing toward the outer aspects of the womb are surprisingly silent. It is amazing how large these tumors may grow without causing either excessive bleeding or other complaints. But if you have even a single walnut-sized fibroid projecting into your uterine cavity, it may cause heavy periods or a life-threatening hemorrhage. Common symptoms due to fibroids are displayed in Table 6.1, although it should be stressed once more that most fibroids are silent.

Cindy was an airline stewardess in her late thirties who came to see me when her fibroid uterus was about as large as a five-month pregnancy, by which time her friends had given up kidding her about the baby. Cindy's only trouble was that some of her periods were slightly heavy and prolonged. Her blood count was normal, and the sonogram I ordered showed that her ovaries were fine, as were her Pap smears. This was during the late 1970s, when the only choices were doing nothing or performing surgery such as myomectomy or hysterectomy. I told Cindy that with her job and with tumors as large as hers, something had to be done. I recommended one of these two operations and remarked that without surgery, sooner or later she was likely to have problems.

Cindy preferred to wait and see. I was certainly not the first gynecologist to nudge her toward an operation, although I may have been the least aggressive, because she stayed with me as a patient. Over the next two or three years, the bleeding gradually got worse and worse, but Cindy's

TABLE 6.1   Symptoms Caused by Fibroids

Excessive Vaginal Bleeding

Heavy periods
Prolonged periods
Bleeding between periods
Bleeding after intercourse (also seen with cancer of the cervix—
    be sure all your recent Pap smears are normal)
Totally irregular bleeding
Anemia-related symptoms: lethargy, dizzy spells, or fatigue on exertion

Abdominal or Pelvic Pressure: Usually Due to Large Fibroids, Grapefruit-Sized or Larger

Abdominal or pelvic tenderness or pain (see discussion in text)
Increasingly painful menstrual cramps
Infertility: if both fallopian tubes are obstructed
Pregnancy-related: miscarriages and premature labor are possible, if unlikely

Miscellaneous Other Symptoms

Pain felt during intercourse
Constipation, rectal pressure
Frequent urination
Possibly backaches, leg pains

attitude was unchanged. She was busy trying out acupuncture, herbal remedies, and changes in her diet—just about anything except surgery. These methods did not work. She began to bleed between her periods and could no longer schedule her flights when she was not going to bleed. By this time, the fibroids were as large as pregnancy of six or seven months' duration; now it was the more outspoken passengers who were kidding her. At this stage, hysterectomy was the better choice, although if the enlargement had been due to a few very large fibroids, myomectomy could still have been tried. We scheduled an operation a few times, but Cindy canceled surgery every time. Some months after the last cancellation, flying into Boston's Logan Airport on a winter afternoon, Cindy began to bleed and then hemorrhaged.

Cindy's colleagues had to pack her underpants with the small hand towels they managed to find on the plane and sent a radio message ahead for an ambulance to meet her at the gate. She was rushed to a nearby hospital, where she was transfused and had an emergency hysterectomy. Cindy recovered from this scary sequence in excellent humor. "I held out as long as I could" was her laconic comment to me, and I saw little point in debating the wisdom of the course she chose. Had she taken care of her fibroids before they reached a huge size, she might have avoided the emergency; had her hemorrhage occurred halfway to London, in the middle of the Atlantic Ocean, she (and her crew, and her passengers) could have had much more profound problems.

I tell the story because it illustrates what fibroids can do. Another patient, a statistician, was luckier. Her fibroids were, in the beginning, almost as large as Cindy's were, but there was less abnormal bleeding. She reached her menopause a few months after I first saw her, two or three years sooner than we expected, and her tumors shrank more than they usually do. When I saw her last, a few years later, she was perfectly well and required virtually no extra care because of her fibroids.

If you have fibroids, you will find that excessive bleeding will be your most common complaint. This may consist of increasingly heavy periods, later followed by bleeding between periods, or even bleeding after intercourse. The flow may become so unpredictable that you never know when the hemorrhage will recur, how long it will last, or how heavy it will be, making it risky to leave your house or apartment. Sooner or later, anemia develops, causing fatigue and dizziness on any exertion. If the anemia is severe, even getting out of bed may become an exhausting project. Such abnormal bleeding demands not reflex hysterectomy but a careful investigation of its cause, and a discussion of treatment options.

Fibroids are surrounded by muscle; they do not bleed themselves. It is almost always the endometrial lining that bleeds, but it is the fibroids that cause the bleeding, usually by enlarging the uterine cavity, so that menstruation takes place from the lining of the substantially enlarged inner surface of the womb. However, even a single fibroid less than an inch across may make you bleed if it projects into your uterine cavity. Again, we blame the victim, the endometrial lining, for causing the bleeding. Overlying or near the fibroid, this lining often shows certain abnormalities such as **hyperplasia**, a condition discussed in Chapter 12, or ulcers, or tiny varicosities of nearby veins. Polyps may also develop; all these may cause excessive bleeding.

Whatever causes the bleeding, the keys to controlling it are *not* curettages, but modern medical treatments or surgery. Medical treatments shrink the fibroids and suppress (or correct) the abnormal growth of the lining, the only tissue capable of bleeding. Surgery may consist of excising the fibroids, with or without **ablating** (removing) most or all of the endometrium. Other, more modern procedures, discussed in Chapter 9, have also become available. These procedures are so successful that, given timely gynecological care of high quality, hysterectomy should be a rarely needed last resort. In simple language, as long as the fibroids have not been neglected, hysterectomy is usually avoidable. However, if individual fibroids have grown very large or there are too many fibroids, treatment becomes more complicated.

Sooner or later, as the fibroids grow, excessive bleeding develops, causing anemia. This in turn may lead to exhaustion and dizzy spells, particularly on exertion. Since the dietary intake of iron, an element essential for making red blood cells, is low in most women, supplementation with iron pills becomes essential. Depending on the rate at which blood is lost, iron alone may or may not reverse the anemia. Fortunately, modern medical treatments are unusually potent in arresting bleeding, and expensive modern drugs can correct anemia much faster than iron tablets alone would. As long as the gynecologist is not presented with the surgical emergency of a seriously hemorrhaging patient, hysterectomy is potentially avoidable.

Anemia is diagnosed with two measurements, called the **hemoglobin** and the **hematocrit.** Hemoglobin levels measure the amount of this oxygen-carrying substance in your blood and require about a spoonful for the test. The result should be above 10 grams per 10 cubic centimeters, or 2 tablespoonfuls; 8 grams or less is worrisome; 5–6 grams or less means that the anemia is severe, calling for urgent action.

The hematocrit, or "crit" as it is usually abbreviated, measures the proportion of blood that consists of blood corpuscles as opposed to plasma, the fluid the corpuscles float in. The crit needs a finger-stick sample of blood only, and should be above 30–35 percent. Levels of less than 25 percent are serious, and below 20 percent the anemia is ominous. If you begin to bleed again, you may need hospital care and possibly transfusions of blood. Each clot you pass means that even less blood is available to your heart, and shock may be just around the corner. With gradual losses of blood, women have been known to survive remarkably severe anemia. Hematocrits as low as 6–10 percent are not unknown, but at this level, women look pale and feel so exhausted that they are barely able to get up to take a few steps. Further bleeding may prove fatal, although this is rare.

It is not difficult to tell if hemorrhage is depleting the volume of blood you need for your heart and your circulation. Extreme tiredness and shortness of breath on activities previously easily tolerated are a reliable clue. You can also count your pulse after five or ten minutes of rest, while lying on your back. The normal rate is 60 to 80 beats a minute—slower in athletic woman, faster in sedentary women. Now sit up suddenly, and take your pulse rate again immediately. If this accelerates by more than 20 or 25 beats a minute from its previous rate, rising to more than 100 or 110 beats a minute, you need medical care urgently. You have lost too much blood, and your circulation has difficulties meeting the demands of exertion as minimal as sitting up suddenly.

With an outright hemorrhage, the flow may be so catastrophic that blood flows out faster than it can be replaced with transfusions. This rare but life-threatening event is usually managed by hysterectomy. In expert hands, there are better ways of avoiding this operation. Many of these methods are relatively new but no longer experimental and, in expert hands, can be recommended as a mainstream procedure. The best-known innovation is **uterine artery embolization**, a procedure that has received much publicity recently. This almost nonsurgical procedure (a thin-walled plastic catheter must be threaded into an artery located in the groin) is described in Chapter 9. While it may be possible to stop even a major hemorrhage with embolization, it may be difficult to find expert gynecologists and radiologists to undertake such treatments in an emergency. As repeatedly emphasized, you may not receive the best care available if you need medical or surgical care urgently and are not already the established patient of a competent gynecologist.

Severe pain is a rare symptom, seen mostly when a fibroid grows too large for its blood supply and the tissue at the center of the fibroid begins to receive less blood than it needs. Deprived of oxygen and nutrients, the fibroid begins to liquefy. Other changes are also possible. For instance, the fibroid may develop layers of calcium-containing deposits; now it can be called a "wombstone." Because they are set in stone, calcified fibroids will not respond well to medical treatments, nor will they shrink much at menopause. However, these fibroids are usually inactive and harmless.

At other times, for unknown reasons, a pedunculated fibroid may twist unexpectedly and abruptly. The torsion cuts off the arterial blood that supplies the oxygen and nutrients all tissues need. This causes sudden degeneration. Toxic breakdown products are soon released, irritating surrounding tissues and causing severe pain. This is a surgical emergency. Unless the tumor is removed, preferably within twelve to twenty-four hours, peritonitis, a serious inflammation of the tissue lining the inside of the abdomen, is likely to set in. If you have large fibroids and develop severe lower abdominal pain, it is essential that you contact your gynecologist for an urgent visit. If this is not feasible, you may need emergency care in the best hospital in your area.

You may develop pressurelike feelings, even abdominal or pelvic pain, particularly if you have larger tumors (in this instance, "larger" means a fibroid uterus larger than a pregnancy of about three months). Other complaints are less frequent. If fibroids push toward the bladder, you may have frequent urination. If one or more fibroids arise from the lower part of the womb or from the cervix and grow large, the pelvis fills up with these tumors and causes pain felt during intercourse. A pedunculated intrauterine fibroid may stimulate the womb to go into labor, complete with rhythmic and painful contractions. As the fibroid is forced into and through the cervix, the pedicle elongates and the fibroid is delivered, at the end of its pedicle, into the upper vagina. The fibroid may even descend through the vagina to appear outside the vaginal lips, still connected to its pedicle. These rare tumors may be removed painlessly, either during an office visit or a short operation.

Fibroids and Pregnancy

Fibroids rarely interfere with conception; infertility due to fibroids is seen mostly when large fibroids block both fallopian tubes. A fibroid on a stalk, lying in the uterine cavity, may act as a natural intrauterine contraceptive device, but this is rare. Numerous fibroids pushing their way into the uterine cavity may cause an otherwise normal pregnancy to abort. The growing pregnancy cannot obtain its usual supply of blood from solid and bloodless fibroids, almost rocklike tumors in areas that usually contain only muscle. Failing to get sufficient blood, the pregnancy may abort, in effect

withering away. Certain other problems may also be encountered: premature labor, bleeding from separation of the afterbirth from its placental
moorings, and the need for a cesarean section. But more often I am impressed with how a huge and extensively misshapen uterus continues to
function reasonably well. There may be some intermittent pain from degenerative changes, but serious problems are rare.

Pregnancy has an impact on the fibroids as well. Increased estrogen levels may increase the size and the metabolic activity of the fibroid—at least
this is the reason gynecologists give for the sometimes dramatic growth of
fibroids in pregnant women. Modern studies with ultrasound scans do not
always support the notion of pregnancy-induced growth; on occasion the
scans show no change, or even show gradual shrinkage.

During pregnancy, more blood may be needed by fibroids than is available. However, fibroids generally have a poor supply of blood, living, as it
were, a hand-to-mouth existence. Fibroids respond by degenerating, an
event that occurs often during pregnancy, particularly to large fibroids
measuring two or three inches across, or larger. The degenerating fibroid
now turns a reddish or salmon-pink color in a process called **red degeneration,** or its center may liquefy.

Premature and abnormal labors are perhaps slightly more frequent than
they are in women without fibroids. However, fibroids usually pose no
substantial problems once the woman passes the first three or four months
of pregnancy. Rarely, the fibroids fill the pelvis and get in the way of normal delivery. If this happens, the baby must be delivered by cesarean section. It is wiser not to remove any fibroids embedded deep in muscle at
the time of a cesarean section unless this is absolutely unavoidable.
Myomectomy at the time of a cesarean section may cause massive, life-
threatening hemorrhage that is manageable only by immediate emergency
hysterectomy.

A thirty-three-year-old woman arrived recently in the prenatal clinic I
was in charge of. She thought she was three months pregnant. She knew
she had fibroids, had previously considered herself infertile, and had given
up on conceiving. In her South American home, hysterectomy was repeatedly urged on her, but she always declined. When she came through the
door of my examining room, she looked about seven months pregnant.
Using ultrasound, we found that in addition to the pregnancy, there were
two large fibroids. The smaller one, measuring four inches in diameter, was

lodged like a rock in her pelvis; it felt like the head of a newborn baby just before delivery. This fibroid was likely to prevent a normal delivery. The pregnancy above looked perfectly well; the fetus seemed about twelve weeks old. But the real tumor sat above the pregnancy. This fibroid was nearly ten inches across, and its center was already liquefied. This meant that much degeneration had already taken place, explaining why she was beginning to feel pain—the real reason for her arrival in my clinic.

Gynecologists cannot offer much during pregnancy with a large fibroid uterus. Should the fibroid degenerate, reassurance and medications for pain are available, but certainly not myomectomy. This woman delivered two or three weeks prematurely, and, as expected, by cesarean section. There were a few other complications, but considering the situation, not many, and none of them serious. The baby was perfectly healthy; her mother was thrilled. I asked her to return to see me two or three months later, to consider having her fibroids remeasured and possibly removed. She obviously thought she'd do better with less gynecological advice: I never saw her again.

The Care of Women with Fibroids

Fibroids are responsible for about one-third of all hysterectomies as well as large numbers of other procedures: curettages (also known as D&Cs,) hysteroscopies, laparoscopies, and myomectomies of various kinds, and a group of modern procedures discussed in Chapter 9. However, this activity is often haphazard, the consequence of customary "wait-and-see" attitudes not appropriate for the modern care of fibroids. If you have been told that you have fibroids, you should sit down with your gynecologist for a detailed discussion and develop a plan. Arrangements should be made for careful monitoring of the fibroids, for dealing with abnormal bleeding, for planning pregnancies, and for discussing the various medical and surgical treatment options available today. If you neglect your fibroids, one possible outcome is emergency surgery that could have been avoided by better planning.

Such a discussion is a rare event. This may be an exaggerated statement, but your dentist has a more complete record of each of your teeth with its fillings (and cavities) than your gynecologist has of your fibroids. This relaxed approach awaits the development of abnormal bleeding, necessitating one or more curettages. These operations, often performed as emergencies, solve little beyond controlling the immediate problem of excessive bleeding. Hysterectomy is the ultimate failure in the care of fibroids. Remarkably often, it is unjustified. The mere presence of fibroids certainly does not call for hysterectomy, nor are moderate enlargements and minor symptoms serious enough to warrant this drastic solution. Hysterectomy may be avoidable using a carefully planned approach, with earlier and better use of known medical and surgical methods.

Whenever I look after younger women with small fibroids, I tell them that if they are heterosexual and sexually active, good contraception is essential, unless, of course, they are trying to conceive. Regular checkups, at intervals of not more than three to four months, are now necessary. These need not be elaborate, expensive examinations. If the patient is well, they can be done in as little as five or ten minutes for a quick update of complaints, a review of contraception, and a rapid pelvic examination. If the fibroids begin to grow, I get a sonogram and a pregnancy test. If the pregnancy test is negative, I cautiously start a discussion I secretly dislike. However, the patient must have this conversation all the same, because under some circumstances her ability to become pregnant may be gradually eroded by her fibroids. To be precise: Fibroids growing in the vicinity of fallopian tubes may occlude them; with both tubes closed, pregnancy is impossible.

If the fibroids grow, some form of treatment, medical or surgical, may become necessary. Either the growing fibroids or the surgery, even if carefully done, may interfere with fertility. Old-fashioned myomectomies are notorious for causing adhesions, discussed elsewhere in this book, particularly in Chapter 10. Unfortunately, such information may make women feel pressured, but it is preferable to deal with these issues well before fertility is impaired. Instead of waiting, for some women a reasonable alternative to myomectomy or to doing nothing may be to start treatment with a new class of drugs called the GnRH agonists, as outlined in Chapter 8. Other drugs, discussed in Chapter 8, may also become available in the near future.

Sara was a social worker, who, at the age of thirty, was told by her gynecologist not to worry about her fibroids. She had just broken off with her fiancé; she had no symptoms, and her fibroids were small. By ultrasound, her womb was slightly enlarged across the top only; all her other measurements were normal. She was asked to return three or four months later, which was a perfectly reasonable way to manage the situation.

However, three months later her father died unexpectedly, and she returned to be examined only when she began to bleed heavily, seven months after her previous examination, by which time her womb was the size of a pregnancy of twelve weeks' duration. This was an unfortunate sequence, which might have been avoided had the gynecologist or his secretary contacted Sara when she failed to arrive for her appointment. Watchful expectancy, the slightly pompous phrase I was taught in medical school, may mean that the disease has a chance to worsen before treatment is started. In this instance, Sara's fertility was at stake, and this was possibly impaired by the delay. Let me emphasize this yet again: Fibroids cannot be neglected. If you have fibroids and are interested in having children, it is even more important to plan carefully.

Fibroids do not often interfere with fertility. However, let us suppose that this happens to just 2–4 percent of all women with medium-sized or larger fibroids. Not discussing fertility-related information with the majority of such women may result in the disservice of withholding essential information from the few who will be affected.

Differential Diagnosis

The idea of a **differential diagnosis** is one of the outstanding features of Western medicine. It is a conscious effort to think through, as logically as possible, all the various conditions that may be responsible for a symptom such as pain or a finding such as a pelvic mass. By deliberately including all the possibilities, no matter how unlikely, physicians can make more accurate diagnoses, particularly when a disease behaves in an unusual or unpredictable way. Too many women are told that they have fibroids when there are none or when the fibroids they do have are tiny and insignificant.

Another condition that enlarges the womb, called **adenomyosis,** discussed in Chapter 7, is often mistaken for fibroids, or the womb may be slightly enlarged from additional layers of muscle laid down during previous pregnancies. It would not be unusual to find all three conditions innocently coexisting, side by side, in a forty-year-old woman with three or four children. This situation would not be dangerous and may cause nothing more than a moderate increase in menstrual flow and a few cramps. A more serious error would be to mistake a small, solid ovarian tumor for a fibroid, because such ovarian tumors are often cancerous.

An ultrasound examination (sonogram) should be reasonably reliable in distinguishing the enlargement produced by fibroids from ovarian cysts. Because they are in extensive use in Obstetrics, women are familiar with sonograms, the other name for ultrasound scans. Vaginal ultrasound, with a thumb-sized scanner in the vagina, does not need a full bladder and is more accurate for small fibroids. Abdominal scans are ideal for medium-size fibroids but need a full bladder. Large tumors may be individually outlined using abdominal ultrasound, but for really large tumors (exceeding the size equivalent to a pregnancy of five months), a CT or MRI scan is required to give pictures that show the entire tumor: For technical reasons, sonograms cannot delineate really large masses. CT and MRI scans are expensive, costing hundreds of dollars. Western medical care is not known for emphasis on saving money; nevertheless, these scans are now used freely. Elaborate investigations such as laparoscopy or hysteroscopy are rarely required, because scans will usually reveal accurately and safely what kind of tumor a woman has. Surgery may still need to be performed, usually because other abnormalities (for instance, irregular bleeding or a possible ovarian mass lying buried among the fibroids) also require investigations.

Occasionally, a "fibroid" turns out to be a solid ovarian tumor. It may be impossible to make this distinction by vaginal examination or by ultrasound, and even more elaborate investigations such as CT and MRI scans, while generally accurate, have occasionally given misleading information. Fear of ovarian cancer is the unspoken specter in much gynecological testing centered on fibroids. Missing an early diagnosis of ovarian cancer in the belief that the mass is actually a fibroid uterus is very rare, but it happens occasionally: One such story was noted in the Introduction. Solid ovarian tumors (as opposed to ovarian cysts) are the usual cause of trouble, because sonograms as well as CT and MRI scans may "read" solid ovarian masses as if they were fibroids. Unfortunately, solid ovarian tumors are often **malignant** (that is, cancerous); memories of such cases justify gynecologists' interest in removing tumors rather than watching them grow.

Maureen Killackey, M.D., a gynecological oncologist previously at Roosevelt Hospital in New York City and now in Cooperstown, N.Y., has studied the problem of misdiagnosis. She came to the conclusion that ultrasound is not as reliable as generally assumed. The older the patient, the more likely that a mass thought to be a harmless fibroid tumor unexpectedly turns out to be a cancerous ovarian mass. Patients over age fifty are at the highest risk of such errors. Bowel and breast cancer that has spread (metastasized) to the ovary is another surprise in store for the unwary gynecologist as well as the unfortunate patient.

Abnormally placed kidneys (so-called pelvic kidneys) and even more rare retro-peritoneal tumors (located behind the sheet of peritoneum at the back of the abdominal or peritoneal cavity) may also mislead physicians who rely solely on their skills doing bimanual examinations. Either an ultrasound or an old-fashioned intravenous **pyelogram** (an x-ray that shows the kidneys, the ureters and the bladder) is more reliable in making these diagnoses.

Practical Matters

Since fibroids can be so troublesome, the patient who has them should educate herself thoroughly about these tumors.

1. A sonogram (or ultrasound scan) is useful because it will verify that fibroids are present, how large they are, and how many there are. On an ultrasound scan, the normal uterus is under 4 or 5 inches in length, less than 2.5 inches transversely and even less from front to back. In young women without children, even these measurements might be abnormally large, suggesting that fibroids (or other problems) are appearing. If there are fibroids, the report should indicate how many there are (unless there are more than four or five, in which case the range in sizes should be given), their location, and their sizes in centimeters or inches. If you undergo such a scan, you should get a copy of the report, and you should file it away for future comparison.

2. With very large fibroids, having an old-fashioned intravenous pyelogram (IVP) is a good idea. Very large fibroids can compress one, or possibly both **ureters**, the fine tubes that carry freshly made urine from the kidneys to the bladder. Partial compression causes the urine to back up above the level of the obstruction, dilating one or both ureters. The pressure or the infections caused by the obstruction may gradually damage the kidneys, ultimately leading to chronic hypertension.

3. If there are symptoms, the woman and her gynecologist must ensure that an unsuspected pregnancy is not responsible for the abnormal bleeding or pain. Even surgical sterilization (including vasectomy) does not guarantee that pregnancy is impossible. As long as the ovaries are in place and functioning, pregnancy is always a possibility, and this should be considered in the differential diagnosis.

4. When there is excessive bleeding, obtaining blood counts and taking iron tablets are generally recommended. Anemia from heavy periods (or other causes) can be debilitating.

5. The presence of abnormal bleeding must be regarded with suspicion, particularly at or past menopause. These days, much abnormal bleeding is the consequence of hormonal treatments; at other times, a definite cause cannot be found. Bleeding between periods is worrisome, and the older the patient, the more suspicious the bleeding. Modern biopsy instruments are soft; a specimen can usually be obtained with minimal or no pain, and the result made available within a few days. Sonograms are also useful: They will show the lining of the womb accurately. An even and thin lining, a few millimeters deep, is reassuring. A thick or irregular lining calls for biopsies (or, possibly, hysteroscopy with curettage) to diagnose precancerous and cancerous changes.

6. Occasionally, the bleeding is caused not by fibroids, but by one or more **polyps**. (These are fleshy, fingerlike growths, attached to the inner surface of the womb and almost always nonmalignant.) Polyps are much easier to remove than fibroids. At times, a hysterectomy is done for fibroids, but the report from the pathologist indicates that the bleeding was actually caused by polyps. These are easily "missed" at curettage but are readily removable by means of hysteroscopy, explaining the modern preference for the latter procedure. There cannot be many gynecologists today who perform curettage without hysteroscopy—I am not sure I'd let a member of my family rely on such obsolete care.

7. A potentially precancerous change, called endometrial hyperplasia, is discussed in Chapter 12. It is rare to come across cancer of the endometrium unexpectedly in premenopausal women; conversely, cancer develops readily and at an earlier age in those massively overweight. Faced with much intermenstrual or other irregular bleeding at any age, the competent gynecologist will perform one of the sampling techniques mentioned above and also listed under diagnostic procedures in Chapter 5.

8. Menopause ends most problems and concerns caused by fibroids. The average woman in the United States reaches her menopause two or three years after the age of fifty. Premature menopause may occur when a woman is in her thirties and forties. If your menstrual pattern has changed, you must ask your gynecologist whether menopause might be imminent; Chapter 14 has more detailed information on this subject.

Thoughts on Observation

Observation (which, in medical terms, means doing nothing except having repeated gynecological examinations every four to six months) is usually fine, except for two important problems. First, although this is rare, an ovarian cancer may develop while the patient is "under observation." The use of serial ultrasound scans has been investigated to help detect such cancers as early as possible. Such scans must be repeated annually, and perhaps more often, to make a real difference. While the risks of developing ovarian cancer are small, the consequences are serious. Ovarian scanning is moderately expensive (if you had to pay for the scans yourself, you might consider them costly). The screening usually detects one case of ovarian cancer per 1,000 scans; about half of these cancers are advanced enough to call into question the usefulness of screening. There is also the possibility of complications if false leads are pursued aggressively. However, many patients undergo such testing and feel that they are getting excellent care. Gynecologists have noticed that women are beginning to ask for ovarian cancer screening. Most likely this has been inspired by articles written by gynecologists and published in popular magazines. Ovarian cancer and its early detection are discussed in Chapter 14.

A second problem with limiting treatment to observation is that the tumors may begin to grow rapidly, a subject that has been discussed already. On the other hand, observation is fine for the woman who has completed her family and does not have large fibroids; it is particularly appropriate if she is close to her mother's or older sister's age at menopause. However, if she plans to continue bearing children, her gynecologist should monitor her for an unexpected spurt in the growth of existing fibroids or the appearance of new crops of fibroids. Frequent checkups are now necessary, at intervals of three to four months. Sonograms will also be needed, probably at intervals of six to twelve months.

If the fibroids are larger than 2 inches across, observation only is still perfectly acceptable, provided the woman understands that there is a chance that she will develop unexpected bleeding or pain. Much depends on an individual's tolerance of these symptoms. If you are a concert pianist or a rising executive, for example, you may not wish to take even small risks because one of your prime concerns will be to avoid emergencies that might interfere with your career.

Treatments

Apart from careful observation, there are three ways of treating women who have fibroids. These are: medical treatments, surgical treatments, and combined medical and surgical treatments. We must now look at the advantages and disadvantages of each of these. Unfortunately, as already stated, in my experience, dietary changes and holistic or counterculture methods have had no effect whatsoever on fibroids.

A Summary of Medical Treatments

Medical treatments cannot cure fibroids, but they can control them so they will not cause complications. The latest, most expensive and most aggressive of these treatments, with GnRH agonists, also called GnRH analogs, are discussed in Chapter 8. These should give you at least six to nine months of relief from symptoms. Longer-range care is also feasible but is more complicated and is also discussed in Chapter 8. However, most fibroids will not need such elaborate (and expensive) treatments.

Iron tablets will enable you to fight anemia but have no influence on the fibroids. Ergot tablets are very old-fashioned and ineffective against bleeding. Ergot cannot be used to diminish uterine bleeding except for a week or two after delivering a baby. I am occasionally dismayed to have women show me a bottle of these tablets, recently prescribed for them, many years after their last delivery.

Abnormal bleeding may respond to the very simple measure of taking antiprostaglandin medications such as Motrin or Anaprox. Today's low-dose BCPs may also be useful, although there is some controversy about using them for this purpose in women with fibroids. Tablets of Provera and injections of Depo-Provera may also be used. Provera is an excellent treatment, likely to provide at least a temporary suppression of the tendency to bleed. Depo-Provera is an effective drug, but it makes for totally irregular and unpredictable bleeding. Depo-Provera was disapproved by the Food and Drug Administration (FDA) some years ago because it caused breast cancer in beagles. More recently, in October 1992, the FDA reversed itself, approving Depo-Provera for contraceptive purposes. Danazol and the newest drugs (called GnRH analogs) are potent medications that interfere with the normal production of hormones. They induce a temporary state of menopause, effectively shrinking fibroids and controlling bleeding.

Remarkable shrinkage of fibroids has been observed in patients using GnRH analogs. The average reduction of size has been about 50 percent, with larger tumors shrinking more than smaller ones. Some tumors have disappeared entirely. GnRH medications may be used in virtually any situation as long as pregnancy and cancer have been "ruled out" and the bleeding is not an outright hemorrhage. Danazol and the GnRH analogs take about ten days to two weeks to take effect. Other hormonal medications work faster but are less effective. If acute bleeding develops, it may be stopped with curettage. Emergency hysterectomy is rare but may be lifesaving.

The latest treatments consist of the GnRH analogs with the addition of other hormonal medications that mitigate the menopausal state: the "add-back" regimens. Medical treatments for fibroids are similar to medical treatments available for endometriosis, and the same treatments can also be used to arrest bleeding due to many other causes. As always, pregnancy and cancer must be "ruled out." Other treatments, designed to prevent the growth of these tumors, are on the horizon; some are already available in Europe; these medications are discussed in Chapter 8.

One other treatment is available but is not in use in the United States. Inserting a progesterone-containing contraceptive device into the womb has been shown to reduce menstrual flow. Such a device is available in the United States; it is called Progestasert. This method of controlling heavy periods is used in Europe. It works best if the patient has had at least one normal delivery—this makes it much easier to insert the device. It also helps if the uterine cavity is not too large or too deformed by fibroids.

Thoughts About Surgery

Surgery should be considered—in other words, discussed, not necessarily performed—if the tumors are large or if symptoms are sufficiently impressive. If the uterus is larger than a twelve- or fourteen-week size pregnancy (five to six inches across), it is generally accepted as sufficient reason for either hysterectomy or myomectomy. However, the fact that this is a gynecological consensus does not mean that you must have an operation, but there is at least a small chance that neglecting tumors this size will lead to complications later.

Fibroid size is a confusing factor in a number of ways. With a normal-sized womb, in a thin patient, small ovarian masses (cysts or solid tumors) are palpable with ease and confidence. Gynecologists therefore assume that they should be able to diagnose ovarian cancer early. There may not be much of a safeguard in this, because by the time ovarian cancer is felt on a vaginal examination, it may be already disseminated and incurable. However, the situation is certainly worse if the fibroids are larger than a three-month pregnancy and the patient prefers not to have surgery. In such a situation, the gynecologist will probably not feel any additional ovarian tumors because they will be obscured by large fibroids, or any changes will be ascribed to new fibroids. If you have a malignant ovarian tumor, this translates into a delayed diagnosis in a situation that does not tolerate procrastination. Most patients with a three-months' pregnancy size fibroid uterus begin to have symptoms, unless the cavity is undisturbed by fibroids safely tucked away, deep within layers of uterine muscle. In practice, it is not at all unusual for gynecologists to simply observe patients who have fibroids of this size with frequent examinations but without more aggressive medical or surgical treatments. However, if you have large fibroids, you must know about adverse developments that are unlikely but serious. The gynecologist's job is to inform you of these risks rather than make decisions for you and have you take risks you do not know about.

If severe enough, symptoms serve clearly as possible indications for surgery. If there are no sudden, acute events, particularly bleeding or pain, there is no emergency. In this scenario, it is up to you to decide how long to defer medical or surgical treatments.

The various operations that are currently used in the management of patients with fibroids are discussed in Chapter 9. Briefly, smaller (under one to two inches in diameter) fibroids projecting into the uterine cavity may be removed through the vagina and the cervix if they cause excessive bleeding: This is called **vaginal** or **trans-cervical myomectomy**. An additional operation called **ablation,** the burning away of all endometrial tissue, may also be appropriate to diminish menstrual flow, but only if you no longer want children. These operations, along with **myolysis, myomectomies** of various kinds, and other procedures such as **uterine artery embolization** are discussed in Chapter 9. Hysterectomy is the last resort.

There are two serious problems with myomectomy you must be aware of: the development of adhesions, and the growth of new fibroids. Adhesions may be a serious problem if you wish to retain your fertility; recurrences may call for further medical or surgical care. Pregnancy occurring after myomectomy may also be complicated; these topics are discussed in Chapter 9.

Combined Medical and Surgical Treatments

Surgery of any kind may be made safer if the fibroids are reduced in size by one of the medications mentioned earlier. The GnRH analogs are regarded as "state-of-the art" medications for this purpose; their advantages are numerous. Blood loss during surgery is less if the fibroids are smaller and the surrounding uterine muscles have been made to shrink by artificial menopause, although the duration of treatment and any subsequent surgery must be carefully timed. While transfusion-related autoimmune deficiency syndrome (AIDS) is very rare, probably less than one case per 250,000 transfusions, the anxiety caused by transfusions may be considerable. The reduced size of the womb may also allow hysterectomy to be undertaken safely by the preferred vaginal route.

Gynecological surgeons have noticed that after starting treatment with GnRH agonists, the timing of surgery is important. If performed within three or four months, the operation may be made easier by the shrinkage of the tumors. A longer delay, of six months or more, may be inadvisable because as they continue to shrink, some fibroids degenerate and, in doing so, cause much fibrosis. In this process, scar tissues are laid down, making myomectomy more difficult, so that while time has been gained, surgical advantages have been lost.

A Note for Young Women with Many (or Large) Fibroids: How to Avoid Hysterectomy

The younger you are, the more fibroids you have, and the larger they are, the more difficult your overall situation. This is because your uterus will probably continue to grow fibroids faster and in larger numbers than other women might experience. Abnormal bleeding and pain (and, much less often, diminished fertility) are the likeliest consequences. However, you have a number of good choices today: medical treatments with one of the GnRH analogs, myomectomy, and surgery such as myolysis and other operations. However, uterine artery embolization is best avoided if continued normal fertility is desired. You will now need to read Chapters 8 and 9, and then consult with an expert gynecologist to help you decide which treatment plan will be best for you.

Questions You Need to Ask About Your Fibroids

Before you are through with your gynecological consultations, you must be familiar with the problems your fibroids may cause. You need not get answers to all of the questions that follow, only to those that apply to you.

1. *How large is my womb, including the fibroids?* If the answer is given in inches or centimeters, ask for a tape measure. Gynecologists have them around to measure pregnant women's abdomens; without a tape measure, you may not have a clear idea what size is being discussed. Anything less than four or five inches from the cervix to the upper end of the womb is barely enlarged. Unless there is very heavy bleeding, even gynecologists do not worry unless the uterus is larger. The size of the womb in all three

dimensions is easier to appreciate if the answer is given in terms of fruits or vegetables: Unless you bleed heavily, do not be too concerned about fibroids until the womb is as large as a grapefruit or a small pineapple.

2. *How many fibroids are there? Or are there too many to be felt individually or to be counted by the sonographer?* As more fibroids are identified, your chances of running into trouble increase. The answer is also important if you are considering myomectomy. Two tumors, each two inches across, are usually easy to remove, unless they are located deep within the womb, in which case they are probably silent and do not need to be removed. If there are crops of fibroids of different sizes, there is a strong possibility that regardless of the surgeon's skills, myomectomy will not be a lasting success. Victor Bonney, a famous British myomectomist, once removed 225 fibroids from one woman in one operation. This sounds wonderfully heroic, but it leads to difficult questions. Did this uterus, after 225 fibroids had been removed from it, stop making them? Common sense as well as expert opinion would say that it did not. Pregnancy may also be hard to achieve after such extensive repairs.

3. *Is there a chance that what I have is not fibroids, but an ovarian tumor?* If there is any doubt, scans are indicated or, much less likely, laparoscopy.

4. *Looking at my records, can you estimate if these fibroids have been growing rapidly over the past few months or over the past year or two?* Rapid growth may mean that there is a pregnancy or that your fibroids have decided to put on a growth spurt. Much less often a rare form of cancer (a sarcoma) is developing. Even if benign (that is, not cancerous), rapidly growing tumors are apt to cause complications sooner rather than later.

5. *Is there any reason to think that these fibroids will interfere with my ability to get pregnant?* This is a difficult question to answer, but for many women, it is the heart of the matter. Investigations with x-rays, ultrasound, CT or MRI scans, or surgery (hysteroscopy, laparoscopy) may show worrisome features. Unfortunately, there is no test that guarantees that anyone's fertility is normal—you can stop using contraceptives and wait to see how soon you get pregnant. If you are a healthy young woman who has regular intercourse without contraception, you should conceive within six months or a year. If you do not, it is time to consider starting an investigation. Infertility may result if both fallopian tubes are compressed as they enter the uterus. Large fibroids distorting the cavity may also cause infertility, although more commonly they either have no adverse effects or cause miscarriages.

6. *Do you think that these fibroids will require surgery in the near future?* This, too, is difficult to predict, except for one simple guide. Fibroids rarely cause trouble "out of the blue." If your fibroids have been harmless for months or years, they may continue to remain silent. Only rapid or gradual growth is likely to change the picture.

7. *If you think that I will need surgery, please explain whether you would recommend myomectomy or hysterectomy, or other kinds of surgery, and give your reasons for your preference.* The gynecologist who tells you that the uterus is there only for childbearing is not likely to be interested in keeping your body intact. You might consider taking notes and matching his or her responses against this (or other) books. Tape-recorders might be more accurate, but they make many people nervous.

8. *How many myomectomies have you done during the last three or four years?* Having done a large number like 50 or 100 is not necessarily a guarantee of quality, but at least it assures you that the gynecologist is familiar with the problems raised by myomectomies. If the answer is 6, or 10, even 15, your gynecologist has at least given you an honest answer but may lack sufficient interest in or experience with this operation.

9. *Would there be any advantage in using drugs such as Depo-Lupron, Synarel, or Zoladex* (trade names for commercially available GnRH agonists) *to shrink my fibroids?* Medications and surgery for fibroids will be discussed in separate chapters. A gynecologist who is not familiar with these drugs is not sufficiently up-to-date to be trusted with anything other than traditional management plans: hysterectomies and perhaps abdominal myomectomies—two old-fashioned solutions you might not need.

· · · 7 · · ·

Endometriosis and Adenomyosis

• Victoria had such terrible menstrual cramps that she regularly missed a few days of high school each month. The kindly old general practitioner who gave her family basic care of decent quality was not willing to prescribe medications strong enough to control the pain, and Victoria suspected that he was not taking her problem seriously. She came to see me with her aunt, who kept reassuring Victoria not to worry about the examination she had never experienced before.

• Pat was a married woman in her late twenties, who stopped her birth control pills in order to get pregnant. She and her husband had always admired large families and were looking forward to starting one of their own. Neither had ever had any medical problems. A year passed and then two. To their increasing disappointment, Pat's periods arrived, regular as clockwork.

• Laura was a linguist, an intense forty-year-old woman who had severe and recurring pains in the pit of her stomach and deep in her pelvis. Every doctor had a different diagnosis and treatment, but the pains kept recurring and were now getting worse and worse. A gynecologist ultimately told her that she probably had a disease called **adenomyosis**, in which the glands of the endometrial lining penetrate deep into the muscles surrounding the uterine cavity. Adenomyosis, he said, usually causes heavy menstrual flow as well as menstrual pains, which Laura certainly had. He recommended hysterectomy as the most reliable treatment but was so casual about the operation that Laura felt she could never trust him.

At **laparoscopy,** an operation in which the woman is anesthetized and the gynecologist takes a thorough look inside her abdomen and pelvis, I found **endometriosis** in all three. This peculiar disease has been diagnosed with increasing frequency and has been responsible for a surging number of hysterectomies. Endometriosis has become a growth industry with expensive new medications and the latest in laparoscopic laser surgery. Much mystery still surrounds endometriosis; unfortunately, short of diseases such as AIDS, severe chronic pelvic pain, and lethal cancers, this illness can be one of the most terrible afflictions imaginable. Women with "endo" can contact the Endometriosis Association, one of the oldest self-help organizations in the United States, whose telephone number is (414) 355-2200. The Endometriosis Association has full-time employees, a newsletter, a hot line, lists of physicians with special expertise, support groups with local chapters, and a wealth of other activities, all providing information and support for sufferers.

Adenomyosis is a disorder of the myometrium, the muscular body of the womb; older texts refer to adenomyosis as internal endometriosis, meaning that the disease affects the internal structure of the womb. As noted, adenomyosis may extend deeply from the endometrial lining of the uterine cavity through layers of muscle, sometimes as far as the outside peritoneal covering of the womb. However, it does not appear anywhere else in the body. There is also an overlap in symptoms: Either disease may cause painful and abnormally heavy periods, but all similarities end there. Most significantly, endometriosis can be treated effectively with hormones, whereas adenomyosis stubbornly resists such treatments. Adenomyosis is probably unrelated to endometriosis; while it may require hysterectomy as treatment, it is (unless it is found in young women) less serious a disease than endometriosis. Adenomyosis will be discussed at the end of this chapter.

Endometriosis—What Is It?

The source of endometriosis is the endometrium, the tissue that lines the cavity inside the womb. This tissue is not meant to appear anywhere else in the body, but with the development of endometriosis, the body makes a startling error: allowing the growth of small islands of endometrial tissue in other sites where it does not belong. Most of these patches of tissue are in the pelvis, where the most frequent symptoms of the disease are pain and infertility. Less often, the patches are outside the pelvis, sometimes occurring as far away as the arms or the legs. If you have endometriosis outside your pelvis, you may develop unusual, even striking symptoms such as coughing up blood during your menstrual periods or getting nosebleeds during your menstrual periods, but these symptoms are rare.

This error of the body, the misplacement of tissue, is very unusual. Thyroid tissue may be found in the neck, a short distance from the thyroid gland itself, but this is a harmless curiosity. A few women have an additional nipple or two, perhaps with breast tissue directly under the extra nipple, located along the **milk ridge** (also called the **nipple line).** This line runs invisibly from the armpits toward the nipples, then down the torso toward the groin; but in a few women, extra nipples are a visible reminder that we descended from mammals with many pairs of breasts to feed a large litter. There are other examples of the misplacement of tissue, but none are major in extent, and serious consequences are rare. Endometriosis is the one important exception to this breakdown of geography. The aberrant patches of endometrium, each usually smaller than a fingertip in size, constitute endometriosis. The condition is readily visible somewhere in the pelvis in at least one woman in twenty, although many more may have a few barely visible areas of endometriosis scattered in their pelvic cavities. If there are no symptoms and the endometriotic patches are barely evident, there is little reason to worry about endometriosis, although gynecologists disagree among themselves on this point.

Another baffling fact has been uncovered recently. If a biopsy is taken from a normal-looking area of peritoneal tissue from healthy adult women and examined with an **electron-microscope** (an instrument that gives much greater magnification than standard microscopes), tiny glands resembling endometriotic tissue may be identified. This does not mean that everyone has barely visible or invisible endometriosis. The significance of the microscopic patches of endometriosis remains unknown, and most experts question the importance of these lesions.

Endometriosis, a major cause of hysterectomy, has been diagnosed with increased frequency in recent years. This may be because the disease appears more often; another explanation may be that the abdominal pains that used to be dismissed are now investigated by gynecologists. In recent years, other conditions leading to hysterectomy have been at stable or declining levels, but according to the National Center for Health Statistics, which lumps these two diseases together, endometriosis and adenomyosis have been the causes of increasing numbers of hysterectomies, currently second only to fibroids.

How and Why Endometriosis Develops

When you menstruate, the more superficial layers of endometrial tissue peel off deeper layers and are sloughed off, a process described in Chapter 5. Menstrual flow consists of blood that has clotted and liquefied again, but it also contains small clusters of endometrial tissue. Uterine contractions, felt as sharp menstrual cramps, force this mixture out of your womb through the cervix and into the vagina. There may also be a smaller amount of backward flow through the fallopian tubes, first noted in the 1920s by the American surgeon John Albertson Sampson. This flow, which spills menstrual blood directly into the pelvic cavity, is a normal occurrence in 70 or 80 percent of women. Sampson named this process **retrograde menstruation**, and thought it was the main cause of endometriosis.

A number of theories attempt to explain the origins of endometriosis, but only a few need be mentioned in detail. The first explanation dates back to Sampson and is based on his belief that with retrograde menstruation, tiny clumps of living endometrial cells are rafted along in the retrograde, or backward, flow of menstrual blood. Sampson observed these clumps spilling into the pelvis and thought they could attach themselves, like barnacles, to various organs there. The clusters of cells would then begin to grow, gradually penetrating deeper and deeper into tissues in which they were embedded, ultimately causing endometriosis. Endometriosis tends to be found most often within two or three inches of the flared, trumpet-like openings of the fallopian tubes near the ovaries. The sequence proposed by Sampson is logical and fits many of the known facts of endometriosis.

Initially, there was bitter opposition to Sampson's ideas. The accepted dogma of the day was another theory, advanced by the famous Viennese gynecologist Robert Meyer, who proposed that within the peritoneal cavity of adult women with endometriosis, small islands of primitive cells persisted, dating back to the time that these women were still embryos growing in the womb. Meyer thought that decades later, the stagnating patches could gradually mature into endometriosis, and he called the process "metaplasia." Sampson, a prominent surgeon from Albany, New York, had an excellent reputation, but his ideas had a hard time standing up against the theory of the famous Viennese gynecologist. Meyer's supporters insisted that the cells in the retrograde flow were no longer alive, could not be implanted, and would not grow, nor could the theory explain the appearance of the disease elsewhere in the body. It was an acrimonious debate, and at least in the beginning, Sampson's ideas were not taken seriously.

Unfortunately for Meyer's theory, no one could ever show that there were such islands of primitive cells to be found in adults, either in the pelvis or elsewhere in the body. In fact, Meyer's theory is very difficult to prove or to disprove, and his ideas about endometriosis survive to this day mostly because of his fame and because he was right about other gynecological issues. However, there is an increasing modern interest in his theory.

A handful of exceptionally rare cases of endometriosis, noted well after Meyer died, seem to support his ideas. For instance, the American expert David Redwine of Bend, Oregon, has found an endometriosis-like area in the pelvis of a female infant who had a crib death; others have reported endometriosis in girls who have not yet menstruated. Endometriosis has appeared in women who, due to congenital defects, were born without a womb, had never menstruated, and clearly had no endometrial tissue to spill. Even more astonishingly, rare cases of endometriosis have developed in the bladders of men with prostate cancer, who were being treated with large doses of the female hormone estrogen. It is difficult, but not impossible, to understand which tissues turned into endometriosis in these men. Women's bodies contain vestigial male organs, and conversely, men possess primitive female organs, including a tiny uterus-like appendage in the prostate. However, it must be admitted that these are speculative and far-fetched ideas, more interesting from theoretical than practical points of view.

Sampson was the first physician to offer a carefully detailed account of endometriosis, and his theory is easier to prove than Meyer's. However, it took a very substantial research effort, carried out over fifty or sixty years after the 1930s, to show that none of the objections raised to Sampson's ideas were valid. The clusters of cells spilled into the pelvis have been shown to be alive. It was shown that they could be implanted and would grow where implanted. Most modern gynecologists believe that Sampson's retrograde menstruation explains many, and perhaps most, instances of endometriosis. Of course, the same disease may be caused by a number of different processes, and Meyer's theory may be just as relevant, or almost as relevant, as Sampson's.

A third theory is much more recent and completes the retrograde menstruation story. It involves the immune system, and it may account for the fact that most women have retrograde menstruation but only a few develop endometriosis. Before we discuss this theory, let us review a few anatomical and demographic facts.

If the cervix remains tightly closed, as often happens if women postpone childbearing, there will be more retrograde menstruation and an increased possibility of developing endometriosis. Congenital abnormalities of the uterus and the vagina, which obstruct the outflow of blood from the uterus into the vagina, also increase the probability of retrograde menstruation, and the chances of developing endometriosis later in life increase. Conversely, if the fallopian tubes are sealed anywhere along their length by tubal infections, endometriosis will most likely not develop. Endometriosis is too eccentric and complicated a disease to follow these rules without deviations, but by and large, the rules hold. Consequently, endometriosis is more frequent in women whose tubes have remained open but who have postponed childbearing until later in life or have never conceived. Thus, we may be able to explain some of the increased frequency of endometriosis by citing the recent tendency of women to postpone childbearing.

The third theory relies on our newly expanded knowledge of immunology, a consequence of the AIDS crisis. Much recent research indicates that it is an impaired immune system that allows endometriosis to develop. One of the many functions of the immune system is to suppress the growth of unusual or foreign tissues, for instance, bacteria or abnormal cells that may be slowly becoming cancerous. If the immune system is functioning properly, skin grafts from randomly selected, incompatible donors will be rejected and destroyed. Skin or a kidney from identical twins carries the identical genetic imprint and is not recognized by the immune system of either twin as foreign tissue. For this reason, a kidney transplant from an identical twin will usually "take," surviving and continuing to function in the other twin. By contrast, bacteria and tissues that appear foreign to the immune system such as cancerous cells and patches of endometriosis will be attacked by scavenging cells of the immune system. Patients infected with HIV, the so-called AIDS virus, in whom the immune system is badly damaged, sooner or later develop recurring infections and tumors that have not been fought off by an intact immune system. In women with endometriosis, the immune system appears to have certain subtle defects that are unrelated to AIDS. If the immune system does not attack earlier patches of endometriosis, the cells survive, and as they continue to grow, endometriosis develops.

In a presentation he gave in New York City, held in the summer of the year 2000, the American endometriosis expert W. Paul Dmowski described how endometriosis has been experimentally observed to appear and disappear in various sites month after month. Dmowski attributed this waxing and waning of patches of endometriosis to fluctuations in the power of the immune system to cope with the disease. Our understanding of the immune system has seen vast improvements because of extensive AIDS-related research. Incidentally, current popular claims to "tone up" or "strengthen" the immune system with over-the-counter medications and herbal supplements are, I believe, much exaggerated. The immune system cannot be boosted the way caffeine or dexedrine give mental faculties a strong charge. Depression, radiation, and certain drugs may lower immunological competence; relaxation and happiness may improve it. However, the herbs that are promoted as boosting the immune system have not been researched; effects attributed to them have probably been exaggerated in an advertising effort to induce you to purchase them.

Endometriosis also shows a tendency to run in families, passed along from mothers to daughters. One recent text cites research according to which the risk of endometriosis is increased sevenfold among the mothers and sisters of women diagnosed with endometriosis. There have also been fanciful notions that the disease was more frequent in women with certain personalities: Driven, career-oriented women who were perfectionists were the customary targets of such theories. Unfortunately, as discussed above, having children later in life may contribute to the development of endometriosis. However, it is bad enough for some women to realize that postponing children or remaining childless (for whatever reason) might promote a serious disease such as endometriosis; there is no need to blame the victim by invoking personality traits as causal factors.

There is another kind of endometriosis, but it is usually little more than a nuisance. It is called **surgical endometriosis,** and it may follow any operation during which endometrial cells are accidentally transplanted by surgical instruments (or the surgeon's gloved fingers) to a new site. Cesarean sections, extensive myomectomies during which a tiny clump of the endometrium is uprooted, and deliveries during which an episiotomy is cut or the skin is torn may all inadvertently lead to surgical endometriosis. The result is an area of tissue just under the skin that becomes swollen and painful during menstrual periods. If the discomfort is marked, simple excision of the affected area usually cures this form of endometriosis.

The Damage Caused by Endometriosis

As Chapter 5 showed, under hormonal influences, normal endometrium evolves through certain phases. These culminate in menstruation, the piecemeal sloughing off of endometrial layers, and the consequent flow of blood. The endometrium of endometriosis responds to the same hormones and follows more or less the same sequence of cyclic changes as endometrium in its normal site. The crucial difference is that normal menstrual flow escapes from the uterus through the cervix, but the blood loosened by menstrual changes in tiny pockets of endometriosis has no escape. It is trapped deep within tissue, forming miniature hemorrhages around each knot of endometriosis. Although much smaller, these hemorrhagic areas resemble the half-purple, half-blue collections of blood within tissue called a black eye, or the similarly discolored finger you smashed in the door of your car a few days ago. The blood is extravasated: That is, it does not circulate within vessels but burrows into tissue, causing swelling and releasing chemicals such as prostaglandins that cause pain. If you suffer from endometriosis, with each menstrual period another scattering of tiny hemorrhages forms deep in your tissues around each pocket of "endo"; in the pelvis this process causes pain and infertility.

If you look at an ovary or area of the peritoneum affected by endometriosis (and your gynecologist may have a photograph or video to show you), most often you will see a few slightly swollen areas surrounding black or chocolate-brown spots, each less than one-fourth inch across in size. These resemble beauty marks or moles, but in fact they are endometriotic deposits. The dark color is that of old blood, still there from the tiny hemorrhage that occurred months or years previously and still visible just below the surface.

Wherever endometriosis occurs, blood wells up within affected tissues with each period. Gradually, adhesions develop—see Figure 10.1. Fallopian tubes slowly become enmeshed in these adhesions, causing infertility and ectopic pregnancies. Ovaries may become enlarged and distended by endometriotic cysts. Bowel and bladder walls are thickened, possibly causing an obstruction. Lungs may collapse, and severe menstrual cramps or chronic pelvic pain may develop, as may mysterious urinary problems. As you can now appreciate, the development of endometriosis may have very serious consequences, although in some women the impact of endometriosis may be minimal.

The Tissues Affected by Endometriosis

Endometriosis commonly involves tissues deep in the pelvis. The ovaries and the **rectovaginal septum**, the thin sheet of tissue that separates the vagina from the rectum, are two typical locations. The peritoneal coverings of the pelvis, particularly around structures called the sacro-uterine ligaments that support the uterus, are perhaps the most common sites of this disease. The bladder may be involved; the fallopian tubes, the small or large bowel, the appendix, and even the deeper ligaments of the pelvic girdle and the spinal column have, at least on rare occasions, developed endometriosis.

A mysterious aspect of endometriosis is the rare appearance of the disease in tissues remote from the pelvis. This may occur almost anywhere in the body: in lungs, skin, bowels, kidneys, and the cavities surrounding the heart (the **pericardium**) and the lungs (the **pleural cavity**). Although endometriosis has been identified in the tissues surrounding and protecting the brain, the brain itself may be the only major organ never involved in endometriosis.

Whatever causes endometriosis in the pelvis can, at least in theory, also cause endometriosis outside the pelvis. The tiny clumps of endometrium thought by Sampson to cause endometriosis are picked up and filtered out of the pelvis by the lymphatic system. Lymphatic fluid belongs to a second circulation, much slower than the circulation of blood, which collects and filters fluid escaping from capillaries into tissues and channels it through a series of lymph nodes. The lymphatics ultimately spill into the bloodstream, so that endometrial cells may wind up circulating through arteries and veins. Thus, the tiny clumps of endometrium originating in retrograde menstruation may swarm through the lymphatics and the bloodstream, causing endometriosis throughout the body.

Endometriosis has been identified in lymph nodes since the early years of the twentieth century, when surgeons hoping to cure cancer began to excise pelvic lymph nodes. On very rare occasions, endometrial cells have also been identified circulating in the bloodstream. In summary, pelvic endometriosis is probably due to Sampson's so-called retrograde menstruation, but possibly due to Meyer's "metaplasia"; extrapelvic endometriosis may be due to Meyer's metaplasia but may follow the spread of clumps of endometrial cells through the lymphatics and blood vessels.

The Symptoms of Pelvic Endometriosis

If you suffer from chronic pelvic pain, a topic discussed in Chapter 10, you will be particularly interested in the unusual story of the symptoms of endometriosis. This disease is unpredictable in a number of ways, the most inexplicable of which is the poor correlation between the extent of the disease and the severity of the symptoms. You may have only two or three small patches of endometriosis in the ligaments supporting the womb, yet you may feel severe, disabling pain, vomiting, and diarrhea with each period. The pain caused by endometriosis may consist of excruciating cramps with every period, lasting well after the period has ended; there may be deep pain with intercourse, or random bouts of severe abdominal pain, or pain when passing bowel movements, or pain on voiding urine. Virtually any abdominal or pelvic pain may be caused by endometriosis. Irregular periods or premenstrual spotting may also be encountered, but they cause much less trouble than the pains. Bladder endometriosis causes symptoms that mimic bladder infections (pain on voiding, frequent voiding) and may also make blood appear in urine at the time of menstrual periods. However, some women with extensive endometriosis involving large areas in the pelvis may mysteriously and unaccountably be entirely free of symptoms.

The gynecological name for painful periods is **dysmenorrhea.** As menstrual flow begins, in most women the cramps begin to subside, but women with endometriosis may continue to feel increasingly unbearable pelvic pain. In addition to disabling menstrual cramps, they may also suffer severe nausea, or vomiting with headaches, even diarrhea, or generalized abdominal pains. These symptoms may combine to produce such devastation, that for the duration of the symptoms, a darkened room, ice packs, medications for pain, and the fervent wish to be left alone are the sufferer's most outstanding needs. Or, to be more accurate, this was the case until the early 1960s, when the first effective treatments for endometriosis began to appear.

Infertility is another symptom of endometriosis, but the relationship of infertility to endometriosis is unclear. If the fallopian tubes are obstructed or extensively damaged by endometriosis or if there are widespread adhesions (discussed in Chapters 10 and 11), infertility is easy to understand. However, some patients are infertile or have difficulty getting pregnant even though their tubes are open. This is usually "explained" by citing abnormalities of the peritoneal fluid, such as its high content of **prostaglandins.** These chemicals are found ubiquitously in tissues and body fluids and have a multiplicity of effects. For instance, painful menstrual cramps and the onset of contractions in labor are both due to prostaglandins. Also, cells have been found in peritoneal fluid that are capable of destroying sperm cells. Intercourse may be less frequent because of pain. Women with endometriosis also have higher-than-average chances of having miscarriages.

The painful intercourse often experienced by women with endometriosis is mostly felt on deep thrusting. Although this is usually at its worst around the time of menstruation, it may be felt at any time, whenever intercourse occurs. The pain is deep, sharp, and gnawing and often prevents intercourse entirely. It is experienced most often by women who have endometriosis of the rectovaginal septum and the nearby ligaments that support the womb. Fortunately, with modern treatments, painful symptoms can improve dramatically.

On very rare occasions, endometriosis can be dangerous enough to create a gynecological emergency. An endometriotic ovarian cyst may rupture, suddenly releasing old, decomposed blood into the abdomen. This happened to a colleague's wife, who, while shopping at a mall, was suddenly doubled over with severe lower abdominal pain. She was brought in by ambulance and underwent surgery within the hour. She was found to have severe endometriosis in one ovary only, causing a large cyst to form. When the cyst ruptured, it spilled at least a pint of old blood into her abdomen. During surgery, the blood and foreign materials were washed out, and the ovary was repaired. At this point, there was no more disease to be seen or felt, and she recovered without trouble. A few years later, she got pregnant and had a baby. She was one more victim of endometriosis in whom the disease had unexpected features.

The irregular bleeding or premenstrual spotting experienced by some women with endometriosis is not well understood. These usually occur with severe endometriosis, in women whose other problems overshadow the irregular bleeding.

Endometriosis is usually encountered in women in their twenties and thirties. However, Donald P. Goldstein, a gynecologist at Harvard University, has investigated the cause of unexplained abdominal pains in teenagers. On laparoscopy, the most precise way of checking the cause of the pain, about one-third of these young women was found to have early endometriosis. Goldstein's work has been corroborated by others, all of whom have taught us that endometriosis may appear at a much earlier age than we assumed. Also, gynecologists generally associate endometriosis with symptoms felt mostly premenstrually and menstrually. The pains investigated by Goldstein appeared with patterns not suggestive of endometriosis. In fact, as already noted, endometriosis produces symptoms capriciously, without following the orderly classifications invented by gynecologists. We shall return to this quandary when we discuss chronic pelvic pain, another problem often caused by endometriosis.

The Unpredictable Severity of Symptoms

I encountered one of the most amazing instances of severe endometriosis that caused barely perceptible symptoms when operating on a woman who was a recent immigrant from the Far East. This woman, then in her late forties, had eight pregnancies and eight children, including a four-year-old girl—not exactly a story of infertility. She came to me for a checkup and mentioned very casually the recent onset of intermittent and vague lower abdominal pains. When I examined her, I found a grapefruit-sized pelvic mass with a pint or two of fluid in her belly. I still remember the sudden shock I felt on feeling this tumor; my first thought was that she had advanced ovarian cancer.

At surgery, two surprises emerged. Rather than cancer, I found one of the worst cases of endometriosis I'd ever seen. Scar tissue surrounded everything; normal structures were not recognizable. This is an ominous and important sign to the surgeon to slow down and methodically identify each organ in order to avoid surgical mishaps. I found the second surprise after well over an hour of laborious dissection: She had a double uterus, located on top of a very peculiar-looking cervix. Loops of bowel were plastered solidly against the top of her womb where the fallopian tubes emerge, but she also had adhesions around her ovaries and the back of her womb. Since her youngest child was barely four years old, I had to presume that her disease started (or got much worse) after that delivery. This woman had no problems with infertility, nor had she had her children late in life— her oldest child was over thirty years old. Despite the large mass in her pelvis, her extensive adhesions, and her severe endometriosis, her symptoms were minimal. Because of the severity of the endometriosis and her age, hysterectomy was performed, and she had an uneventful recovery. With disease as widespread as hers, hysterectomy was, I thought, a reasonable choice.

This disparity between the extent of disease and the severity of its symptoms is one of the most striking and unsolved peculiarities of endometriosis. With most diseases that produce symptoms, a simple rule applies: The worse the disease, the more pronounced the symptoms. The woman I just described contradicted this notion impressively. Another patient I saw the same year experienced the opposite. She was a New York businesswoman in her early thirties who had excruciatingly severe menstrual pains with each of her periods. Laparoscopy the year before had shown no abnormalities. When she became my patient, I repeated the laparoscopy and found four or five tiny but distinct patches of endometriosis in her pelvis. Medical treatment with GnRH agonists (outlined in Chapter 9) virtually eliminated her symptoms. The symptoms felt by these two women tell me that we understand endometriosis much less well than we understand other diseases.[1]

The Symptoms of Endometriosis Outside the Pelvis

The symptoms of endometriosis outside the pelvis depend on the organ involved, and they may be very striking. For instance, endometriosis of the colon may cause bowel obstruction. If the lungs are involved, the woman may cough up spoonfuls of blood with each period. The inexplicable entrance of air into the space around the lungs may cause the dramatic collapse of a lung, with sudden pain in the chest and severe shortness of breath. These are rare emergencies that must be treated surgically, preferably by abdominal or thoracic surgical specialists as opposed to gynecological surgeons.

Endometriosis of the lining of the nose (the nasal mucosa) is an exceptionally rare condition; it causes a theatrically embarrassing symptom: nosebleeds with menstrual periods. Skin endometriosis may develop spontaneously, or it may be implanted inadvertently during surgery such as a cesarean section or myomectomy. A tiny tuft of endometrium sticks to the surgeon's glove and is brushed off a few seconds later. Unintentionally transplanted, the cells now begin to grow under the skin, soon causing a tender swelling. The painful mass is most troublesome during and after menstruation. Endometriosis in other sites causes symptoms that are not necessarily more pronounced during menstruation. For instance, bowel endometriosis will slowly thicken bowel walls and, if severe enough, may

---

[1]There is also the contrarian view: that it is not endometriosis that causes infertility but that voluntarily delayed fertility causes endometriosis. We have already noted that delaying childbearing allows the cervix to remain tightly closed and thus leads to retrograde menstruation. The recurrent showering of pelvic surfaces with clumps of endometrial cells may promote the development of endometriosis. The appearance of this disease in teenagers whose cervix or vagina is blocked, obstructing the flow of menstrual blood in this direction, also supports this view. Dilating the cervix with minor surgery called a Dilatation and Curettage (D&C) does not diminish this possibility, because the cervix closes down rapidly following artificial dilatation—only the delivery of a baby results in a permanently wider cervical canal.

cause intestinal obstruction. Some women have recurring monthly symptoms to warn them that something ominous is developing; others are free of problems until a surgical emergency develops.

The Diagnosis of Endometriosis

Severe endometriosis usually creates small lumps and masses that may be felt during a careful bimanual examination. The same examination, however carefully performed, is not sensitive enough to tell if you have minimal endometriosis, because your gynecologist's fingers may not detect anything abnormal. Tenderness on pelvic examination is reported by most women with this disease, and even a slight wince during the examination may be taken as evidence of endometriosis. However, many other pelvic diseases cause pain, and in a few women, the examination itself may be painful. Thus, the exact cause of the pain may remain obscure. Even if the gynecologist feels abnormalities and suspects endometriosis, other diseases such as a chronic tubal infection may be found, or possibly no disease at all will be discovered. Extremely rarely, a totally unexpected condition such as ovarian cancer is found. For these reasons, laparoscopy is essential in making a definitive diagnosis. In the language spoken by physicians, laparoscopy is the "gold standard" in the diagnosis of endometriosis.

Endometriosis is usually diagnosed in one of three ways. In some patients, infertility calls for an investigation, which culminates in the laparoscopic diagnosis of endometriosis. Other women undergo laparoscopy because of painful periods or pelvic pain. Finally, the disease may be found accidentally, when a surgeon (or gynecologist) performs some other operation, such as appendectomy or tubal ligation and finds endometriosis.

Ultrasound scans are not the best way of looking for possible endometriosis. If the scan is negative, you may still have a few small areas of this disease in your pelvis that are perfectly capable of causing much pain. In this case, the so-called negative scan was an expensive way to acquire misleading information. A few experts may be willing to diagnose endometriosis from the appearance of characteristic small cystic cavities in the ovaries and the pelvis. Glen Hofmann, an endocrinologist previously at the Mt. Sinai Medical Center in New York City, where I interviewed him, but currently working in Cincinnati, diagnoses endometriosis with confidence from ultrasound scans by recognizing tiny cysts—tissue damage caused by the disease. However, this level of expertise cannot be matched by most sonographers. The role of the even more expensive CT and MRI scans in the diagnosis of endometriosis is not well defined, although MRI scans appear promising. Unfortunately, if the endometriosis is microscopic, the scan may be misleadingly negative. If there is damage, for instance, some measurable abnormality such as a cyst measuring an inch in diameter, most scans will note the cyst but will not be able to ascertain its cause. Thus, laparoscopy will usually be required as the next (and almost definitive) step for the accurate diagnosis of the disease, for assessing the severity of the disease, and, above all, to start surgical treatment. The phrase "almost definitive" is slightly confusing. As we have seen, endometriosis behind the peritoneal lining is invisible. It would be very complicated and risky to cut into these tissues looking for a site to biopsy; this cannot be done. One practical way to make this diagnosis would be to treat the woman as if she had endometriosis—in other words, have her undergo a therapeutic trial. If her symptoms disappeared, you could deduce that she had endometriosis.

A relatively new test, called CA 125, is often ordered for gynecological patients who might have endometriosis or ovarian cancer. This test measures the levels of a protein, also called a "tumor marker," in blood. CA 125 was originally thought to be released by ovarian cancer cells only, but then it was found to be elevated in a host of other conditions, including endometriosis, tubal infections, fibroids, certain cancers, and pregnancy. It even fluctuates during menstrual cycles. The test is not expensive, but unfortunately, it is not as useful as hoped. CA 125 levels increase dramatically in the presence of certain common forms of ovarian cancer, very high levels usually indicating widespread disease. If the test is negative, not much has been excluded with certainty. If positive, your gynecologist may still need to perform laparoscopy to learn if there is a disease in the pelvis. The use of this test is discussed further in Chapter 14, which deals with ovarian cancer and related matters.

Endometriosis is usually diagnosed by means of laparoscopy. In the course of this operation, areas usually involved by endometriosis are carefully inspected for evidence of this disease. Small, deeply colored nodules (almost like black beauty spots) scattered on the surface of various pelvic organs are characteristic of endometriosis. However, during the last ten years, gynecologists have discovered unexpected additional details about

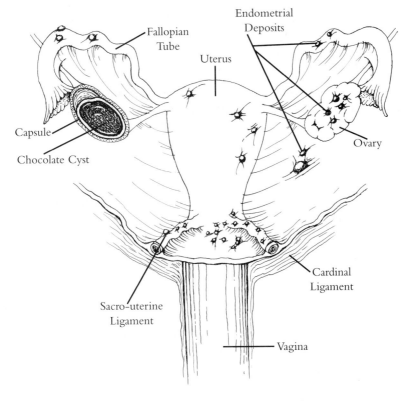

FIGURE 7.1   Endometriosis (posterior view of internal organs)

endometriosis. Any abnormality of the peritoneum, whether consisting of colorless, yellowish, or white streaks, or tiny cystic areas or apertures, or scarred-looking areas, may show endometriosis if examined under a microscope. Even normal-looking but tented up, raised peritoneal tissues may show endometriosis a fraction of an inch underneath the superficial layers. David Redwine, one of the best-known American experts, thinks that there may be a gradual maturation in the appearance of endometriosis, from colorless, white, or yellow scarring to its mature appearance as black or chocolate-brown nodules. Redwine believes that endometriosis may be missed because surgeons look for what *they* recognize as evidence of endometriosis, the deeply colored nodules, but remain oblivious of the significance of more subtle signs. I have heard similar observations from other experts, raising the possibility that even expensively obtained laparoscopic information may be erroneous.

It is impossible for you to know the depth of your gynecologist's expertise with minimal or subtle signs of endometriosis, and it may feel awkward to display your knowledge of this information. Tactful but pointed questions about the laparoscopic diagnosis of endometriosis should resolve this difficulty. Examples of such questions will be found at the end of the chapter.

Minimal endometriosis raises other difficulties. If there are no symptoms, the tiny patches may not be a sufficient justification for aggressive treatment. There is a lingering quandary here: Is it possible that if left untreated, these tiny patches may progress into full-blown endometriosis, invading and damaging tissues some years later? At this point, we simply don't know; it is difficult to be sure. British and Belgian research shows that such invasive progression may occur, and this is the standard view of most endometriosis experts. However, as already noted, in some women the patches seem to move around, appearing in some areas but disappearing in others. Attacked by the immune system, patches of endometriosis may disappear. Should the immune system falter, the patches may thrive exuberantly, producing symptoms.

As is the case with fibroids, endometriosis rarely turns cancerous. The usual frequency cited is well under .5 percent, or less than one woman in 200 with endometriosis. The fear of cancer should not be used to push women toward hysterectomy. However, a word of caution has been voiced by Robert Scully, a highly regarded pathologist from Boston. Scully reminds gynecologists that endometriosis, the disease, is composed of relatively normal endometrial tissue in unexpected sites. We know that the prolonged use of estrogens without progesterone may cause a cancerous change in such tissues, a subject discussed in Chapter 12. These ideas may be speculative and such tragic events rare, but they are important if you have endometriosis, particularly if you have already had a hysterectomy and your ovaries were removed. Under these circumstances, gynecologists customarily do not worry about endometrial cancer and are apt to use estrogen without balancing it with a progesterone-like drug. Scully advises the combined use of these two drugs in women who have had a hysterectomy for endometriosis, particularly if some of the endometriotic tissue was impossible to remove and was therefore left behind.

The severity of endometriosis is usually assessed in one of two ways. The surgeon in charge of the operation may, depending on what is found, describe it as "minimal," "mild," "moderate," or "severe." There should also be a full description of his or her findings in the surgical notes, particularly in a detailed, dictated (and therefore typewritten, and legible), operative note. I generally offer a copy of this to my patients. Should they need it a few years later, the operative report should be readily available.

There is a more scientific classification of endometriosis, originally devised by the American Fertility Society, now called the American Society for Reproductive Medicine. This classification has grown more and more complicated over the years but is used whenever a more objective and thoroughly descriptive idea of the severity of the disease is required. The main value of this complex classification is in research, comparing the improvements brought by different operations and drugs.

The Treatment of Endometriosis

The treatment of endometriosis is not a cut-and-dried, highly standardized set of prescriptions and procedures. Much depends on the severity of the disease as noted during laparoscopy: Endometriosis may be so minimal that it causes barely any concern, but it can also be a devastatingly widespread and damaging disease. Your age, your desire for children, your temperament, and your ability to follow complex regimens of medications or accept surgery all influence your treatment plan. The training, skills, and intelligence of your gynecologist are also important factors in determining which medical and surgical approaches will be used. Ideally, your treatment should be undertaken by a member of the American Society for Reproductive Medicine, but such perfectionism may be impractical, except in the vicinity of large medical centers. If you need surgery, members of the American Society of Gynecological Laparoscopists have excellent qualifications, although any gynecologist with laparoscopic skills may do equally well. At the least, as noted in the Introduction, he or she should be a Fellow of the American College of Obstetricians and Gynecologists. Finally, because many of the treatments we'll discuss are expensive as well as prolonged, your insurance (or the lack of it) will also influence your care.

Like fibroids, endometriosis may be managed in four distinctly different ways. Once diagnosed, it may be observed without treatment, a method a few gynecologists may recommend for minimal endometriosis. The growth of fibroids is easy to track with pelvic examinations and sonograms; but endometriosis may worsen with neither the woman nor her gynecologist appreciating the gravity of the situation. However, the diagnosis is usually made during laparoscopy. The gynecologist who undertakes your first laparoscopy should be skilled not only with diagnosing this disease but should be ready to commence medical or surgical treatment should endometriosis be found. Chapter 8 lists the medications, and Chapter 9 lists the various operations available.

There is no agreement on the need for treatment in women who have no serious symptoms but are found to have minimal endometriosis. In any patient in whom the preservation of fertility is an important consideration, I recommend treatment. Some of the minimal patches may gradually turn more extensive, and there is no convenient way to track this without repeated laparoscopies—this would clearly be neither cost-effective nor practical as a long-term plan of management. A good way to treat minimal endometriosis in teenagers and young women involves two steps. First, immediately after endometriosis has been identified, most deposits can be excised or vaporized. After successful surgery, most experts are concerned about recurrences and recommend further treatments to prevent these. The old-fashioned way is to prescribe the standard low-dose birth control pills: These are cheap, easy to use, and can be taken for months or years, possibly until the woman wishes to become pregnant. The other treatment for endometriosis is complicated as well as expensive: the class of drugs known as the GnRH agonists, and the more recent GnRH antagonists, all of which induce temporary (and reversible) menopause, also known as "pseudomenopause."

Medical treatments, mainly antiprostaglandin drugs and BCPs, are appropriate if laparoscopy has not been performed and the diagnosis is still uncertain. It is not appropriate if the gynecologist's bimanual examination or scans of the pelvis show masses, cysts, or other abnormalities: Medical treatments cannot dissolve these. Another disadvantage of medical treatments is that these cannot cure endometriosis but can merely suppress it temporarily. However, GnRH analogs may offer long-lasting relief from pain. Surgery is more aggressive, but essential if the disease has caused structural damage: cysts, adhesions, damage to fallopian tubes, obstructed organs. Surgery may help with infertility and pelvic pain. Definitive, long-lasting cure is only feasible if the womb and the ovaries, as well as all visible endometriosis, are excised or vaporized with cautery or laser beams. Fortunately, this is almost always avoidable. Finally, most gynecologists combine medical and surgical treatments in an extended plan of management.

Endometriosis thought to be moderate or severe either by symptoms or surgical findings needs treatment. The use of the hormone testosterone dates back to the decades when there was no effective treatment for endometriosis; this treatment is now obsolete. Another older treatment now obsolete is the use of the older, large-dose birth control pills. Other drugs such as Provera tablets, Depo-Provera injections, and danazol are in use, but they have been largely supplanted by the GnRH analogs or agonists. Some gynecologists precede surgical treatment with GnRH agonists; others precede and follow surgical treatment with a variety of medical regimens.

How to Avoid Hysterectomy for Endometriosis

Hysterectomy is rarely an absolute necessity when endometriosis is the sole reason for the operation. Modern surgery excises or otherwise removes all (or most) diseased tissues; medical regimens allow the suppression of endometriosis for six months, and, using the so-called "add-back" regimens, for much longer. Surgery that leaves healthy tissues intact but eliminates troublesome patches of endometriosis is used in preference to hysterectomy with removal of the ovaries and tubes. Much more often, particularly when childbearing is no longer an issue, patients may get discouraged with the continued need for medical attention that endometriosis often necessitates. The prospect of ten or fifteen years of elaborate and expensive hormonal treatments is not something to be taken lightly, and no woman should feel guilty for preferring hysterectomy. During this operation, all affected tissues should be removed, more often with, but possibly without, removing the ovaries and tubes. Nonemergency surgery (if and when you decide to have this) is a choice you should think through carefully and discuss in detail with your gynecologist well before you are admitted to a hospital.

143

Pregnancy and Endometriosis

We have already discussed the tangled connections between endometriosis and infertility. Most gynecologists believe that once pregnancy is achieved, the symptoms of endometriosis are greatly relieved, certainly throughout the pregnancy and possibly for months or longer after delivery. This, of course, does not help if the endometriosis prevents pregnancy or if pregnancy is not desired when endometriosis is diagnosed. Women anxious to conceive will be happy to hear that there is good evidence that fertility improves after surgery, but the effects of medical treatment are less clear-cut.

Adenomyosis

In adenomyosis, the endometrial tissue begins to spread from the inner lining of the womb, tiny tentacles reaching deeper and deeper into the muscular layers. Ultimately, adenomyosis may reach the outer surface of the uterus, becoming visible as fine, yellow-white scar tissue, a delicate tracery seen on uterine peritoneal coverings.

Unlike endometriosis, a disease usually first detected in women during their twenties and thirties, adenomyosis typically affects women who have had children, when they are in their late thirties, forties, or fifties. These women, who usually had normal periods before, now begin to notice unpleasant symptoms. The periods are heavier, last longer, and are more painful than before. When they consult with a gynecologist, the womb is found to be slightly enlarged. Adenomyosis may also be suspected from the characteristic spongy feel of the uterus on examination. Not infrequently, fibroids are diagnosed; in fact, both diseases may exist side by side in the same womb. If ultrasound scans are performed, fibroids usually appear different from adenomyosis, but minimal adenomyosis may go undetected. MRI scans are more valuable but also more expensive.

Unlike endometriosis, adenomyosis does not respond to hormones, probably because the abnormal tissues lack receptors, the tiny structures that hormones lock onto before a biochemical response is activated. Receptors are detectable only by means of elaborate electron-microscopic studies; these are not easily available in most hospitals.

Good medical treatments are available: Motrin, Advil, Aleve, Naprosyn, and similar antiprostaglandin drugs may help. If the only symptom is the "midline" dysmenorrhea felt in the middle of the pelvis premenstrually and menstrually, low-dose BCPs may be tried, but only if there are no medical reasons against the use of these medications. I must add that most of my patients were not helped by BCPs. All these matters are outlined in Chapter 8.

If symptoms are severe and the intermittent use of pain medications brings no relief, hysterectomy may be the only solution. However, the mere presence of adenomyosis is not by itself a good reason for surgery. Many cases of adenomyosis are discovered "accidentally," when hysterectomy is done for some other reason, and the pathologist identifies patches of adenomyosis in the uterus. This tells us that adenomyosis is often a painless condition.

Adenomyosis has not received the same intense attention that endometriosis has. Sampson's observations led to scores of research projects, and the docility with which endometriosis responds to hormonal managements has attracted dozens of investigators since the 1920s. Gynecologists understand at least some aspects of endometriosis reasonably well and have helped women overcome this peculiar disease. Adenomyosis has remained more incomprehensible and enigmatic than endometriosis; but perhaps because infertility is rarely a problem and because hysterectomy relieves all its manifestations, this disease has not caused as much havoc as endometriosis.

Every rule has exceptions. Rarely, young women are found to have a severe case of adenomyosis. This is particularly upsetting, because unlike fibroids, which can be excised one by one, adenomyosis usually has no distinct borders and is therefore difficult to remove. Most gynecologists have seen so few instances of severe adenomyosis in women still in their twenties or early thirties that they lack expertise in treating it. If you are such a patient, you need an experienced gynecologist to advise you—probably an expert in the treatment of endometriosis, even if these two diseases are dissimilar.

Questions You Must Ask If You Are Told You May Have Endometriosis

Before Laparoscopy

1. *I have read that endometriosis may look unusual and may be missed at laparoscopy. Is this true? What can you do to make sure that this will not happen to*

me? (Endometriosis has been "missed"—left undiagnosed—by gynecologists not sufficiently familiar with modern ideas about the laparoscopic appearance of this disease.) It would not be diplomatic to ask your surgeon about atypical endometriosis, implying that you may know this disease better than he or she does. You may simply tell your surgeon that you have read that not all endometriosis looks black or chocolate-brown and assess the reaction this information elicits. Members of the American Society for Reproductive Medicine are unlikely to make this error, but this rough rule of thumb does not take into account competent surgeons whose routine work does not warrant membership in the society.

2. *If you find endometriosis, will you be able to begin to treat me then and there, or will you refer me elsewhere for surgical treatment?* It is much better to have the procedure done by a gynecologist skilled with laparoscopic laser surgery. However, due to the frequency of the disease and the relative scarcity of equipment and specialists, this may not be possible except in or near large urban (or suburban) medical centers. For help with the selection of hospitals and specialists, refer to the Introduction. You can also write to or call the American Society for Reproductive Medicine for a referral. Their address and other details are in the Resources section at the end of the book.

After Laparoscopy

1. *How severe is my endometriosis? Is it minimal, mild, moderate, or severe? Which organs are involved? Would you later give me a copy of your dictated surgical note, so that I can file it among my medical records?*

2. *Do you plan to follow the laparoscopy with hormone treatments?* The most recommended drugs are expensive, costing hundreds of dollars a month and are usually prescribed for six months. "Add-back" treatments, described elsewhere, may prolong treatment; some insurance plans cover these costs. The gynecologist who forgets to discuss details such as these is not a great communicator. Much more troublesome is the fact that the United States is alone among major Western powers in having tens of millions of uninsured or underinsured men, women, and children. The quality of health care available to these people is often inferior (although Medicaid, at least in New York, will pay for GnRH agonists).

If your financial and insurance circumstances do not allow the use of the latest and the best treatments, all is not lost. The BCPs are, by expert consensus, not as effective against endometriosis as the GnRH agonists, or the equally expensive treatment with danazol, but they may provide good relief of symptoms. Other hormonal medications, for instance, medroxyprogesterone acetate (Provera) and others can also be used. Similarly, diseased tissues can be removed and healthy tissues can be preserved with conventional surgery using scalpels almost as well as with laser surgery. However, without laparoscopy and laser surgery, you will have to accept laparotomy, the old-fashioned way of opening the abdomen. Laparotomy is an effective operation, but it will leave you with a longer scar, either horizontal (the "bikini cut") or vertical, and more adhesions. If you desire to retain your fertility, you must know that adhesions are more extensive and more difficult to treat after laparotomy.

... 8 ...

Medical Treatments for Fibroids, Endometriosis, and Abnormal Uterine Bleeding

It was not a pregnancy an ex-patient of mine we'll call Judy would ever forget. Around the fifth month, her husband abruptly deserted her for a younger woman. This left Judy, who had just turned thirty-seven, to cope with a large house she could ill afford as well as the care of her two young children and her newly established business as a computer consultant. Judy delivered without trouble in Connecticut, where she'd moved the year before, in the care of another gynecologist, but a month later she began to hemorrhage. She underwent an emergency curettage and received a transfusion of three or four pints of blood. Judy also consumed a purseful of iron preparations and tried birth control pills (BCPs) and Provera tablets, yet the bleeding continued.

After another curettage, she was still spotting and bleeding heavily enough for hysterectomy to be discussed. When she called me in New York, she had just started taking Ergotrate, a drug that controls bleeding from a relaxed womb by forcing its muscles to contract powerfully, thereby stopping the flow of blood. Unfortunately, ergot preparations, familiar to women who suffer from migrainous headaches, are only useful for a week or so after delivery, and I was not optimistic that they would help. The pre-scription also made me question the quality of the gynecological care Judy was receiving. Meanwhile, the bleeding kept recurring. Judy was now deal-ing with upset customers, potential housekeepers, and a divorce lawyer, and she thought that a hysterectomy would be the last straw. I agreed to see her early the next morning before my other patients were due to arrive.

Blood tests, a sonogram, and the hysteroscopy I performed revealed no clues about the cause of the trouble. At the time, I was considering an in-vestigation of danazol, a drug that was then one of the standard treatments for endometriosis, to shrink fibroids. Danazol (also known by its brand name, Danocrine) stops bleeding by causing temporary menopause. Dana-zol changes the endometrium, the tissue that bleeds, from a lush and thick layer of tissue, engorged with blood vessels, into a thin, parchment-like sheet of tissue with no discernible arteries or veins. As a last measure, and after a detailed discussion, Judy began to take danazol.

As the drug took effect, Judy's milk dried up and her breasts became smaller. Hot flushes appeared, but, to her delight, the bleeding ceased. At last she could begin to take charge of her life—at which she excelled—without the distractions of gynecological visits, not to mention the dreaded hysterectomy. Four months later, we stopped the danazol, the arti-ficial menopause slowly disappeared, and Judy's normal periods returned. We never learned why the bleeding occurred. (Doctors often understand these events less well than they let on. Symptoms often appear and disap-pear mysteriously, without anyone understanding why. I am familiar with intense psychic turmoil wrecking menstrual periods but have no reason to think that Judy's bleeding was caused by her marital disaster.) Bleeding can be arrested with much better drugs today, but the episode stayed with me for nearly twenty years: This was the first time I had staved off hysterec-tomy by inducing temporary menopause. Then it was an experimental treatment that some of my colleagues discouraged; today, with better drugs, it is mainstream gynecology.

Controlling Diseases with Medications

This chapter deals with medical (that is, nonsurgical) treatments for certain diseases. Fibroids, endometriosis, and bleeding problems are entirely dissimilar from each other as diseases: Fibroids are potato-like tumors usually locked deep in the muscles of the womb. Endometriosis is a subtle and painful infiltration of mostly pelvic tissues by tiny pockets of endometrium, the tissue that lines the uterine cavity. Bleeding usually originates in some abnormality of the lining of the womb, although fibroids and endometriosis may also play a part. In spite of these differences, medical treatments for these problems almost always involve hormones in various combinations. I can add chronic pelvic pain (CPP) to the above list. CPP is an enigmatic problem to most women, and often to their physicians; CPP can be included because it may be caused by endometriosis, whose medical treatment is detailed in this chapter.

Dissimilar as they appear, these diseases receive similar treatments because they share one feature: All the organs and tissues involved are extremely sensitive to hormones. With estrogen and progesterone coursing through pelvic blood vessels, these tissues thrive. Deprived of the same hormones by menopause or by drugs that induce menopause, the same tissues **atrophy**. This word is often disliked by women who associate it with aridity and senility, but "hibernation" would be a more accurate description: If the hormones reappear, the tissues recover completely.

Hysterectomy used to be the solution for many instances of these diseases, but this is no longer true—at least not without a full discussion of treatment options. The unusual responsiveness of women's pelvic tissues to hormones (and to being deprived of hormones) allows us to try a variety of medical treatments instead. However, before any medical treatment is undertaken, we must be sure that neither malignancy nor pregnancy is responsible for the symptoms. The uses of smears, biopsies, pregnancy tests, and various scans and operations to rule out cancer have been discussed in Chapter 5.

This section discusses the medical treatments available for treating fibroids, endometriosis, and abnormal bleeding from the womb, along with certain treatments prescribed for women suffering from chronic pelvic pain. The medications we'll discuss include estrogenic and progesterone-like medications as well as combinations of the same hormones known as birth control pills. Alternately, drugs that induce a temporary (reversible) menopausal state may be used.

The information provided will enable you to consider these drugs confidently. Some medications will be noted by their brand name—the name used by the manufacturer of the drug to distinguish its product and the name usually most familiar to women. This name will appear with its first letter capitalized (e.g., Provera or Tylenol). The generic names of chemicals (e.g., medroxyprogesterone, or estrogen, or estradiol) are printed in lower-case letters. After discussing these medications individually, we'll discuss their use for women with abnormal bleeding, fibroids, endometriosis, and chronic pelvic pain.

Estrogens and Estrogenic Medications

From their early teens until the mid-forties, women's bodies overflow with estrogens. These are the decades during which women ovulate, and the mature ovary is a ceaseless and dynamic producer of the basic hormones estrogen and progesterone. This, of course, is a simplification. The main hormone during the years noted is called estradiol, but there are dozens of estrogen-like compounds produced all over the body. Estrogens are derived from androgens, testosterone-like hormones swirling around in women; men's organs also produce various estrogens; all kinds of tissues (skin, brain, liver, bone, vessels, and so forth) are in the metabolic loop as producers and consumers of estrogens. All the same, pelvic tissues in women are extraordinarily sensitive to estrogen, a veritable and potent growth hormone to all pelvic organs and tissues, and a hormone whose absence drastically slows, even shuts down the life-sustaining activities of the same organs.

Except for menopausal years, women are rarely short of estrogen. The main reason estrogen is prescribed during these years of sexual maturity is that estrogen prepares tissues for the arrival of progesterone; estrogen facilitates and potentiates the effects of the latter hormone. As a practical example, progesterone-only birth control pills are less effective and more difficult to use than combined estrogen-progesterone birth control pills.

Estrogens alone, without progesterone, may be used in the control of heavy bleeding, but only for the unusually heavy bleeding a few young teenagers may develop as sexual maturation (and ovulation) commences. Combined medications, mostly as birth control pills, are commonly used during and after teenage years; this use will be discussed shortly in the sections that deal with BCPs and menopausal uses.

Estrogens stimulate the growth of endometriotic and fibroid cells, as well as precancerous (or cancerous) tissues in the endometrium and possibly the breasts. For this reason, estrogens are not used in the management of fibroids and endometriosis unless they are combined with a progesterone-like medication, called a progestin. The use of estrogens after recovery from breast cancer is highly contentious, with cautious physicians not prescribing them after treatment for breast cancer; most gynecologists avoid estrogens forever after endometrial cancer has been diagnosed.

If you have, or have ever had, fibroids and endometriosis, and the drug you are taking contains estrogen, check the details with your gynecologist or your pharmacist. The insert that accompanies your medication may also have relevant information. The exact dose of hormones used and the presence or absence of a progestin are important. If you have had a hysterectomy for fibroids, estrogens can be used without a progestational addition. After myomectomy, these hormones are probably best avoided, except in low doses. If the surgery was for endometriosis, read the section on the add-back regimens and the estrogen threshold hypothesis in this chapter.

Estrogens are invaluable in mitigating menopausal symptoms and in preventing postmenopausal osteoporosis and, probably, heart disease. Most medical experts believe that except for the aftermath of uterine and breast cancer, contraindications are few and the benefits of taking estrogen (usually referred to as estrogen replacement therapy, or ERT) outweigh the disadvantages. A much-quoted article from Massachusetts General Hospital in Boston, published in 1989 by internist Gail Greendale and GYN endocrinologist Isaac Schiff, reported that female internists were much more likely to prescribe hormone replacement therapy (HRT) than were male internists. Gynecologists were unanimous believers in HRT, regardless of their gender. However, the story of hormone replacement therapy has been a regular roller-coaster ride, with the latest studies always conflicting with yesterday's expert opinions, a subject further discussed in Chapter 14.

Estrogens are usually prescribed under brand names such as Premarin, Estrace, Ogen, and a handful of other preparations. Skin patches (Estraderm, Climara, and others) and estrogen-containing vaginal creams may also be used. Injections and pellets of estrogen implanted under the skin are not in widespread use in the United States; an estrogen-containing vaginal ring is currently available.

Since these hormones are made in fatty tissues as well as the ovaries, very heavy women, whose bodies make substantial amounts of estrogen, are at an increased risk of developing endometrial cancer, gallbladder disease, and breast cancer. Obesity is usually accompanied by abnormal lipid values and may also lead to arteriosclerotic heart disease. Conversely, obese women are protected from osteoporosis. Thin women, who generally have lower levels of estrogens, have less endometrial and breast cancer but more osteoporosis.

Progesterone and Progestins

Progesterone has two major purposes: protecting pregnancy by suppressing contractions of the uterine muscles and balancing estrogen in the uterus and the endometrium, and probably the breasts. Unlike estrogen, natural progesterone is ineffective when swallowed. However, it is available for vaginal use in suppositories (a fact well known to some PMS sufferers) and by injection. Since suppositories and injections are inconvenient, synthetic progesterone-like drugs called progestins have been developed. Provera and the progestins in BCPs are by far the most often used and best-known progestins. BCPs not only prevent conception but have a host of other uses; the most important of these, from the point of view of women with irregular, heavy, or otherwise abnormal bleeding, is the facility with which synthetic BCPs moderate, suppress, or regulate uterine bleeding. Natural hormones cannot be prescribed to achieve the same effect month after month—a mysterious contradiction. A "micronized" progesterone tablet called Prometrium has been introduced recently, synthesized from a vegetable source; it remains to be seen how popular it will become.

The progestational medications most often used are Provera and its long-acting, injectable counterpart called Depo-Provera; Megace is used more by oncologists than by gynecologists; the progestational mini-BCPs Micronor and Ovrette are less popular than their combined counterparts that contain estrogen as well as progesterone. Finally, there is a progesterone-containing intrauterine contraceptive device (IUCD) called Progestasert.

The chemical name of Provera is medroxyprogesterone acetate, usually abbreviated to MPA. Progesterone and drugs such as MPA are anti-estrogenic; by far the most frequent reason for prescribing them is to counter the irregular bleeding caused by estrogen without progesterone and the slight but definite tendency of prolonged estrogen treatment to lead to endometrial cancer.

Provera is available in three doses: tablets of 2.5, 5, or 10 mgm. Because of their adverse effects on serum lipids, the dose in long-term users may be reduced to 5, or even 2.5 mgm daily. While better in terms of the heart, we do not yet know how protective the lower doses are against endometrial cancer. For even better care, the levels of lipids circulating in the blood may be monitored by a physician familiar with these matters, usually an internist.

Progestins should not be used after clots have developed in leg veins (thrombophlebitis) and after thromboembolic episodes, cerebral hemorrhage, or breast cancer, or in patients who are pregnant or are having a miscarriage. Hypersensitivity to progestins is rare.

Provera: Side Effects

The side effects of any drug are difficult to assess. An amazing number of drugs are described as causing headaches and dizzy spells; it is at least possible that the diseases for which the drugs were prescribed, and the anxieties and uncertainties connected with the need for treatment, are responsible for these symptoms. Textbooks describe an unusually long list of possible side effects attributed to Provera. How many of these are caused by Provera and how many are coincidental may be debated endlessly without certainty. Progestins including Provera may cause depression, fluid retention, breakthrough bleeding, venous thrombosis, and thromboembolic diseases, allergic reactions, and adverse effects on the eyes. In practice, only the first three are seen with any frequency, and at least some research has also questioned depression as a side effect of progesterone. If these drugs caused depression, PMS sufferers, who often use very large doses for the relief of symptoms including depression, should have noticed this effect. This has not been reported, demonstrating the unusually tenuous nature of our knowledge of drugs and their side effects.

The use of Provera for fibroids and the bleeding abnormalities that appear in women who do not ovulate cannot result in a cure; rather, it is a useful treatment that may last months, even a year or two. But sooner or later, the bleeding may start again. Also, a few patients do not respond at all and continue to bleed despite Provera. If this is the case, other medical or surgical treatments must be considered. Among medical treatments, menopause-inducing GnRH analogs stand out because of their reliability in stopping bleeding. Surgical treatments will be discussed in Chapter 9, mostly under the rubric of hysteroscopic surgery: surgery performed while looking into the uterine cavity.

Depo-Provera

Depo-Provera contains MPA, the same medication contained in Provera, but it is given by injection, with the hormone present in a suspension of tiny crystals. At the standard dose of 150 mgm every three months, it will remain effective for at least three months after being injected. Double doses will last at least six months. However, once injected, no medication can be removed from the body. For this reason, the 300-mgm dose was never used in the United States.

During the 1960s, Depo-Provera was used in the United States as a contraceptive agent. Two effects were noted: Instead of menstruating, some women on Depo-Provera spotted or bled intermittently. Others noticed a mild depression, discussed earlier. The major advantage was that after Depo-Provera was injected, there was no need for contraception for at least three months: Pregnancies were all but unknown among women using Depo-Provera. In developing countries, the 300-mgm injection every six months provided more cost-effective contraception.

Subsequently, it was found that beagles receiving large doses of Depo-Provera grew breast cancers, a finding that led to a ban on the use of this drug from the FDA. This ruling made for some confusion, since Depo-Provera was at the same time thought to be a reasonably effective palliative for endometrial cancer. Whatever the significance of this finding, the use of Depo-Provera was much curtailed. Your gynecologist may be willing to prescribe Depo-Provera to treat abnormal bleeding patterns, but more likely he or she will not. The reluctance to use this medication concerns the frequency of breast cancer, medicolegal considerations, and, most of all, the availability of other, more effective medications. After all, one problem with Depo-Provera has always been that it made women bleed irregularly, even if lightly—an improvement from heavy flow, but hardly a cure.

In October 1992, the FDA reversed itself and approved the use of Depo-Provera as an injectable contraceptive. In the wake of that ruling, "Depo" is beginning to be used more extensively as a contraceptive in the United

States. However, "unlabeled" uses, for purposes not approved by the FDA, are at the discretion of the prescribing physician.

Depo-Provera should *not* be used for women who have had previous episodes of thrombophlebitis, thromboembolic disease, and strokes. Hypersensitivity to Provera or Depo-Provera is rare. It must be avoided in women who are or who may be pregnant, and particularly in women who are going through a miscarriage or have vaginal bleeding of unknown cause. Depo-Provera must be avoided in women who have, or have had, breast cancer.

The Birth Control Pills

The birth control pills, also called oral contraceptives (and abbreviated to BCPs, OCs and OCPs) are not really pills, which by definition have a hard, smooth, glossy shell surrounding the medication. They are tablets, but the word "pill" has displaced the more correct term. Today's BCPs are "low-dose," with a small fraction of the weight (and the hormonal activity) of Enovid, the first BCP, marketed about forty years ago. Most BCPs consist of combinations of two "female" hormones: one estrogen-like, or estrogenic; the other progesterone-like, or progestational. The estrogenic component is usually 20 or 35 micrograms (20 or 35 times one-millionth of a gram, abbreviated to mcg) of such a hormone, and 0.1 to 1 milligram (one-thousandth of a gram, abbreviated to mgm) of a progesterone-like hormone, also called a progestin, in each tablet. BCPs are as sold as 21-day or 28-day packages; the latter have seven so-called "dummy pills" for days 22 through 28. These pills have no hormonal content; they are there to help women continue the convenient one-pill-every-day routine without stopping on certain days.

Before World War II, when estrogens were first identified, they were extracted from the urine of pregnant women. Soon afterwards, DES, that infamous hormone, was produced in a laboratory. After World War II, when they began to be prescribed, estrogens were made from the urine of pregnant mares; later, other estrogens were synthesized but were difficult to use without progesterone. Natural progestrone is not absorbed from the intestinal tract when swallowed; it has to be given by injections or used as vaginal suppositories or creams. The scientific breakthrough of the BCPs consisted of developing hormones that could be produced on a large scale through chemical synthesis, manufactured in laboratories and later in factories, and developing hormones that worked when swallowed. Today's estrogens and progestins are all synthetic, factory-made from plant precursors. The original precursor was the tuber of the Mexican yam; today's precursors are trade secrets not shared with anyone.

Well over thirty BCP combinations are available today, a dizzying number if you try to assess which is the most suitable preparation for you. Excluding, for the moment, progesterone-only minipills, the differences between competing formulations are relatively unimportant, stressed more by manufacturers and the advertisers they retain, jockeying for higher sales, than by women or by physicians. Because of their striking effect on the endometrial lining, these pills can be used not only for contraception but also for regulating bleeding patterns—let us remember that almost all bleeding originates in the endometrium. When taken to control abnormal bleeding, the older formulations, which contain a fixed amount of hormones in each tablet, are easier to use. The newer preparations, called "biphasic" or "triphasic," contain fluctuating amounts of hormones from week to week and are better avoided. Swallowing tablets with no hormonal content is, in effect, the same as ceasing to take hormones. You may recall that it is the drop in hormone levels in the blood that produces normal periods; stopping the tablets or taking tablets without hormonal contents produce the (usually light) periods you get while taking BCPs.

BCPs work mostly by preventing ovulation: the monthly release of an egg cell from an ovary. The minuscule amounts of hormones just noted are enough to convince the brain centers responsible for the regulation of ovulation that the hormones originated from a normal pregnancy. These centers are programmed to cease their ovulation-inducing hormonal commands during pregnancies; duped by synthetic hormones that mimic a pregnancy, they now cease producing the hormonal commands to ovulate. The BCPs have many other effects as well, but most of these concern contraception and not the control of bleeding, which is our focus here.

BCPs are, of course, in widespread use as contraceptives. They are also used to help women with painful periods and to correct abnormal bleeding. When used to check bleeding, we rely on the hormonal stimulation provided by the BCPs, which results in the steady growth of the endometrium. As this layer grows, tissues are regenerated and bleeding vessels are sealed, stopping the bleeding. When the tablets in a packet are finished, the hormone levels drop abruptly, and (as happens with normal menstruation) a period follows. If bleeding can be controlled with BCPs, there is usually no reason to operate. However, I have often counseled patients whose gynecologists recommended hysterectomy as treatment for excessive bleeding without trying these extremely effective medications first. As long as you are a healthy nonsmoker and have not had illnesses that preclude the use of the BCPs, today's low-dose pills are safe even past the age of thirty-five.

Noncontraceptive uses of the BCPs include the treatment of endometriosis, mittelschmerz (ovulatory, or midcycle pain), painful periods, and bleeding problems. Much less often they are used to prevent pregnancy after intercourse or rape, to treat acne, or to prevent ovarian cysts and possibly prevent PMS. Occasionally I see them recommended as effective treatments for chronic pelvic pain—I only wish such a simple therapy could work! If your CPP is associated with severe menstrual pains, you might be suffering from endometriosis; this may be one of the best reasons for trying BCPs.

Other Benefits of Birth Control Pill Use

In addition to effective contraception and less painful periods, the BCPs have numerous other benefits. Tubal infections and ovarian cysts as well as benign breast cysts and ovarian and endometrial cancer are all less frequent among women who are taking, or have taken, BCPs. Because the periods of women taking BCPs are light, they will reduce a woman's chances of becoming anemic. Thus, the use of BCPs can contribute to better health and, indirectly, to fewer hysterectomies. Other women find that they begin to put on weight or develop migraines, or find that their headaches worsen while they are taking BCPs. There are also limited (and energetically debated) statistics showing that the BCPs may contribute, in a very minor way, to the development of breast or cervical cancer. Most experts do not consider these realistic objections to BCP use. BCPs have been approved as contraceptives by governmental agencies and are in widespread use throughout the world, in some countries without such niceties as medical supervision or prescriptions.

However, BCPs have also caused major complications, such as myocardial infarctions (coronaries, or heart attacks), strokes, thromboembolic complications (blood clots), and liver and gallbladder diseases. Elizabeth McConnell, M.D., a well-known American expert on contraception, thinks that the BCPs have received an unfair assessment from the media. Her view is that it was mostly the older preparations, with larger doses of hormones, that caused most serious complications. Based on current medical literature, it appears that she is correct—modern, low-dose BCPs appear to be safe. However, we certainly do not have a method of birth control that is entirely safe, 100-percent effective, convenient to use, and affordable. Condoms and diaphragms with abortion as a backup seem to come closest, but many will not find this solution acceptable.

The Disadvantages of the BCPs

The Food and Drug Administration (FDA) prohibits the use of these drugs in women who have had thrombophlebitis (clots in leg or pelvic veins), thromboembolic disease, strokes or heart disease, cancer of the breast or other estrogen-dependent tumors, pregnancy, and certain liver tumors. In smokers at any age (particularly in women over the age of thirty-five) or in the presence of diabetes, hypertension, and diseases of the gallbladder and the arteries and veins (for instance, migraine and varicose veins) the pills are not a good choice. Major complications such as thromboembolic diseases are rare, occurring in a few women in every group of 100,000 users annually. However, these complications are serious and potentially fatal. When the blood in a calf or thigh vein forms a clot, also called a **thrombus**, it usually adheres to the inner wall of the vein and is gradually absorbed—there may be no symptoms at all. If it becomes detached, the bloodstream promptly carries it to the lungs. If large enough, it cuts off the circulation through one or both lungs, causing a sudden emergency. This usually causes severe shortness of breath, blood may be coughed up, or, in worst-case scenarios, the patient dies before effective help can be summoned.

BCPs should not be used in women whose endometrial lining shows a change called **hyperplasia**. This is an estrogen-induced condition, diagnosed after a biopsy has been taken or a curettage performed; certain varieties of hyperplasia may become cancerous. Women with these problems may need hysterectomy, although lesser grades may be managed with progesterone-like drugs such as Provera or Megace, as long as stimulation from estrogen is avoided. Endometrial hyperplasias are discussed in Chapter 12.

Practical Points to Consider

The BCPs are used in one of two ways for endometriosis and bleeding disorders: in a cyclic fashion and continuously. **Cyclic use** means that the BCPs are taken for 21 days, followed by 7 days without them or 7 days of so-called dummy tablets that contain no hormones, only inert ingredients. **Continuous use** means that hormones are taken daily, without interruption. All gynecologists have their preferences, and it cannot be claimed with any certainty that one method is superior to the other. If the desired response (relief from pain in endometriosis or diminished bleeding) is not obtained, the usual response is to increase the dose. As Robert Kistner has shown, this is feasible for some months, but sooner or later breakthrough bleeding will usually occur. If the response to BCPs is unsatisfactory, other medical or surgical treatments must be considered.

A discussion of the side effects and complications of the use of the BCPs, a far-reaching and complex subject, is not possible here. By federal law, each package of BCPs must contain a patient package insert. This insert includes a detailed account of side effects and complications. Also, magazine articles and popular books often address this subject. *Our Bodies, Ourselves for the New Century: A Book by and for Women Written by the Boston Women's Health Book Collective* (Touchstone Books/Simon and Schuster, 1998) has a distinctly feminist point of view, pulls no punches, and contains an extensive and balanced account of this and related topics. I recommend it.

The medications we have discussed so far are all growth-promoting hormones for various tissues. If used for too long, day after day at the same fixed dose, they may result in atrophy, one of the vagaries of the way many hormones work. Nevertheless, under ordinary circumstances, hormones are doers—they make things happen. We now come to other hormones that do the opposite: They shut down metabolic activities, making women menopausal. This is not a step lightly undertaken, and it should occur only in response to major illnesses with widespread repercussions. The first of these drugs is danazol, whose trade name is Danocrine.

Danazol

During the 1970s and the early 1980s, new medications began to be used for endometriosis and for fibroids. These caused temporary menopause:

not exactly a desired state, but one that relieved the symptoms of endometriosis and fibroids and even put an effective end to abnormal bleeding. Menopause without hormonal replacement results in symptoms such as hot flashes, flattened breasts, diminished vaginal secretions, and possibly lessened interest in sexual activity. Normal periods are replaced by no periods at all or, more often, by irregular but scanty bouts of bleeding, because the endometrial lining has become inactive and thin. When the new drugs are stopped, the artificial menopause wears off, usually within two or three weeks. Remarkably, the beneficial effects on the disease for which the new drugs were prescribed may persist for a while after the medications have been discontinued, a topic we'll return to shortly.

The first of the new drugs was danazol, also known by its brand name, Danocrine. Danazol is a complex drug to describe. It suppresses the mid-cycle surge of hormones that cause ovulation, causing menopause. It has properties described as androgenic (masculinizing, for instance, promoting the growth of hair) and anabolic (building muscle and bone mass). It is an expensive drug to use; Depending on the dose required to produce the desired effect, two, three, or four capsules, or 400, 600, or 800 mgm each day, may be needed. Either Danocrine or the substantially less expensive generic danazol may be used. The cost of treatment may range from less than $100 to over $300 a month, depending on the dose, the pharmacy, and your choice of generic or brand-name medication. Danazol is usually taken for six, or possibly nine, months; then it is stopped. Experts consider danazol to be almost as effective as the newer hormonal medications, a group usually referred to as the GnRH analogs or agonists, which are described in the next section, but the drawbacks of danazol are more pronounced. For this reason, the use of danazol has declined sharply during the 1990s.

Disadvantages

Danazol has serious and unavoidable side effects. This drug may cause unfavorable (if temporary) changes in blood lipid levels. Although some of the so-called anabolic effects (familiar from the use of steroids by athletes) are potentially useful, and in particular bone mass is not lost, the weight gain experienced by some women is a disadvantage. Androgenic effects—the drug's tendency to lead to the growth of male-type, dark hair in places such as the upper lip, hair that will not ever disappear—are not welcomed by women either. Because of these disadvantages, the GnRH analogs are preferred to danazol. Some women find that the so-called cure is worse than the disease and will not tolerate either of these medications; others are happy that at last a medication has been found to relieve their symptoms. Unfortunately, neither danazol nor any of the GnRH agonists offer a cure. Rather, they control the disease as long as they are being taken and for a few weeks or months after they have been stopped, when the salutary effects of the medications have not yet worn off.

Danazol was first used in the treatment of endometriosis and fibroids and, much less often, for severe breast pains due to fibrocystic disease. Danazol must not be used during pregnancy and breast-feeding. Ovulation is unlikely to occur in women taking this drug; nevertheless, the makers recommend additional nonhormonal contraception. Severe hypertension and liver and kidney disease are good reasons for *not* using danazol.

Side Effects

Side effects from danazol are numerous. Weight gain; irregular bleeding or spotting; hot flashes; diminished libido; fluid retention; decreased breast size; and growth of hair on the face, between the breasts, on the nipples, and in the midline of the lower abdomen have all been noted. One patient was a mezzosoprano but became a contralto because of danazol—she was not pleased with the change. Other women have complained of headaches and acne or have noticed oily skin. In summary, the side effects are considerable, but the symptoms of endometriosis may be so severe that any medication promising help is welcomed.

Taking Danazol

Danazol must be started during or just after a period, following a negative pregnancy test. Barrier contraception is recommended even though patients are unlikely to conceive while taking danazol. As already noted, the standard dose of danazol is two to four 200-mgm capsules a day. Some gynecologists start danazol at 400 mgm a day and increase this dose if the response (usually defined as the lessening of pain from endometriosis) is not sufficient. Others start the drug at 800 mgm a day and diminish this dose when the desired effect has been achieved. When the effects of danazol wear off, endometriosis symptoms may return rapidly, but it may take months (or even years) before serious symptoms recur. Danazol is not in current use for shrinking fibroids.

The next treatment to be approved for use was another group of medications that artificially and temporarily induced a menopausal state in women. These medications were referred to by two equally cumbersome names: the GnRH analogs or the GnRH agonists.

The GnRH Analogs

• Analogue (analog): That which is analogous to, or corresponds with, some other thing. *Webster's New International Dictionary,* Second Edition, The Merriam Company, 1957.

• Agonist: A prime mover. *Dorland's Illustrated Medical Dictionary,* W. B. Saunders Company, 1988.

The hormone responsible for initiating each new menstrual cycle is called gonadotropin releasing hormone, usually abbreviated to GnRH. The identification of this hormone in 1971 was an advance of such importance that in 1977 it was awarded the Nobel Prize in medicine. GnRH can be found not only in humans and all other mammals but also further down the tree of evolution, for instance, in fish. In women, GnRH activates cells in the pituitary gland to produce two other hormones, follicle stimulating hormone (FSH) and luteinizing hormone (LH). These are released into blood, that soup of a myriad of ingredients, to be carried to the ovaries. FSH and LH carry messages that ultimately result in ovulation: the release of a fertilizable ovum, or egg cell, from either ovary. In men, GnRH does something similar but different. Again, the pituitary gland produces FSH and LH, but in men there is no need for the precise synchronization and careful balancing of hormones there is in women. Instead, FSH is essential to enable testicular tissue to make sperm cells, and LH to maintain testosterone levels, keeping male genitals functional. The healthy male has a steady output of GnRH, FSH, and LH, and produces millions of sperm cells, swarming and waiting for one to fertilize the single ovum, carefully crafted by the female with the help of the same hormones.

Research indicates that a plentiful supply of GnRH is responsible for the dominant sexual activity and brilliant colors of the male of an African species of fish, the *cichlid*. The chance arrival of larger and more colorful males is a threatening event to smaller male fish. This misfortune inhibits the production of the hormone, leading to a loss of sexual potency, plainer colors, and submissiveness. Such patterns of secretion of the sex hormones evolved millions of years ago. This ancient drama shows that in the *cichlid,* psychologically stressful events may have profound physical consequences—a story we'll return to in another context: that of chronic pelvic pain.

Released into the bloodstream in periodic spurts, natural GnRH is exceptionally short-lived, lasting only a few minutes. This is all it needs, since it has to travel a short distance, from the arcuate nucleus, a collection of nerve cells in the base of the brain, to the pituitary, located about an inch further down. The composition of natural GnRH may be chemically altered in a laboratory. Minor changes of its formula result in the synthesis of much more durable hormones, called the GnRH analogs. Analogs of GnRH are either agonists, which promote a sequence of hormonal events, or antagonists, which retard or inhibit the same events. The two terms *analog* and *agonist* are used interchangeably in gynecological writings, a confusing practice made possible by the fact that all the analogs released for commercial use to date have been agonists. Over 2,000 chemicals with an agonistic action have been synthesized, but only a few are in clinical use today. They are expensive drugs to use. GnRH antagonists are slowly being accepted and used, but their tendency to cause allergic reactions has, at least to date, dimmed their promise.

When receiving a medication that provides a continuously and unfailingly high level of stimulation with a GnRH agonist, as opposed to the hourly spurts it is used to, the pituitary at first responds by releasing high levels of FSH and LH. This stimulates the ovaries, which may swell, and increases libido. GnRH is a temporary aphrodisiac, but as the brain gets used to the high levels of this hormone, it no longer responds with increased libido. Therefore, GnRH cannot be used effectively for this purpose.

Continued stimulation by natural or synthetic GnRH has a striking effect. After a week or two of nonstop stimulation, the pituitary gives up, as if disgusted with the relentless prodding. The entire chain of hormonal events now shuts down, very much as if the ovaries (or testicles) were removed. In women, FSH and LH levels diminish sharply, the all-important midcycle surge of LH is lost, ovulation ceases, and a temporary menopause sets in. In men who receive a GnRH analog, in addition to shrunken genitals, impotence and hot flashes have been noted. Previously thought to occur in women only, men's hot flashes follow the loss of male hormones rather than estrogens. Fortunately, in women and in men, all side effects disappear within ten to fourteen days after the drug causing them has been stopped. If menopause were about to commence when treatment with a GnRH agonist was started, artificial menopause would, as the drug wore off, change imperceptibly into natural menopause.

The newfound ability to use GnRH in a mode of continuous stimulation (as opposed to the cyclic release of spurts) was a breakthrough in the medical treatment of many conditions. One of the first to be treated was precocious puberty, the sexual maturation of children well before the age of eight (for girls) or nine (for boys). This is a rare condition, involving five to seven girls for every boy. The premature appearance of hormones causes the cessation of growth, with consequent short stature, as well as the arrival of sexual maturity. In girls, pubic hair appears, the breasts develop, and ovulation follows. For instance, one young South American girl with precocious puberty delivered a child at the record age of five years and seven months. Before the GnRH analogs became available, treatments for this condition were much less effective.

In men, prostate cancer and benign enlargements of the prostate were found to be treatable with GnRH agonists. Endometriosis and fibroids were next. Expert gynecologists started the treatment of these conditions well before the FDA officially approved the use of the GnRH analogs for such purposes. A range of other possible uses followed. GnRH analogs are used in the treatment of male and female infertility. For instance, they may be used to induce ovulation in women who have ovaries with multiple cysts, a condition that may result in irregular periods, obesity, excessive hair growth, and infertility. The ability of these chemicals to stop uterine hemorrhage is now used with confidence by physicians who were, a few years ago, barely aware of the existence of these substances. This use alone promises to reduce the need for hysterectomy among women whose bleeding does not respond to other treatments. Finally, research shows promise that drugs resembling GnRH may become useful in treating endometrial and perhaps other cancers in women.

In combination with other hormones, GnRH analogs are used extensively with techniques of assisted reproduction, the current name for the numerous procedures that have been developed to simplify and replace in vitro fertilization. GnRH agonists are also used to thin the endometrium before surgical procedures are undertaken in the uterine cavity, because a thin lining makes for less bloody and more effective surgery. There are other uses, including, for example, helping women with PMS or excessive hair growth. There may be other uses in contraceptive research and in the treatment of certain rare menstrual disorders such as **premenstrual edema**, the massive premenstrual gain in weight experienced by a few women.

Treatment with GnRH Analogs

The next topic is a very basic aspect of treatment with GnRH analogs. The effect of GnRH analogs on fibroids, endometriosis, and the endometrium is striking. For instance, fibroids shrink by an average of 50 percent after three or four months of treatment. GnRH agonists also cause a profound melting away, or atrophy, of most endometriotic tissues. Heavy bleeding diminishes, to be replaced with intermittent, light spotting, or no bleeding at all. However, the underlying diseases are *not* cured permanently; instead, there is a potent suppression of disease at least as long as the medications, usually given for six months, remain effective. Within three months of stopping the GnRH analogs, the fibroid tumors return to almost their pre-treatment size. Endometriosis often responds better than fibroids, with endometriotic tissue continuing to hibernate well after the effects of the medications wear off.

Infertility, an enormous concern for many, may be due to endometriosis or, much less often, to fibroids. Using the new drugs may be helpful, although surgery is much more effective in restoring fertility and eliminating fibroids.

If one of the GnRH agonists is used to stop excessive bleeding, depending on the cause of the bleeding it may also recur as the medication wears off; but if this happens, surgical methods are available to treat this. And, as Judy's story showed in the beginning of this chapter, heavy flow does not necessarily recur.

Side Effects

The bad news is that the side effects of the GnRH analogs may be profoundly disconcerting, and to some women, the treatment may be almost as bad, or worse, than the disease. Symptoms start a week or two after the drug is started and in the beginning reflect the stimulant effects of the agonist used. There may be breast tenderness, increased libido, headaches, and dramatic mood swings. The ovaries enlarge, possibly causing bloating or abdominal pain. As the drug becomes effective, these sensations diminish, to be replaced by the intended effect: that of a temporary, reversible menopause. Ovulation is inhibited, estrogen levels in the bloodstream diminish, and menopause starts.

You may recall from Chapter 5 that during sexually mature years, the most important estrogen is estradiol. Hot flashes may appear with low menopausal levels of estradiol. A dry vagina, slightly flattened breasts, diminished libido, and intermittent, usually slight spotting or bleeding may also be noticed. Heavy bleeding is possible, but rare.

Before you despair, I must emphasize the variable effects of low estradiol levels. Many women have used these drugs without the marked symptoms just described. Also, the latest improvement in the use of the GnRH agonists, called the add-back regimens, go a long way toward minimizing side effects. They also enable gynecologists to use the GnRH analogs for longer periods of treatment. One or two courses of medication, each lasting six months, may not be a definite solution for a thirty-five- or forty-year-old woman with endometriosis or fibroids. Courses lasting a year or two, each producing a long period of relief even after the effects of the drug wear off, are much more promising.

The add-back regimens are used by an increasing number of gynecologists. As research continues and new regimens are developed, even better control of these stubborn diseases and treatment side effects will become possible. The add-back regimens are described in the concluding section of this chapter.

GnRH analogs can be used by virtually all women. Allergic reactions are exceptionally rare. However, a few women cannot tolerate the hot flashes and other symptoms of artificial menopause, which may be severe. Now the medication must be allowed to wear off, or one of the add-back regimens must be discussed.

Currently Available GnRH Analogs

Leuprolide, released under the trade name Lupron, was the first GnRH agonist released for use in the United States. Originally approved by the FDA for the treatment of prostate cancer only, Lupron rapidly began to be researched and used for women with two other conditions: endometriosis and fibroids. At first, Lupron had to be given by daily injections to produce a temporary menopause. The daily shots were too cumbersome, and "depot" formulations (small storehouses of the medication) were soon developed. These were active for one month and were called LupronDepot, but almost everyone called the shots Depo-Lupron. More recently, a formulation containing a supply sufficient for three months became available; this is still called Depo-Lupron. In much the same way sustained-release capsules are made, depot preparations consist of vast numbers of tiny, almost microscopically small spheres, each containing a small amount of medication embedded in polymer. The microspheres are gradually absorbed by the deep muscles into which they were injected, slowly releasing the contained medication.

Depo-Lupron is given by injection, once a month or once every three months, self-administered or given by the gynecologist's nurse. Each injection contains 3.75 or 11.25 mgm of the medication. The current cost of the most popular injection, of 3.75 mgm a month, is over $300 at most pharmacies. Some insurance plans cover this; in New York State Medicaid pays for Depo-Lupron.

Nafarelin was the next drug to be released, this time primarily for the management of endometriosis. Nafarelin appeared with the trade name Synarel and was designed to be used as a nasal spray. Women take a dose of 200 mcg per spray once or twice a day, into one or both nostrils, giving a daily dose of 400–800 mcg. About one woman in ten develops an irritation of the nasal mucosa, called **rhinitis**, which may interfere with the continued use of Synarel. The cost of nafarelin (Synarel) is in the same range as the cost of leuprolide (Lupron Depot, or Depo-Lupron). Another GnRH preparation called Zoladex is also available.

Synarel or **Depo-Lupron**? Physician and patient preferences determine which drug is to be used, but Depo-Lupron has been used much more extensively than Synarel. Synarel can be stopped at any time, and its effect wears off rapidly, usually within a week or two, a major advantage. The effects of Depo-Lupron continue for about four to six weeks after the injection was given. Some gynecologists start the patient on Synarel. If the woman tolerates the drug, the doctor may offer to continue treatment with either drug. Synarel may be slightly better because the dose is easier to vary, from 400 mcg to 600 mcg to 800 mcg a day, these representing two, three, or four nasal sprays a day. The effects due to low estrogen levels (the so-called hypo-estrogenic state) are easier to adjust with a slight change in dosage. Also, Synarel does not depress estradiol levels as sharply as Depo-Lupron does, possibly giving women fewer menopausal symptoms. On the other hand, Depo-Lupron has the advantage of avoiding the need for nasal sprays, eliminating the possibility of inflammation and irritation of the tissues lining the nasal passages.

Fibroids shrink remarkably within three months of using Depo-Lupron or Synarel. Once these medications take effect, and for four to six weeks past the time when the drugs wear off, the fibroids stay inactive and do not grow. Women thus stand to gain at least seven or eight months of relief from their symptoms. Endometriosis improves more than fibroids do, although larger endometriotic cysts, measuring over one inch across, do not usually disappear and therefore need surgical care.

The Add-Back Regimens and the Estrogen Threshold Hypothesis

During the late 1980s, danazol and the GnRH analogs were the best drugs available for the treatment of endometriosis; a few gynecologists used them for fibroids. However, as mentioned, they usually produced menopausal and other symptoms that some found difficult to tolerate and were unacceptable to others. Danazol had anabolic activities already noted, limiting its use to courses lasting six to nine months at most. The GnRH analogs had another major disadvantage: Due to concerns about osteoporosis, the loss of bone, these medications could not be used for more than six months. When the effects of any of these drugs wore off, fibroids began to grow back. Endometriosis was slower to reappear, but it too had a tendency to emerge again gradually. Thus, hysterectomy could be held off, but only temporarily. With one or two added well-spaced courses, a few more years of relief were obtainable, at least in theory. However, neither gynecologists nor women had reason to be pleased with the long-term use of these medications. The drugs were thought to be useful mostly as a preparation for surgery and in women who were assumed to be within a few years of the arrival of their spontaneous menopause.

The latest advance in the treatment of endometriosis and fibroids consists of a subtle manipulation of hormonal treatments. This promises to avoid menopausal side effects and to extend the use of the drugs to much longer spells of time. The new management is the add-back regimen, so called because it gives back to the patient carefully selected levels of estrogen and progesterone. The estrogen threshold hypothesis explains the rationale of this seemingly paradoxical sequence, the *removal* of the hormones on which the existence of the disease depends, followed by the *giving back* of smaller amounts of similar hormones.

In a way, the method is like first using your air conditioner to cool down your bedroom, and then running your heating system and your air conditioner simultaneously to achieve an ideal temperature as long as you wish. However irrational (and expensive) this routine might appear, a low but precisely regulated level of estradiol works well. Moreover, it has been tested in a large numbers of patients, with many years of successful and continuous use—in principle, the combination may be used indefinitely. In this context you may recall that BCPs were initially limited to monthly courses but not exceeding two years, at which point they were cautiously stopped for a few months. As side effects and complications were discovered, the dose was reduced. Gynecologists now prescribe BCPs for years on end, often past the previously accepted maximum age of thirty-five years.

Consider a patient aged forty-five, who undergoes hysterectomy for severe endometriosis. One or two patches of endometriosis prove so difficult to remove that they are left behind. Her ovaries (and fallopian tubes) are also removed to prevent the regrowth of endometriosis in areas from which it could not be removed. The woman returns to her gynecologist, complaining of severe hot flashes. To treat this and to prevent osteoporosis, she is now cautiously given a low daily dose of estrogen. Surprisingly, her endometriosis does not recur. The dose she takes is high enough to treat menopausal symptoms and prevent osteoporosis, but insufficient to reactivate her endometriosis.

Two Harvard Medical School gynecologists, Andrew J. Friedman and Robert L. Barbieri, devised a similar sequence for women taking the GnRH analogs. The add-back regimens reflect and stem from their ideas about the potential of the hormonal control of gynecological disease. The add-back regimen was the subject of a program televised primarily for American gynecologists (but available to anyone tuned to the channel) one Sunday morning in April 1992. Early in the program, Dr. Barbieri recalled that his first use of the regimen followed the refusal of a young woman to stop using the GnRH agonists. This twenty-five-year-old woman had se-vere endometriosis that did not respond well to other treatments. Her first six months on the GnRH agonists were apparently the first pain-free six months of her life since she had developed the disease. Robert Barbieri re-called the older experience just recounted, that of the forty-five-year-old woman with endometriosis who was given a small dose of estrogen after her ovaries had been removed. Barbieri and Friedman duplicated this hor-monal situation, except for one detail. They prescribed estrogen for a woman who still had her ovaries, although these organs were temporarily inactivated by the GnRH analogs.

Another plan evolved to treat fibroids. This may have occurred because fibroids were known to be unusually sensitive to estrogen levels, and there was a practical advantage, too: It is easy to measure the effects of any treat-ment on fibroids. A cheap, safe, and noninvasive (i.e., nonsurgical) ultra-sound scan of the pelvis tells the story precisely. To track endometriosis, re-peated laparoscopies would be necessary, clearly not a reasonable idea. However, the responses of these two diseases to the GnRH agonists appear to be virtually identical. The add-back regimens have now been investi-gated in large numbers of women in the management of fibroids and as treatment for endometriosis. The GnRH agonists are also effective against PMS (although, it seems to me, at a high price).

After three months of treatment with GnRH analog, there is a substan-tial shrinkage of the fibroids, usually to about half their previous size. The addition of estrogen and Provera decreases menopausal symptoms to a tol-erable level. Even more important is the fact that with a little estrogen avail-able to bones, osteoporosis will not develop, thus minimizing the danger of bone loss. With the add-back regimens, long-term control of fibroids, en-dometriosis, and other diseases such as CPP has become a possibility.

This idea was investigated by Andrew Friedman, who continued the treatment of five women with uterine fibroids for over two years. As re-ported in the journal *Fertility and Sterility* in 1989, these women gave themselves daily injections of Lupron, a GnRH analog, for three months. For the next twenty-four months of the study, they took daily injections of Lupron as well as daily doses of Premarin and Provera. These hormones, as you will read in Chapter 14, are perhaps the most frequently used estrogens and progestins prescribed for menopausal women as hormone replace-ments. The hot flashes disappeared in four women when they took 0.625

mgm of Premarin (a small, oval yellow pill familiar to many women). These women all had a monthly menstrual flow, analogous to a pain-free period.

There were no bone losses, at least when measured by single photon absorptiometry, a method no longer considered accurate enough to be useful. However, at the levels noted, Premarin was already known to be adequate in preventing postmenopausal osteoporosis. The paper included the customary disclaimers, including the need for better investigations of bone loss and the general necessity of further studies. But for the first time ever, the growth of fibroids was artificially inhibited for over two years.

Anyone with access to a competent gynecologist can avail herself of the standard course lasting six months. Experts as well as good gynecologists are all using add-back regimens. Using a GnRH analog with estrogens and progestins, and perhaps other medications to prevent osteoporosis or to promote the repair of bone damage caused by osteoporosis, a large number of add-back regimens are feasible. One problem is that it is impossible to know which treatment will emerge as the best possible regimen—there are too many combinations being used. The add-back regimens are now widely available as gynecological treatments. Other drugs and combinations are also being researched, combining hormones with medications used in the treatment of osteoporosis.

According to the estrogen threshold hypothesis, after menopause, with estradiol levels around 20 picograms (one billionth of a gram) per one cubic cm of blood, estrogen-dependent cells (including bone, fibroids, and endometriotic tissues) go into hibernation. Hot flashes and other menopausal symptoms then become prominent. At levels of 100 picograms, the same tissues thrive, and there is neither bone loss nor other symptoms. Levels of 30–50 picograms appear high enough to protect bone and prevent menopausal symptoms but not high enough to allow the resurgence of endometriosis. The key feature, the maintenance of serum estradiol levels within a narrow range, is not particularly difficult to achieve, but it does need the patient's cooperation. Serum estradiol levels are easily available in most laboratories, and the cost, in the range of $75 per test, is modest considering the beneficial effects. It may also be possible to use clinical signposts and avoid biochemical tests. For instance, the dose just sufficient to do away with hot flashes may be the right dose to protect heart and bones.

New treatments are customarily tested under carefully observed conditions, by independent groups of investigators, before being adopted for more widespread use. Such work is proceeding now. The usual progression in using new treatments is from expert pioneers to specialists to general use. In this instance, the add-back regimens, new when the first edition of this book appeared, are no longer the province of the pioneers and a few specialists; virtually all gynecologists and endocrinologists use them.

You should not have any problems locating a physician skilled with using the GnRH agonists. Members of the American Society for Reproductive Medicine are familiar with these drugs. Many of their members work as gynecological endocrinologists; others are affiliated with units that provide in vitro fertilization and similar technologies for women with fertility-related problems.

Disadvantages of the Add-Back Regimens and When Not to Use Them

The small possibility of allergies to the GnRH analogs has been discussed already. Endometrial cancer will probably not develop while a woman is on this treatment; in fact, there is some evidence that the GnRH analogs may retard the growth of endometrial cancer. But sooner or later, some patient using recommended add-back therapy will be found to have a sarcomatous growth. **Sarcomas** are cancerous tumors developing deep within tissues such as fibroids, discussed in Chapter 6. At least one such occurrence has been reported already, the "tipoff" being the continued growth of a fibroid uterus while using a GnRH analog. It is impossible to be sure if the delay in treating this sarcomatous tumor made a difference in the outcome, but it is unlikely to have been helpful. Unfortunately, on rare occasions, not removing an organ may have adverse consequences.

The materials in this chapter consist of highly sophisticated but forced manipulations of normal female functions, replacing them with artificially maintained hormonal states. It would be better if these diseases could be treated with less dictatorial regimens; so far, no such treatments have been devised. However, the potential demise of an aggressive surgical treatment and its replacement with a medical regimen represent a breakthrough. I cannot say how realistic it might be to hope for simpler treatment schedules in the future.

With the new treatments discussed, you are entirely dependent on the skills of experts. The book outlines ways of assuring yourself of gynecological expertise. If you are wary of high-technology expertise, you still have the choice of the more standard surgical treatments described earlier.

Finally, a word about GnRH antagonists. These drugs are still being researched. Initial problems encountered include allergic reactions.

The Treatment of Specific Diseases

1. The Treatment of Endometriosis. The BCPs were, in the early 1960s, the first effective treatment for endometriosis. Robert Kistner, a gynecologist from Harvard University, first described and popularized this use. Women took the BCPs every day without a break, in increasingly large doses, for up to nine months. The dose Kistner introduced was very large by today's standards, and Kistner's regimen doubled the already-large dose every few months, whenever his patients developed breakthrough bleeding; an occasional and usually minor BCP side effect consisting of vaginal spotting or intermittent bleeding. The response of the endometrium to the uninterrupted and gradually increasing doses of hormones was interesting: Instead of continuing to grow, the endometrium began to hibernate, became thin and inactive, rarely bleeding heavily. Amazingly, none of Kistner's patients developed any of the serious complications ascribed to the high-dose Enovid tablets then in current use, even though the Kistner regimen called for exceptionally high doses, unheard of since then. Most of the women were delighted, because for the first time, they had a drug that relieved the symptoms of endometriosis.

These days, experts prefer newer medications for endometriosis, particularly the GnRH agonists. For women who have minimal or mild endometriosis, the BCPs offer definite advantages. They are reasonably priced, whereas the newer drugs are very expensive. BCPs can also be used year after year; this is infinitely more complicated with the newer medications. Experts disagree about the need to treat minimal endometriosis, some preferring a wait-and-see attitude; others are concerned that if left untreated, the disease might get worse and slowly begin to interfere with fertility. I favor the use of the BCPs, but only after the larger and more accessible deposits of endometriosis have been surgically treated: excised, cauterized, or vaporized. Depending on the severity of the endometriosis, it may be better to use the GnRH agonists for a few months first. Surgery (laser or other methods) should come next, to deal with adhesions, larger cysts, and nodules, perhaps returning for three months to the GnRH agonists. Finally, women might be switched to the BCPs to keep the disease in check at a reasonable cost and with minimal inconvenience.

There are enormous variations across the land in gynecologists' choices for the treatment of endometriosis; approaches different from those outlined here may be equally good. If in doubt, the Endometriosis Association in Milwaukee may be contacted; their telephone number is (414) 355-2200. If you join their approximately 9,000 members, among other benefits, they will send you their list of gynecologists they recommend.

2. The Treatment of Fibroids. According to many experts, the estrogen in the BCPs stimulates the growth of fibroids. If you have small fibroids and control of abnormal bleeding is desired, today's low-dose BCPs might be very effective. However, not every gynecologist will be willing to prescribe them, and it is difficult to know how long this treatment might remain effective. The use of the BCPs in women with fibroids calls for frequent checkups to watch for an unexpected spurt in growth. In the presence of larger fibroids (over two inches across), the BCPs are probably best avoided. Age is not as much a limitation as previously believed. In healthy, thin, nonsmoking women, BCPs are probably safe until menopause arrives, and perhaps longer.

The first and most simple way to reduce menstrual flow in women with fibroids is to try any of the standard antiprostaglandin medications available without a prescription: Advil, Aleve, Motrin, Anaprox, Naprosyn—the names change slowly from year to year. Newer drugs are Vioxx and Celebrex: Originally released for arthritis, they are increasingly used as generic pain-relieving medications. You must remember the unwieldy name "antiprostaglandin," and the fact that these medications tend to irritate the lining of your stomach. If you are prone to ulcerlike symptoms, use these medications cautiously, or swallow with milk, even antacids, and preferably on a full stomach.

Fibroids may be made to shrink by means of GnRH agonist medications. Some of the problems that come with this treatment have been outlined already—menopausal symptoms. These can be reversed through the use of add-back hormones; but now you are in a high-technology area, dependent on potent medications until you reach your menopause. GnRH agonists cannot make your fibroids disappear, although this has happened inadvertently: Fibroids have very little blood supply, and they may begin to decay because of shrunken vessels during artificial menopause. More commonly, after the GnRH agonists are stopped, the fibroids slowly resume their previous size.

Other drugs are under development and investigation to prevent fibroids. Writing in the journal *The Female Patient* in May 2000, Director Nelson H. Stringer of the Fibroid Uterine Treatment Center at the University of Chicago has reported research involving two promising medications: Pirfenidone and Tibolone. The first of these, Pirfenidone, seems the more remarkable: It appears to be capable of interfering with the production of certain constituents of cells essential for the growth of fibroids. Thus, it may come to be used, if and when it is released for such use in the United States, to prevent the growth of fibroid tumors. The second drug, Tibolone, is a steroid medication that might at some future date find a niche as an improved add-back medication used in combination with a GnRH agonists.

3. The Treatment of Bleeding Abnormalities. BCPs are remarkably effective and are widely used to control abnormal bleeding due to a condition called **anovulation**, discussed in Chapter 13. Anovulation is one of the most frequent causes of irregular bleeding when women reach their forties and fifties. Dysfunctional uterine bleeding (DUB) is another name for the same condition. Any of the standard low-dose pills should work for DUB. If BCPs do not work—in other words, if you continue to bleed excessively—the careful gynecologist will need to ask about missed tablets, the most common cause of irregular spotting and bleeding. He or she should again consider other diseases such as an undiagnosed fibroid tumor, a malignancy, and polyps, and perhaps an unsuspected pregnancy before increasing the dose.

The daily dose may be increased from a tablet containing 20 to 35 mcg of estrogen, or from 35 to 50 mcg. It may be more convenient (and certainly cheaper) to double up on a supply already in your possession, but remember that biphasic or triphasic tablets are difficult to simply "double up": These tablets have fluctuating hormone levels, and doubling up may cause added fluctuations. It all depends which tablet has been doubled. This unevenness may cause intermittent spotting or bleeding: exactly the problem you are trying to treat. There is no such problem with monophasic pills with 21 pills to a package: if you double *any* of the tablets, you'll double the dose.

Continued bleeding in the face of increased doses should spark a renewed search for fibroids, polyps, and cancer. If hysteroscopy, an operation in which a gynecologist looks up through the cervix to inspect the lining of the womb, has not yet been done, now is the time to schedule this procedure.

Provera is also used to control abnormal bleeding. The administration of 10 mgm (or even more) of Provera every day, week after week, or even month after month, may at least temporarily control abnormal bleeding due to anovulation and fibroids. This is an excellent temporizing measure, but after a few months it is likely to fail, allowing the bleeding to start again.

4. The Treatment of Chronic Pelvic Pain. BCPs are excellent for mittelschmerz, which is ovulatory, or midcycle pain, and for menstrual pains. If you have noticed an accentuation of your symptoms during your cycle, premenstrually and menstrually, BCPs are worth trying. It might be best to try one of the monophasic BCPs continuously first, taking a hormone-containing tablet every single day for three months, although most gynecologists are more familiar with the customary cyclic use: three weeks on, one week off.

Although much progress has been made, chronic pelvic pain is a poorly understood condition. It may be caused by a variety of diseases; often it is impossible to know for certain what exactly causes the pain. Endometriosis is a frequent culprit. This disease may be diagnosed by means of laparoscopy; another approach is to try treating the patient as if she had endometriosis, and await results. This complex regimen is discussed in Chapters 10 and 11.

Most women I have seen with CPP did not respond well to treatment with BCPs, but this may be because those who were helped no longer had any need to enroll in a CPP Clinic. Relief from BCPs indicates that the CPP may be due to endometriosis, in which case excellent and much better treatments are available: the GnRH agonists. GnRH agonists with or without add-back are under intense research scrutiny; preliminary reports indicate substantial success from their use. GnRH agonists are used in the treatment of CPP exactly the same way they are used to shrink fibroids or alleviate endometriosis-related problems.

$\cdots$ 9 $\cdots$

Surgical Treatments for Fibroids, Endometriosis, and Abnormal Uterine Bleeding

If medical treatments fail or are not right for you, surgery becomes your next, and possibly last, defense against hysterectomy. To avert this operation, you must become familiar with a number of gynecological operations. Hysterectomy and myomectomy, the piecemeal removal of fibroids, both date from the middle of the nineteenth century and are thus over 150 years old; most other gynecological procedures in current use were developed during the last fifty years. Much more recently, an inventive surgical genie must have emerged surreptitiously out of some ancient lamp, because over half a dozen new operations capable of replacing hysterectomy have appeared. All these operations destroy the endometrial lining—the tissue that bleeds heavily in women who have fibroids or suffer from excessive bleeding due to many other causes—but they leave the womb largely intact. Richard Soderstrom is a distinguished professor of OB/GYN from Seattle, whose interests have included many aspects of laparoscopic and hysteroscopic surgery, particularly those related to the safety of these operations. Soderstrom has edited the annual Technology issues of *Contemporary OB/GYN* for the past decade. In the April 15, 2000, issue Soderstrom stated unequivocally that **endometrial ablation**, an operation that vaporizes endometrium, could potentially replace one-third of American hysterectomies. Ablating procedures have been available for over twenty years and have improved over the years; why they have not reduced hysterectomy numbers is a conjectural topic addressed throughout this book. The latest treatment for fibroids is different again: It is a procedure performed by specialist radiologists that eliminates abdominal or pelvic surgery entirely. Called **uterine artery embolization**, the name is usually abbreviated to UAE.

First things first. You will not be able to participate in your care intelligently unless you understand what these operations can and cannot do, how they impact your fertility, and how often they fail. Most of these operations work well, but in a few cases, hysterectomy has to be performed eventually in spite of everything that has been done to avoid it. And as stated before, you should not rush into accepting any surgery, including the very latest, safest, and least painful operation, without careful prior questioning. Modern treatments have given us absolutely enormous potential for eliminating hysterectomies, but this does not automatically mean that lesser surgery is needed. Instead of undergoing an unnecessary hysterectomy for a few small and harmless fibroids, there is no point in having the very latest and best, but equally unnecessary, laparoscopic laser myomectomy for the same harmless and benign tumors. Before any elective surgery is scheduled, you must be satisfied that the operation is unmistakably needed—the main theme of this book.

Some of today's operations, such as curettage and radical hysterectomy, date back to the nineteenth century. Laparoscopy and hysteroscopy came into everyday use during the 1960s and 1970s, when the amazingly bright light produced by modern fiber-optic systems and ingenious operating instruments began to enable gynecologists to replace laparotomy with laparoscopy. Laparotomy usually requires an incision measuring three to five inches in length; laparoscopy needs one or more small incisions, well under half an inch long. Laparoscopy is ideal for much gynecological surgery: It causes less pain and fewer adhesions than laparotomy. During the last fifteen years, hysteroscopy and laparoscopy have been combined with miniaturized operating instruments, computers, and technical advances such as lasers. The essence of the new approach is that instead of removing entire organs, such as the uterus, surgeons can meticulously remove diseased areas only. Fibroids, endometriotic areas, adhesions, and abnormal endometrium can be cut away, vaporized, or frozen, leaving the ovaries and the womb in place. Operations that offer women the most are hysteroscopic surgery, various myomectomies, and laparoscopic surgery.

Another operation, a traditional curettage, usually referred to as a D&C, may also be offered to you. However, except when treating miscarriages and major hemorrhages, old-fashioned curettages have very limited value. In women who are not suffering from some pregnancy-related complication, curettage must be combined with hysteroscopy. Putting it bluntly, and bearing in mind the two exceptions noted above, I would not trust a gynecologist old-fashioned enough to perform curettage without also performing hysteroscopy to provide anything more than basic, routine care—for instance, emptying the uterine cavity after a miscarriage.

Before specific operations are discussed, a few principles must be understood:

1. Bleeding may be caused by a number of diseases, but it is almost always the endometrial lining that bleeds. Once cancer and pregnancy have been excluded, most bleeding can be halted at least temporarily by medical means, discussed in the previous chapter. Surgery, discussed in this chapter, usually provides a permanent solution. Endometrial ablation is the most practical way to reduce or eliminate uterine bleeding through surgery, *regardless of its cause.*

2. Fibroids can be made to shrink with medications, but this is mainly a temporary effect. Fibroids can be excised, or lysed, or made to decay through surgery, most practically through myomectomy.

3. Endometriosis can be treated with medications. Endometriosis surgery may be performed abdominally, by means of old-fashioned laparotomies or through modern laparoscopic treatments.

Let us now consider the range of operations available.

Dilatation and Curettage (D&C)

Curettages are excellent for stopping heavy bleeding, but they are overused. Since nothing is irretrievably lost in the process and costs are not exorbitant, unnecessary curettages have not excited nearly as much indignation as unnecessary hysterectomies.

Who needs curettage? If you are bleeding rapidly, using tampon after tampon or pad after pad (a situation most often encountered in women who are miscarrying), you need a D&C. A heavy hemorrhage may also follow a delivery or be caused by fibroids, cancer, or polyps. If medications or surgery such as curettage cannot control the hemorrhage, hysterectomy will be lifesaving surgery. However, these desperate situations are rare. Curettage is used too often for other purposes, such as diagnosing cancer or fibroids. There are better ways of achieving these objectives; they are described in Chapter 5. Curettage is also used to control bouts of excessive bleeding: This it does only temporarily, and the curettage can often be avoided with a variety of drugs.

Curettage, also known as a "scraping out," is very simple. General or local anesthesia is used to ensure you will not feel any pain. Next, the cervical canal is opened by passing metal dilators of gradually increasing diameters through it; afterward, the uterine cavity is curetted, or scraped out, until the bleeding stops. If the problem is caused by a miscarriage, curettage may be combined with vacuum curettage, also known as suction curettage; this consists of suctioning the cavity until it is empty. At this point, the bleeding usually stops, and the operation has been completed.

The curette is a small, sharp, horseshoe-shaped instrument, invented by the French gynecologist Joseph Recamier in 1843. Curettage may be completed in as little as ten to fifteen minutes and has a double purpose. It arrests the bleeding by scraping out the tissues that are the source of the bleeding. Next, when the tissues removed are stained and examined under a microscope, information may be obtained about the cause of the bleeding, including an essential detail: the presence (or absence) of cancer and precancerous conditions of the endometrium.

Nonemergency curettages may be done in a gynecologist's office under local anesthesia or under general anesthesia. Previously, they required a two-day hospital stay, but with steadily increasing pressures to economize, for healthy women they are usually performed in ambulatory surgical units. This means that if you are scheduled to have a D&C, you walk into the unit where the operation is scheduled. Some hours later you walk out, although you should be told that you are not supposed to drive yourself home.

Curettages are more useful in stopping heavy bleeding than in providing a diagnosis. They are overused in the sense that there are easier ways of obtaining tissue to be examined under a microscope and because there are excellent medical treatments for stopping bleeding and regulating cycles. Curettages are also far from error-proof: Even competent surgeons have relied on curettage and have missed diagnosing polyps, small fibroids, even cancer. Some experts estimate that one-fourth to one-third of these operations result in the wrong diagnosis! Diseases may have been "missed" (overlooked) because curettages are done by feel only. Operating inside the womb, the surgeon cannot see the areas being curetted. A small cancer, located in a corner where the fallopian tube enters the cavity, is easy to miss. Also, old-fashioned curettage (without hysteroscopy) cannot remove fibroids or polyps, except by accident.

The woman who has had repeated curettages and now "needs" a hysterectomy—not an unusual sequence—may be a victim of poor gynecological care. I knew one such woman whose successful business took up so much time that she neglected routine gynecological needs. In two years, she had six emergency curettages in various cities for heavy bleeding, always in the middle of the night but never resulting in a good diagnosis or a cure. She was proud that she always signed out of the hospital the morning after the curettage and promptly continued to take care of her business. Although her circumstances were partly responsible for her inefficient care, she could not know (and was not told until the last operation) that the curettages were unlikely to diagnose and cure the cause of the bleeding. The first time the woman had a planned, nonemergency curettage, another gynecologist first did a minor procedure called hysteroscopy. The polyp that caused all her bleeding was easy to see, it was removed without effort, and the hemorrhages never recurred.

Hysteroscopy

Who needs hysteroscopy? Virtually everyone who undergoes curettage may benefit from diagnostic **hysteroscopy**. During this operation, the gynecologist inserts a telescope-like instrument through the vagina and the cervix to look at the inner walls of the cervix and womb. Depending on the size of the cervical opening (larger in women who have had at least one normal delivery) and the width of the instrument, dilating the canal may not be necessary or minimal dilatation only may be required. Diseases

TABLE 9.1   Common Reasons for Diagnostic Hysteroscopy

Abnormal bleeding, including postmenopausal bleeding
Abnormal bleeding due to fibroids and polyps
Investigation of infertility
Finding and removing intrauterine contraceptive devices (IUCDs)
The investigation of congenital abnormalities of the uterus

that have escaped detection during curettage are readily recognized during hysteroscopy. The surgery may be done in the gynecologist's office, thereby avoiding the risks of anesthesia and the costs of a hospital stay. It should not be done if the woman is pregnant (or miscarrying), and it is more difficult (or impossible) in the presence of heavy bleeding, which obscures vision.

Diagnostic hysteroscopy yields so much information that it should always be available whenever curettage is scheduled. If your gynecologist is recommending curettage without hysteroscopy, find out why. Since you are going to have an operation, you might as well derive the most benefit from it. If your gynecologist is not experienced with hysteroscopy but you are otherwise satisfied with him or her, ask to have a colleague with hysteroscopic skills assist with the procedure. In larger hospitals, there should not be any difficulty arranging this, possibly without a direct charge to you, as a courtesy from one gynecologist to another. Curettage is easily performed after hysteroscopy; this step is important to enable a pathologist to stain tissues that were removed during curettage with special dyes and to examine the tiny shreds of tissue under a microscope.

Sharon, a nurse who worked in my office, provided an excellent example of the value of hysteroscopy. The cause of her abnormal bleeding became apparent within seconds of starting the procedure: There was a long-forgotten intrauterine contraceptive device (IUCD) in her womb. Sharon was embarrassed to admit she thought it had been removed six or seven years before. A recent ultrasound had failed to notice the device, which often throws a very faint shadow only. It is difficult to practice medicine without trusting all the reports that come pouring in, yet once in a while, deceptive or incomplete information causes a lot of trouble before the mistake is recognized.

So far the discussion has been about diagnostic hysteroscopy, during which the surgeon looks at the inner walls of the womb. Only the most simple surgery, such as curettage or the removal of polyps or contraceptive devices, may be undertaken during diagnostic hysteroscopy. For the past ten or fifteen years, instruments have been available to perform much more elaborate surgery inside the uterine cavity. This is called **operative hysteroscopy** or **hysteroscopic surgery**; it is one of the newest and best ways of staving off hysterectomy in the treatment of many uterine diseases that cause heavy bleeding.

Hysteroscopic Surgery

Who needs hysteroscopic surgery? Any woman with abnormal bleeding or infertility who is scheduled for a curettage or hysteroscopy may benefit from hysteroscopic intrauterine surgery. Ideally, whoever undertakes hysteroscopy should be able to remove small fibroids and polyps as well as intrauterine contraceptive devices that could not be removed in the gynecologist's office. More elaborate surgery may also be undertaken, but this needs additional measures: deeper anesthesia, laparoscopy to help avoid missteps, a blood bank, nurses, and surgical assistants

Working at St. Luke's Hospital Center–Woman's Hospital on Manhattan's Upper West Side, Robert S. Neuwirth produced a gynecological breakthrough in 1976 when he showed that myomectomy could be done without a large abdominal incision. Approaching fibroids through the vagina and the cervix, using an instrument called a **resectoscope** that he modified from urological instruments used on men's enlarged prostate glands, Neuwirth shaved and cauterized away small to medium-sized fibroids projecting into the uterine cavity. **Submucous** or **transcervical myomectomy**, as the surgery is called, is only feasible before the fibroids (and the womb) grow too large. This means that you need high-quality

TABLE 9.2   Common Reasons for Hysteroscopic Surgery

Excessive uterine bleeding that does not respond to hormonal or other treatments
To stop all bleeding by freezing, heating, or ablating the endometrium
To remove polyps, selected fibroids, and IUCDs
To divide intrauterine adhesions
To repair certain congenital anomalies

gynecological care well before surgery becomes necessary: If the fibroids get too large, it becomes much more difficult (and risky, or impossible) to attempt this operation. If submucous resection cannot be performed, myomectomy or other modern operations may become unavoidable, converting a high-technology but relatively safe operation into major surgery.

The next development came from Milton H. Goldrath of Detroit, who introduced a new way of dealing with vaginal bleeding without resorting to hysterectomy in 1981. Goldrath devised an apparatus for "ablating" the endometrium with light rays from a laser. **Ablation** means burning away or vaporizing all or most of the endometrial layer, sharply reducing the amount of menstrual flow without endangering the womb or the ovaries. However, while tubal ligations are potentially reversible (although not without new problems), ablation irreversibly destroys tissues essential for carrying a pregnancy.

At first, ablation was used primarily in women too ill to undergo abdominal surgery. For instance, an overweight, hypertensive, and diabetic patient is not a good candidate for surgery because her chances of complications are high. Avoiding the large incision and the extensive dissection required by hysterectomy lowers her risks substantially. If there are no features that suggest malignancy, a very important proviso, the new procedure avoids hysterectomy by removing only the part that bleeds: the endometrium.

Rollerball ablation, the next technology to be developed, is another effective choice; it uses heat produced by electricity to burn away the endometrial layer. Then, as more powerful lasers were developed and gynecologists became confident using them, other uses appeared. For instance, in addition to ablating endometrial surfaces, fibroids could be vaporized during the same operation. Women who were good surgical risks but who were anxious to avoid hysterectomy were happy with the new operation. Endometrial ablation is now available not only for heavy bleeding but also for reasons that are increasingly "cosmetic." For instance, it has been proposed as contraceptive surgery. (As already noted, a normal endometrial layer is essential for pregnancy.)

Going one giant step further, it has also been mentioned for possible use in athletes and women engaged in high-powered business activities and for women who simply do not wish to be bothered by menstrual periods. There may not be much demand for elaborate surgery for these unusual reasons today, and responsible gynecologists I know are not happy with these new and possibly frivolous uses. However, it has happened before that surgery condemned for some legitimate reason was later resurrected. Aggressive merchandising and promotion may also prevail. In a few years' time, women may be able to arrange endometrial ablation through sleek saleswomen working in elegant boutiques in fashionable stores, along with face-lifts, liposuction, and the sculpting of more fashionable breasts. This is not a recommendation; it is, perhaps, an anxious appraisal of future possibilities you might want to know about.

Meanwhile, another choice replacing hysterectomy for excessive bleeding has become available. A device called Thermachoice, also developed by Robert Neuwirth, ablates endometrium by means of heat applied through a balloon introduced through the cervix and then distended with water heated to 75 or 80 degrees Centigrade, or about 175 degrees Fahrenheit. Other procedures still in development ablate endometrium by freezing it or by heating the endometrial layer directly by means of hot saline circulating freely within the uterine cavity or through the use of **thermistors**, which are metallic strips electrically heated to temperatures high enough to destroy the endometrial layer. As of December 2000, only Thermachoice had been approved by the FDA for use in the United States.

The major complication of all intrauterine surgery is **perforation**, the term used to describe the damage that occurs when a surgical instrument such as a curette, a forceps, or a hysteroscope is inadvertently punched through the muscular walls of the womb, creating a small hole. Perforation may result from surgical incompetence (there are horrifying but well-documented accounts from the 1950s of inexperienced abortionists removing foot after foot of small bowel instead of the pregnancy), but even experts with excellent skills may cause a perforation. If the walls of the womb are thin or the cervix is unusually tight, it is relatively easy to force the tip of the hysteroscope inadvertently through the walls of the womb. If adjacent vessels or organs are not damaged, perforations may heal without trouble. Damage to uterine blood vessels causes bleeding and necessitates emergency surgery, possibly including hysterectomy; damage to bowel requires elaborate repair. To avoid these problems, your gynecologist should be as experienced as possible at intrauterine surgery, including hysteroscopy.

To prevent perforations or at least to be able to identify (and treat) them immediately, it is advantageous to have an assistant look at the outside of

the womb while the surgeon works on the inside. This is achieved with another operation called laparoscopy, the next procedure to be discussed.

Laparoscopy

Laparoscopy consists of looking into the abdomen with a telescopic instrument called the **laparoscope**. This is inserted through an incision that
may be only about one-fourth inch long, just below the navel. General
anesthesia is used, although some enthusiasts have succeeded with sedation
and local anesthesia only. At laparoscopy, a panoramic view of internal organs may be obtained, giving the surgeon in charge the best chance of
making an accurate diagnosis. Like hysteroscopy, laparoscopy has also been
adapted for more extensive surgical work. Modern laparoscopic surgery for
fibroids and endometriosis is discussed following the next section on conventional gynecological surgery.

Myomectomy

As mentioned previously, one of the earliest alternatives to hysterectomy
performed to deal with fibroids was **myomectomy**, the piecemeal removal of fibroids from the womb through an incision made below the
navel. If your fibroids are not too large, the incision may be made through
a transverse (that is, bikini-line) incision; if larger than a five-month pregnancy, the esthetically less pleasing vertical incision may have to be made
to allow better access to the larger tumor. The operation usually leaves a
scarred but functioning womb.

First attempted by mid-nineteenth-century surgeons such as Amussat in
France and Washington Lee Atlee in this country, abdominal myomectomy
became better known and available to women eighty or ninety years later
through the efforts of two men. Isadore C. Rubin, a Russian-born and
American-educated gynecologist, popularized the operation in the United
States. A Londoner, Victor Bonney, a gentle and brilliant but slightly eccentric surgeon, also had a strong interest in preventing the unnecessary
excision of ovaries as well as wombs. Bonney in particular became a
world-famous proponent of abdominal myomectomy. Rubin and Bonney

gradually persuaded their colleagues that this operation had much to offer to women. Myomectomy, often removing numerous fibroids from a greatly enlarged and disfigured uterus, became reasonably successful in averting hysterectomies.

A word of caution is in order: Operating for small fibroids that cause little or no trouble is probably the most frequent form of unnecessary surgery inflicted on women. If the fibroids are large or cause symptoms, only myomectomy and uterine artery embolization are available to avoid hysterectomy. This is emphatically not the case if individual tumors are smaller than an inch or two in diameter, are located toward the outer surface of the womb, and cause no symptoms.

Until recently, myomectomy was used mostly in the treatment of large fibroids. Even when considered for women with these tumors, staid gynecological opinion usually confined the operation to women whose main intent was the preservation of their potential to bear children. Consequently, myomectomies were done much less frequently than were hysterectomies. However, there were always a few enthusiasts who preferred myomectomy, some publishing their experiences with over 1,000 of these operations.

During a cocktail-party conversation some years ago, a very elegant woman of about forty, on hearing of my occupation, pulled me into a corner to find out why three senior gynecologists all urged her not to bother with myomectomy but to have a "definitive cure" with hysterectomy. She came to see me as a patient later. At surgery, I found what I expected from my previous examination: a womb of normal size, surmounted by a single but huge fibroid, attached to the womb with a short stalk. It took about thirty minutes to open and close the abdomen, but not more than thirty seconds to remove the tumor. I still cannot fathom why my predecessors were so dogmatic. One of them, a famous New York gynecologist, was so set against myomectomy that he spent more time advising her against this "gamble" than on the rest of the consultation.

There is a resurgence of interest in myomectomy. Without much doubt, this is due, at least in part, to women's insistence on avoiding hysterectomy. Many older gynecologists did not believe in myomectomy, some using this operation in as little as 5 percent of all surgery performed for fibroids, but recent statistics show more extensive use. One excellent feature of myomectomy is that it may improve fertility—but only if the fibroids were responsible for the failure to conceive or the tendency to miscarry and if there are no other problems with fertility.

Myomectomy may be done three different ways: hysteroscopically, abdominally, or by laparoscopy. Newer operations include **myolysis, cryomyolysis,** and **uterine artery embolization**—these will be discussed later.

Hysteroscopic myomectomy removes fibroids with instruments inserted through the vagina and the cervix. It is ideal if the fibroids project into the uterine cavity and are small (for instance, less than an inch or two across). The larger these fibroids, and the larger the cavity, the more difficult the operation. If the fibroid is pedunculated (attached by means of a stalk), hysteroscopic myomectomy is easy: The stalk is divided and the fibroid is removed. If it is hanging through the cervix, it may even be cut off without anesthesia; there are no nerve fibers in the stalk to send pain messages to the brain. Alternately, the stalk may be twisted until it shreds and breaks—this may cause cramps, but minor discomfort may be preferable to surgery. My practice has always been to explain my plan but to offer to stop immediately should the patient ask me to quit the procedure; this has almost never happened.

Abdominal myomectomy starts with **laparotomy**, the generic term for opening the abdomen through an incision usually longer than two inches. Fibroids deep in muscle must be shelled out one by one, each being removed like the seed from a ripe avocado. The process is easy in one woman and unpredictably difficult in the next. Even in competent hands, myomectomy may be a more difficult operation than hysterectomy, requiring transfusions of blood; at other times—as noted above—it may be easy to perform.

Myomectomy has many disadvantages. On rare occasions, with very large tumors, there may be so much bleeding that emergency hysterectomy becomes unavoidable. Serious infections during the first few days after surgery may also call for hysterectomy. However, in over thirty-five years of learning, doing, and teaching these operations as well as going to conferences where complications are discussed, I have come across only a handful of such cases. With modern antibiotics and methods of shrinking fibroids preoperatively, these disasters should be even less frequent. Nevertheless, your surgeon will probably ask you to sign, in addition to the consent for the myomectomy, a consent for a hysterectomy that is valid under emergency conditions only. Gynecologists will not operate without this consent, lest they be sued for doing in an emergency exactly what you were specifically trying to avoid.

The most serious disadvantage of myomectomy is recurrence. It may be impossible to excise every tiny tumor deep within the womb, and new tumors may begin to grow after all visible and palpable tumors have been excised. Thus, myomectomy cannot be guaranteed to provide a permanent cure. Even if the surgeon removes every single fibroid that can be felt or seen, other tiny tumors, neither visible nor palpable during surgery, may be inevitably left behind, and these may become evident years after myomectomy. Overall, 15–20 percent of women undergoing myomectomy will need repeat surgery some time later. Most of these will be for excising newly emerged fibroids, but a few operations may be necessitated by bowel obstruction caused by the adhesions that follow most myomectomies. In short, most women will not need another operation, but a few others will need more surgery.

It is not difficult to make an intelligent guess about the chances of fibroids recurring after myomectomy. If you are in your late twenties, if a pelvic examination or scan identifies numerous fibroids, and if fibroids run in your family, then you face a difficult choice. Unfortunately, your womb has a pronounced tendency to form fibroids, and this is not changed by surgery. If you behave passively in this situation, you can sit back, do nothing, and hope to complete your family before the enlargement of your tumors begins to cause serious trouble, and you can then await the onset of menopause. If you are more of an activist, you have a number of strategies to delay adverse developments.

As you can see, myomectomy remains a good choice, but it has its share of problems. A better choice would be medical treatment with GnRH analogs for three months, followed by myomectomy, and then a return to the GnRH analogs for another three to six months. The use of add-back hormones, discussed in Chapter 8, is another option. These treatments offer the best possible chance of suppressing the tendency of your womb to develop fibroids. As also discussed in Chapter 8, new drugs that suppress the tendency to grow fibroids are already available in Europe; within a few years the FDA will probably approve some of these drugs for use in the United States.

Contrary to established (but older) expert opinion, the older woman with a few fibroids is an excellent candidate for myomectomy: She will soon reach her menopause, at which time whatever fibroids were not re-moved will shrink spontaneously.

Myomectomy has another serious disadvantage: The badly scarred womb may not be able to withstand the stretching caused by pregnancy. If the scar through which a fibroid was removed gives way and opens up, the womb bursts; this is called **uterine rupture**. Although this complication is rare, it causes a life-threatening emergency that requires immediate surgery. Rupture usually occurs during the later months of pregnancy, al-though it may occur during the second trimester—a major disaster, be-cause the immature fetus usually dies. If you become pregnant after my-omectomy, it is essential that the details of the surgery be made available to your obstetrician as early as possible. The easiest way is to tell your gyne-cologist (who may or may not practice obstetrics when you need it) that you would like to have a copy of the dictated operative note after my-omectomy, before (or soon after) you are discharged from the hospital. (Only an exceptionally old-fashioned doctor will object to this request.) The report must be filed in a safe place so it remains easily available when needed.

If you are about to have a myomectomy, you should discuss your plans for future pregnancies with the surgeon. *Your surgery should be performed by someone thoroughly familiar with these operations.* There is nothing wrong with asking the surgeon how many of these he or she has done in the last two or three years. If the number is under ten or fifteen, you are dealing with an honest surgeon, but one possibly not experienced enough for this op-eration crucial for your childbearing potential.

Another major problem with myomectomies has been mentioned al-ready: the tendency to form adhesions after this operation. In spite of ex-tensive research, only one method has been found to limit (and, unfortu-nately, not to eliminate) this tendency: the use of surgical barriers, materials that limit postoperative adhesion formation. Pirfenidone, a medication mentioned in Chapter 8, has been shown in Europe to inhibit the forma-tion of adhesions as well as fibroids, but since this new drug is not yet avail-able in the United States for fibroids, it can hardly be recommended to prevent adhesions.

Laparoscopic myomectomy will be discussed shortly with other la-paroscopic operations.

Hysterectomy for Fibroids

Hysterectomy remains a choice, particularly for women who keep growing new fibroids and who have suffered from much bleeding and pain. Regardless of surgical skills, some women form many adhesions after intraabdominal surgery, and a second or third myomectomy may become unusually difficult in these women. Others may find that there are too many side effects to the medical treatments we have discussed or that they are prohibitively expensive. Hysterectomy has an advantage not to be casually dismissed: Once performed, women will not have any further problems with bleeding, pain, recurrences of fibroids, or indeed any other gynecological problem involving the womb (but not the ovaries). Hysterectomy that is needed as well as accepted should not be regarded as a failure any more than a cesarean section performed for good reason is a failure.

Indications for Hysterectomy—Fibroids

The American College of Obstetricians and Gynecologists has elaborate criteria (indications) for hysterectomy, originally presented in its Technical Bulletin No. 192, dated May 1994. This document has been replaced by ACOG's Practice Bulletin No. 16, dated May 2000 and published in ACOG's Compendium of Selected Publications for 2001. Unlike its predecessor, the new bulletin does not give elaborate details of clinical circumstances warranting surgery. Significantly, ACOG neither lists large uterine size as an indication for hysterectomy, nor does it recommend myomectomy for the preservation of fertility only. The bulletin states that "hysterectomy remains the most common treatment for leiomymas because it is the only treatment that provides a cure and eliminates the possibility of recurrence." However, because women are interested in alternative treatments, the bulletin reviews medical and surgical treatment, discussing myomectomy, ablating procedures, and uterine artery embolization

The new bulletin gives ACOG's reasons for favoring hysterectomy but retreats from earlier (and old-fashioned) indications. It also accepts alternative treatments. However, as shown in the early chapters of this book, official guidelines have been flouted in the past and are likely to be disreguarded again. The new guidelines will not lead to fewer hysterectomies.

Performed for fibroids, hysterectomy does not call for the removal of the ovaries. Elective excision of the ovaries is an option with a complicated set of advantages and disadvantages, discussed in Chapter 14.

Hysterectomy for Endometriosis

Hysterectomy with excision of both ovaries was for many years the standard cure, particularly for older women with extensive disease. For these women, this operation was a reasonable choice. If low-dose hormone replacement therapy (estrogen *and* progesterone) is accepted, this sequence gets good results with the least need for either medical surveillance or further treatments. Hysterectomy conserving at least one ovary is another choice, but the chances of recurrence of "endo" are higher than they are with both ovaries excised. If you wish to avoid hysterectomy altogether, the next choice is to remove as much diseased tissue as possible, conserving the womb and the ovaries. This is best done laparoscopically, provided an expert surgeon is available to perform the operation. However, chances of a recurrence are higher with such conservative surgery. You can circumvent this with a variety of hormonal medications, but these increase your needs for medical supervision including complex treatments.

Laparoscopic Surgery

Laparoscopic surgery is the newest arrival on the surgical scene. In the beginning, laparoscopy was undertaken for observing only, to diagnose illness, or to make sure that there was no disease. Instruments were next developed for burning or banding fallopian tubes, and contraceptive surgery became the choice of millions of women. With better instruments, the damage caused by tubal (ectopic) pregnancies could also be repaired through laparoscopic surgery. The field expanded into laparoscopic gallbladder and colon surgery, laparoscopic infertility surgery, and the laparoscopic removal of ovarian cysts. Hysterectomy and gynecological cancer surgery have also been undertaken through the laparoscope. However, the technical wizardry of laparoscopic surgery ought not blind you to the fact that it is perhaps even more likely to be abused than old-fashioned abdominal surgery. The latest and trendiest forms of laparoscopic surgery, namely laparoscopic hysterectomy, laparoscopically-assisted vaginal hysterectomy (LAVH), and videolaparoscopy may be easy operations to "sell" to women. They sound modern and promise few complications, with the avoidance of long (and painful) incisions. But remember: If you do not need the operation, the surgeon will benefit more from the operation than you will.

The past decades have brought a deluge of mail directed at general surgeons and gynecologists, offering expert instruction in laparoscopic (and hysteroscopic) laser surgery. However, there are profound disagreements over much of this surgery, viewed as excessive by some and as a boon to patients by others. **Laparoscopic cholecystectomy** (the excision of the gallbladder), for example, may be unnecessary almost as often as laparoscopic hysterectomy. If the surgery is described as "easy" and "safe" (or if it *is* easy and safe), it becomes easy and safe to recommend the operation to patients whose need for it is dubious.

The excitement displayed at medical meetings that teach (and promote) laparoscopic surgery is usually centered on complex equipment and technical skills, and these are impressive. Good reasons to have the surgery tend to received lip service or none at all. This had its own perverse logic: The courses offer to teach the gynecologist how to perform the operation, not when to do it. Perhaps it is assumed that gynecologists already know when to undertake a hysterectomy, an assumption I am reluctant to take for granted.

Laparoscopic Hysterectomy

In **laparoscopic hysterectomy**, the ligaments that keep the womb in place are divided through the laparoscope, using one or more small incisions, after which the womb is removed through the opened upper vagina. The ovaries may be removed or left behind. There is much less postoperative pain, and the hospital stay is much shorter. If the past is any guide to the future, laparoscopic hysterectomy may become an everyday procedure. Today, it is—or should be—performed by experts only. More important, as always, women have to watch out for themselves. The excitement of keyhole surgery and seductive references to lasers and "almost complication-free" surgery ought not blind anyone to the fact that there must be good reason to operate in the first place.

Laparoscopic hysterectomy may be done in a variety of ways, but the particulars and differences are of more interest to gynecologists than to women. The cutting, for instance, was first done using lasers; then miniaturized scissors were found to be easier to use. An instrument called the "Harmonic Scalpel" is another recent innovation; this uses ultrasound energy.

Laparoscopically Assisted Vaginal Hysterectomy

Laparoscopically assisted vaginal hysterectomy (LAVH) is another recent development, over ten years old now. LAVH is a conventional vaginal hysterectomy, parts of which are performed laparoscopically. It is technically less demanding than laparoscopic hysterectomy. There is an ongoing and scholarly debate about the appropriateness of LAVH. The annual Technology issue of *Contemporary OB/GYN*, dated April 15, 2000, contains such an exchange. One well-known and prestigious panelist wrote that he thought LAVH was expensive and difficult; his opponent, also possessing excellent qualifications, deemed it safe and cost-effective. Your temperament will probably determine your reaction to such a discourse: You may be indignant that LAVH was allowed to become popular without prior inquiry, or you may feel that the dissent is part of a democratic process, evidence of healthy skepticism and scientific debate that will improve care.

Videolaparoscopy is an unusually elaborate surgical setup, consisting of laparoscopy with multiple small incisions. A miniature camera is used to project a televised picture of the pelvis onto a screen; the display may be watched by the entire surgical team, the husband, or anyone authorized by the patient and accepted by the surgeon. Zoom equipment gives a panoramic view or a focused-down, enlarged view of areas about to be operated on. Other openings are used to insert a variety of laparoscopic instruments; for instance, laser rays may be used to burn away pockets of endometriosis. Using yet other instruments, fibroids may be excised or fallopian tubes damaged by infections may be repaired.

Laparoscopic myomectomy is difficult to discuss without unusually technical details. There are numerous rules and exceptions, and they vary from surgeon to surgeon. This operation is ideal for medium-sized fibroids located toward the middle or outer aspects of the wall of the womb—but of course these are fibroids usually not in much need of surgery in the first place. If the tumors are small, the virtuoso work of laparoscopic myomectomy is probably wasted on tumors that might never need removal. If the tumors are large, the operation—mostly the essential part of closing the defect left behind when the fibroid has been removed—is too difficult except for experts. If fertility is to be preserved, the closure must be meticulously done, and this is difficult through small laparoscopic incisions. Only one guideline can be offered for this operation: It should be done by a genuine expert, ideally someone involved in researching and teaching laparoscopic myomectomy at a large and prestigious hospital. If you have no access to a real expert, laparotomy may serve you better.

Laparoscopic Endometriosis Surgery

The essence of laparoscopic surgery for endometriosis consists of using a variety of laser rays to vaporize, or burn, pockets of endometriosis wherever feasible without damaging nearby structures such as the ureters. Endometriotic ovarian cysts are eliminated, adhesions are divided, fallopian tubes are repaired, and normal anatomy is restored. However, normal tissues are retained. Drugs may be used before and after such surgery to suppress endometriosis; these details vary from surgeon to surgeon.

There is increasing concern that laparoscopic surgery and videolaparoscopy may not be the wonderful advances their adherents believe they are. Roy Pitkin, a respected gynecologist and senior editor of the journal *Obstetrics and Gynecology,* has questioned the explosion in the use of these techniques in a 1992 editorial. Entitled "Operative Laparoscopy: Surgical Advance or Technical Gimmick?" the editorial is strongly reminiscent of Norman Miller's article, "Hysterectomy: Therapeutic Necessity or Surgical Racket?" with which Chapter 1 of this book opened. There are expert surgeons involved in laparoscopic surgery, but there are also serious misgivings that too many gynecologists have leaped onto the bandwagon, attended a course or two, and now feel ready to start using this exceptionally elaborate technology.

Extensive research is warranted before recommending laparoscopic hysterectomy or videolaparoscopic surgery to anyone. The major advantages are less postoperative pain—something to be taken very seriously, particularly in view of questions about the quality of nursing care in many hospitals—and fewer adhesions. However, there are many ways to improve postoperative pain relief; PCA, or patient-controlled analgesia, is but one of many recent improvements. Other advantages are cosmetic and fiscal. The cosmetic advantage is that instead of a large scar, there are two or three much smaller incisions. The fiscal advantage is that you will spend two or three days in the hospital instead of four to six days. In return for these, you are giving up the safeguards that have been built into old-fashioned, laparotomy-based surgery over the last 150 years.

Before agreeing to have complicated laparoscopic or hysteroscopic procedures performed on a member of my family, I would question the prospective surgeon diplomatically but very closely about his or her training. Older gynecologists who are skilled enough to teach these procedures would be my first choice. Much younger gynecologists trained for at least six months by experts would be my second choice. Gynecologists who attended one or more courses that teach advanced techniques would come last—and only if they have acquitted themselves well with the surgery planned over the years. Unfortunately, you cannot discover these details without virtually cross-examining your surgeon about the details of his or her training and subsequent experience.

One of the new words in vogue among hospital administrators is *credentialing*. To be credentialed means that a physician had been found to possess sufficient knowledge, training, and experience to undertake a procedure. Gynecologists in training must be credentialed to do simple procedures such as circumcisions and curettages; later, they must be credentialed to undertake more complex procedures. You should know this word, because there is a relatively easy way to start questioning gynecologists about their experience with laparoscopic surgery. Instead of a searching but personal question, you can begin by asking about credentialing practices at their hospitals. In due course, it will be easier to ask about personal experiences they have had with the procedure you (or someone you care about) is supposed to undergo.

Myolysis and Cryomyolysis

These procedures are not widely available in the United States. They consist of heating or freezing fibroids with probes inserted deep into each fibroid under laparoscopic guidance. Either heating or freezing fibroids (by means of electrocoagulation or by freezing with liquid nitrogen) causes necrosis, the gradual decay of tissues. The best-known American proponent of myolysis is Herbert Goldfarb of Montclair, New Jersey, who learned the operation in Europe.

Uterine Artery Embolization (UAE)

Embolization procedures were first used as a desperate experiment, to control severe hemorrhage after delivering a baby and for certain cases of severe gynecological bleeding. The theory was that if the flow of blood to the womb is interrupted, it cannot continue to bleed—much as a tourniquet stops a hemorrhage. More recently, UAE procedures have been widely reported as popular treatments for fibroids even though the number of such procedures performed is relatively small.

UAE is performed by a skilled radiologist who starts by making a tiny opening into an artery in the patient's groin. This is done under local anesthesia, giving as much intravenous sedation as needed. The radiologist next passes a fine catheter (tube) up into the patient's abdomen. Using radiological guidance (that unfortunately irradiates the ovaries to some extent), the catheter is threaded into uterine arteries that supply blood to the womb—first on one side, then the other. Tiny polyvinyl pellets or similar substances are next injected into both uterine arteries, and these immediately obstruct the flow of blood to the womb. The process is called embolization; its effects depend on the loss of oxygen and nutrients that all tissues need to survive and without which all tissues decay. There is a certain unpredictability to this process: If too much tissue decays, layers of healthy muscle might die, ovaries have been known to be damaged, and at least one patient has died of massive sepsis after UAE.

UAE is perhaps no longer experimental, but it is far from acceptance as an established, mainstream treatment. The advantages of UAE consist of the avoidance of surgery, the high proportion, about 85 percent, of women who are happy with the procedure, the appreciable shrinkage of uterine size after UAE, and diminished menstrual flow. The disadvantages consist of undergoing a procedure about which much has to be learned. For instance, gynecologists have a precise statistical idea of the likelihood that a woman will die because of her hysterectomy; depending on various circumstances, this will happen to one woman in 1,000 or perhaps 1,200 hysterectomies. Less precise but somewhat similar information is available for ablation procedures, but the mortality of UAE, while probably low, is unknown. Major complications appear to be rare, but are different from hysterectomy complications. About 2 percent of women who choose UAE need hysterectomy to treat certain complications.

One little-discussed problem with EUA is that it is difficult or impossible to know in advance how much myometrium (womb muscle) will be lost with this procedure. If continued fertility is desired, UAE cannot be recommended. Women have conceived and delivered after UAE, but serious problems have also been encountered. Uterine rupture in particular is a major and worrisome possibility: If too much muscle is lost, the remaining layers may prove too weak to hold a pregnancy safely for nine months.

Indications for Surgery: Myomectomy and Hysterectomy

If fibroids are very large, grow at an alarming rate, or cause heavy bleeding, hysterectomy is an acceptable solution—provided the patient understands and agrees with the gynecologist's reasoning. Myomectomy, possibly excising numerous fibroids, is another choice. Smaller fibroids, particularly if they do not cause symptoms, are emphatically not indications for hysterectomy or myomectomy. Surgery that removes three or four fibroids, each measuring under an inch in diameter, from the outer surface of the uterus, is probably unnecessary surgery. To be more precise: There may be some purpose in removing these small tumors from the womb of a young woman undergoing surgery for some other reason, in order to prevent problems later, but I would not recommend undertaking surgery primarily for such tumors.

Chronic Pelvic Pain: An Overview

The two women who were leaving the hospital didn't even glance at me as I entered the elevator. I was wearing a raincoat instead of my customary white coat; they were engaged in an intimate conversation. I recognized them because they were enrolled in the hospital's Chronic Pelvic Pain Clinic, which I started at St. Luke's Hospital Center–Woman's Hospital (now part of St. Luke's–Roosevelt Hospital Center) in 1976. The clinic opened because my staff and I took care of many women with chronic and severe pelvic pain as well as numerous other poorly understood symptoms, and I realized that we had neither an honest diagnosis nor effective treatments for most of them. My plan was to investigate all their complaints carefully to find out what caused them and to improve their care.

"It's been killing me forever," said the first one, a nurse at a nearby home for the elderly. "They all have different ideas, but nothing helps the pain. All they do is give me Tylenol with codeine. All it does is get me constipated." She glanced at her new friend sheepishly as the personal confession slipped out, but the other woman was too involved in the exchange to worry about this lapse.

"Yeah, I know," said the second, a heavyset woman who was always trying to make ends meet with welfare checks. With an occasional (and underpaid) job, two hyperactive toddlers, and a live-in boyfriend who roughed her up every few weeks, her life was a succession of crises. "I've been trying to get a hysterectomy for months now, but they keep changing their minds. With me, no one really listens; it's antibiotics, antibiotics, antibiotics all the time. I may have to go and try another hospital if I don't get relief real soon. Sometimes it's so bad I think I'll go crazy if somebody doesn't help me." They got off the elevator ahead of me and walked out into the rain, deep in conversation.

Chronic pelvic pain (**CPP**) is a complicated subject. The cause of the pain is often obscure, and most women find that effective treatments are difficult to come by. Even hysterectomy, which many women view as the last desperate resort, may not provide permanent relief. Recent research shows that at least some chronic pelvic pain may originate not from gynecological conditions but from nearby organs such as bowel and bladder; hysterectomy cannot be expected to cure such pains. Experts are generally against cutting out organs that look healthy to ease pain, although recent years have seen less rigidity against hysterectomy for chronic pelvic pain. At a different level, and depending on his or her training, the average gynecologist may be for or against hysterectomy for pain relief. New evidence collected during the 1990s, first in Belgium and later in California, indicates that endometriosis, an unusual disease discussed in Chapter 7, may be the secret cause of much CPP. These women may be treated with medications effective against endometriosis, as outlined in Chapter 8, with substantial relief from chronic pain.

During the early 1970s, CPP was barely a footnote in the annals of gynecology. CPP attracted little research, textbooks had no chapters to help young gynecologists, professional meetings never addressed this unrecognized problem. By the 1990s, there was a drastic change, with widespread attention paid to the ravages levied by CPP. New ideas and treatments are currently published month after month, symposia abound, and arguments rage about the effectiveness of the new treatments. Meanwhile, regardless of professional debates, and because surgery is so familiar and straightforward, exasperated women continue to hope that after hysterectomy their lives will return to normal.

CPP is a frequent cause of hysterectomy in the United States, particularly among American women of African descent in Southern and Western states. About 70,000 of these operations are performed annually in the

United States in search of relief from pelvic pain. This is a considerable number, particularly considering the uncertainty that the operation will succeed. Since only women with at least moderately severe and long-standing pelvic pain undergo hysterectomy, the number of women with CPP must be much larger—a topic we'll return to shortly. If you are considering hysterectomy to alleviate CPP, read this book carefully before signing the consent form.

Chronic Pelvic Pain: What It Is, What It Does

Gynecologists are usually successful when treating women with acute lower abdominal or pelvic pain because the cause of the pain is often fairly easy to pinpoint. For instance, infections and tubal ("ectopic") pregnancies are frequent culprits. With or without an accurate diagnosis, treatment usually relieves the pain, and the encounter between the patient and her gynecologist is likely to be satisfying to both. Most often the pain just disappears without much certainty about its cause; such an outcome is also satisfactory, although it leaves many women wondering about the cause of the troublesome symptoms they recently endured.

CPP is much more difficult to deal with. Whatever might be the cause of the pain, various treatments are tried but they rarely bring relief. The pain is often severe, often interfering constantly with usual activities. It keeps recurring, shifting from the center of the pelvis to the sides, higher into the abdomen, to the back, to the upper thighs. Within a few months of suffering (three to six months is the semiofficial definition for CPP), other complaints appear, including headaches, deep pain with intercourse, and often a chronic, life-sapping lethargy. Palpitations shake the chest, a bleak nervousness ruins the day, insomnia replaces sleep. There may be so many symptoms plaguing women with CPP that they lose the joy of life they had before and begin a ceaseless search for relief.

There is often a pattern to this search. In the beginning, women suffering from CPP consult a series of gynecologists; then internists for the headaches, palpitations, and lethargy; surgeons for the abdominal pains; orthopedists for the backaches; and neurologists for the dizzy spells. These practitioners produce all kinds of plausible-sounding diagnoses; however, none of their treatments brings relief. A friend recommends a female gynecologist, whose ideas turn out to be neither different nor any more helpful. The chiropractor and the acupuncturist don't help, but a trusted friend recommends **transcutaneous electric nerve stimulation** (**TENS**). The little box that gives the TENS is held in place against the skin of the lower abdomen with a belt. It burns the skin slightly and works for two or three weeks, then its effects fade. Surgery may be tried next. Laparoscopy is first, but reveals only a few adhesions or a small fibroid or two. The adhesions are divided, the fibroids excised; sooner or later, ovarian cysts are found and removed, perhaps followed by the appendix. Even hysterectomy may be performed, but in many women the pains stubbornly return, and in a few they may get worse.

One such patient I got to know was Dolores, a beautician who owned a busy salon on Manhattan's Upper West Side. Dolores had already had a hysterectomy in an effort to rid herself of pain. Within a few months, the pains were back, worse than ever. Now Dolores was told that the pains were due to adhesions that formed after the hysterectomy. To her disgust, neither the surgeon who had originally performed the hysterectomy nor other gynecologists seemed to be eager to schedule surgery to cut the adhesions. Because she had already spent large sums she could ill afford on gynecological care, Dolores felt confused and angry at this lack of interest. No one seemed to be taking her seriously any more. Worse, she began hearing thinly veiled suggestions that it was all in her head, and once she was referred to a psychiatrist. This infuriated her so much that she stormed out of the doctor's office, slamming the door behind her.

Women with CPP resent such ideas intensely. Meanwhile, their existence often continues to descend into an abyss of stubborn symptoms, numerous diagnoses, and useless treatments. Fortunately, not everyone is so profoundly affected, but short of cancer and endometriosis, and perhaps another poorly understood gynecological condition, namely, severe PMS, there are few other gynecological conditions as capable of ruining a woman's life as CPP. I have seen husbands and lovers leave, children neglected, and more than a few divorces, bankruptcies, and failed careers among CPP sufferers. Worst of all, during the 1970s and the 1980s, when many treatments available today were still unknown, a few women were so sharply affected that they had a nervous breakdown and needed extended psychiatric care before they recovered.

Data from the United States as well as from the United Kingdom show that pelvic pain is one of the most common reasons for a visit to the gynecologist. Robert C. Reiter, a gynecologist from Iowa City and an expert on pelvic pain, cites a study from San Diego, which shows that almost 10 percent of all GYN clinic visits are due to CPP. Other experts from the United Kingdom and from the United States give higher percentages. In Britain, half of all laparoscopies are undertaken because of pain, acute as well as chronic. In the United States, this figure has been reported at the almost-identical level of 40 percent. Reiter estimates that 20 percent of all American laparoscopies are undertaken because of CPP.

Based on a Gallup poll of nearly 18,000 households conducted in the United States in 1994, experts consider that 15 percent of American women suffer from CPP; some estimate the total to exceed 9 million women. Such figures seem inflated, part of the hype that permeates many official statements. Also, the numbers depend on the definitions used. For instance, if women with severe menstrual cramps over the past six months are included, the figures and percentages increase substantially. While sympathetic to women with these symptoms that are, at least usually, not difficult to treat, my professional interests have been focused on women with *severe* CPP, women whose pains and other complaints are stubborn and serious enough to be a recurring and often ruinous part of their lives. If your menstrual problems are severe and have not been improved by treatments, you may have endometriosis or adenomyosis, or you may have CPP. Fortunately, there are new and successful treatments for all these problems, although many of the treatments are complicated, and you may have to assert yourself to get the health-care system to pay serious attention to your symptoms.

In my experience, about one woman in thirty has severe CPP, often poorly investigated and undiagnosed. Sadly, I have found in listening to these women, that many have simply given up on gynecologists, often not even bothering to mention their symptoms. Through bitter experience, they have found that regardless of their symptoms and complaints, only more tests and more useless treatments will follow. However, I believe that a quiet revolution has occurred in the gynecological understanding of CPP. We now have a better understanding of CPP symptoms as well as better treatments; this revolution will bring much relief to CPP sufferers.

In medical school, I was not taught much about chronic pelvic pain. The only causes ever mentioned were **acute** or **chronic salpingitis**, these being infections of the fallopian tubes. Later, as a young doctor, I assumed that the women I saw suffering from CPP indeed suffered from some form of salpingitis. I treated them with antibiotics and pain medications, but most often I never saw them again. Early in any young doctor's career there is much hope and optimism as well as a measure of innocence; you are a fountainhead of much recently acquired knowledge but may not recognize areas of remarkable ignorance. It was thus all too easy for me not to notice that few women who had CPP improved with the treatments my professors had recommended so authoritatively just a few years before.

During the early 1970s, after I went into practice in New York, I began attending to the same women month after month. Soon I noted that CPP was a frequent problem whose treatment was rarely successful, and I began to wonder why the pains obstinately returned to plague the women again and again. Also, the frequency and severity of the headaches and lethargy made no sense to me. These are not standard gynecological complaints; I heard them rarely from my other patients. I thought that their presence implied the need to search for other diseases. The mystery was that despite many consultations and a profusion of diagnoses that sounded likely, few women were helped. Listening to the women in my Pelvic Pain Clinic I was amazed at how much these women had suffered and was dismayed by the conflicting (and, it seemed to me, often confused and even condescending) gynecological advice they had received.

The women were usually desperate to find out what the trouble was but received only a series of implausible and occasionally irresponsible diagnoses from their gynecologists. Also, they often appeared to be severely depressed. Not unreasonably, they attributed this to their years of suffering and the chaotic succession of diagnoses and ineffective treatments.

In the course of setting up a pelvic pain clinic, I arranged for a standard medical evaluation. This included a careful investigation of all complaints, followed by laparoscopy to check the health of internal organs. To understand the emotional content of the situation our patients found themselves in, I also arranged interviews with social workers, psychologists, and psychiatrists. I knew that the women might resent the psychological probing, but the severity of the headaches and physical exhaustion told me that very likely something I did not understand was happening to them. I explained that I planned to leave no stone unturned in search of the cause of their complaints and asked them to accept the interviews.

206

Much of the resentment my request caused was due to women feeling that no one, including me, seemed to believe the full extent of their sufferings. Many were tormented by their pain and other complaints and seemed to be demoralized and deeply depressed. I explained that I knew they had many serious symptoms, that I did not doubt that their suffering was genuine, and that I accepted the fact that they faced many long-standing and unresolved medical problems. I thought they might have something to gain from a low-pressure interview, almost always with another woman, either a social worker or a psychologist, to understand the way they felt about their impasse with the medical profession.

The women in the CPP clinic generally feared that a serious gynecological disease would be discovered as the cause of their complaints. When laparoscopy showed normal organs, as was often the case, many improved, at least for a while, on hearing the good news. There was little enthusiasm for psychological discussions. The women hoped that gynecological treatments would solve their problems completely. As they saw it, my job was to sort out what ailed them, and to fix it as rapidly as possible. Unfortunately, this hope was rarely fulfilled during the 1970s, although this unsatisfactory situation has improved substantially in recent years.

The contents of this chapter are often complicated, and I am concerned that the ideas that follow are difficult to present in an easily comprehensible manner. Table 10.1 presents a key to "navigating" the maze of CPP. While simplified, the approach it outlines will help you chart a logical, intelligent, and successful course.

Chronic Pelvic Pain and Laparoscopy

In the mid-1960s, the laparoscope came into widespread use in the United States. The introduction of this instrument was perhaps the most useful gynecological development of the decade. For the first time, gynecologists could check the accuracy of their diagnoses relatively easily by means of laparoscopy, a brief abdominal operation that may be done in as little as twenty minutes and needs a hospital (or ambulatory surgical center) stay of a few hours only. A few enthusiasts performed the surgery in an office setting, the main advantage only consisting of reduced costs. Laparoscopy allows the surgeon to take a thorough look at all pelvic and many abdominal

TABLE 10.1   A Plan of Action for Women with CPP

If you have pelvic pain symptoms but you also suffer from constipation, possibly alternating with diarrhea, flatulence, and stabbing abdominal pains, read the section on irritable bowel syndrome in this chapter. You may need a family physician, an internist, or a gastroenterologist to help you.

If you have pelvic symptoms but you also need to urinate urgently and frequently; if, for instance, your sleep is repeatedly interrupted, night after night, because your bladder seems to fill up too fast, read the section on chronic interstitial cystitis in this chapter. Instead of a gynecologist, you may need urological attention.

If you have severe headaches, lethargy, backaches, and many other problems, you probably have CPP as part of a chronic pain syndrome. Unless money is no problem and you have excellent physicians, you should entrust your care to a pain clinic.

If you have never had laparoscopy, a type of surgery to be discussed shortly, consider undergoing this procedure. However, first review your situation with an experienced gynecologist. If your current gynecologist cannot find at least thirty minutes to do this with you, find one who can. This gynecologist should be willing to listen to you and examine you carefully, perform laparoscopy, and try a course of menopause-inducing medications to see how much you might improve. Another approach might be to try the same medications without undergoing laparoscopy first, as discussed later in this chapter.

Be skeptical if anyone attributes your symptoms to small fibroids, to ovarian cysts that are less than two inches across, or to a retroverted womb. These are unlikely causes of severe pain, another topic we'll return to shortly.

If you have been diagnosed as suffering from fibromyalgia, chronic headaches, irritable bowel syndrome, and depression, your nervous system may misperceive pain. Effective treatments are beginning to be developed for these problems women commonly suffer from, but you'll need a neurologist to make this diagnosis and provide care for it.

organs. The ovaries, fallopian tubes and the womb; and much of the bowel, usually including the appendix, the liver, and the gallbladder are all visible through the laparoscope.

Two Swedish gynecologists, Lennart Jacobson and Lars Weström, were the first to study the diagnosis of acute salpingitis by means of laparoscopy. The results were first reported in late 1969 in the *American Journal of Obstetrics and Gynecology,* the most academic source of OB/GYN information, and were unexpected and interesting enough to be discussed in detail. Working at the University of Lund, Jacobson and Weström analyzed over 900 operations, most of which were laparoscopies, performed during the 1960s. They reported that only 65 percent of the diagnoses of acute salpingitis were correct. Twelve percent of the patients had a variety of other conditions; 23 percent had no disease at all. One immediate benefit of this approach was that the 12 percent with other, unsuspected diseases could now receive correct treatment without further delay. And, of course, the 23 percent whose internal organs were normal could safely be sent home (although without a diagnosis), instead of receiving days of unnecessary and expensive intravenous antibiotic treatments in the hospital.

It was an eye-opening experience for me to read that one-third of these 900-odd diagnoses of acute salpingitis (also called **pelvic inflammatory disease,** or **PID**) made by experienced Swedish gynecologists were plainly wrong. The standard professional pontifications had covered up, certainly for the patients and possibly for the physicians, how erroneous some of the confident diagnoses were. A second uncomfortable thought occurred to me almost immediately. Was it possible that the diagnoses of salpingitis in CPP patients were equally dubious?

Numerous studies of CPP patients have shown that neither a careful vaginal examination nor investigations such as sonograms were accurate in producing a reliable diagnosis. Laparoscopy, on the other hand, was often useful in determining what was happening to various organs that were thought to be diseased and responsible for the pain. The results of a number of studies may be summarized as follows: Some CPP patients were found to be suffering from visible endometriosis, and I will return to the significance of the word "visible" in this sentence. Other women were found to have adhesions—a condition we'll also discuss in due course, shown in Figure 10.1. Many women had minor abnormalities such as small fibroids that could not be regarded as the cause of severe and often complex symptoms, and in others, all pelvic organs appeared to be normal. Salpingitis, so commonly diagnosed in women with CPP, was rarely seen through the laparoscope. Only too often, what was found at surgery did not correlate well with the women's complaints.

It is important to understand these unexpected and unusual findings. The care of women with endometriosis, relatively straightforward and usually successful, is outlined elsewhere in this book. Women with endometriosis do not remain CPP patients for long because modern treatments usually produce a striking improvement. If treatments do not help, endometriosis must be discounted as the main cause of the pain; these women now belong in the third group, with no identifiable disease to explain their symptoms.

The treatment of women with adhesions and no other disease (or women with neither adhesions nor any apparent disease) is not easy or straightforward. Inexperienced gynecologists may be left with no distinct plan of management and the women with little hope of reliable treatment. While this leaves a large group of women who have no clear explanation for their symptoms, a number of possibilities remain:

- It is possible to hold the adhesions responsible for the pain and to effect a cure by dividing them. This approach works for some women only. The operation is called **adhesiolysis**, and it will be discussed shortly.
- These women may have endometriosis existing invisibly, deep in pelvic tissues, behind organs that have been inspected and found to be normal. This possibility calls for a so-called therapeutic trial: treating the woman for three months as if she had endometriosis and awaiting her response.
- The women may have engorged pelvic veins, also called varicosities, or the "pelvic congestion syndrome," as the cause of their pains. British experts recommend hysterectomy as the best treatment, but the therapeutic trial described above should also work for women whose symptoms might be caused in this fashion.
- They may have diseases that are not of gynecological origin, discussed later in this chapter. These women must be evaluated by a number of other specialists to understand the cause (or causes) of their symptoms. This is best done through a pain clinic.
- Recent thinking indicates that these women may be suffering from a newly discovered form of **neuropathy**, an abnormality of the nerves that conduct pain impulses from the spine to the brain. Neuropathy is an "overreading" of pain impulses, resulting in a sharply increased perception of pain. For instance, whereas a healthy woman might, in response to bowel activity, feel only a vague lower abdominal pressure that she barely notices, an affected woman might register the identical activity as excruciating pain, and cry out, in genuine distress. Unfortunately, the unusual notion of neuropathy is more familiar to neurologists than to gynecologists. It is supported by basic research, and also by the frequency with which women who have CPP also suffer from other prob-

lems that involve pain such as fibromyalgia, headaches, backaches, and the irritable bowel syndrome, to name the most common such problems. Neuropathy and other recently minted diagnoses such as **"pain processing disorder"** may appear ethereal abstractions, but they have been successfully treated with medications such as gabapentin (Neurontin), discussed in the following chapter.

Neuropathies may be a revolutionary new idea; meanwhile, they also present serious difficulties in our understanding of diseases and the symptoms they produce. If the notion is correct, virtually any acute disease that caused severe pain once might later cause severe (and inexplicable) chronic pain. And even if this sequence is correct, excising the organ originally responsible for pain may not succeed in relieving pain permanently. Hysterectomy for CPP is the example gynecologists are most familiar with, an example we'll discuss in Chapter 11.

This brings us to a contentious topic: attributing pain to conditions that physicians consider coincidental, benign, and probably not the cause of symptoms—for instance, claiming that small fibroid tumors, or simple, small ovarian cysts, or retroversion cause CPP.

There are many scientific reasons gynecologists cite to prove that small fibroids cannot cause the ravages of CPP. Except for the remote possibility of neuropathy, there is no mechanism for small fibroids to cause complex symptoms. It has taken doctors nearly 150 years to understand that cause-effect relationships are often not simple. If you believe that your apparently insignificant abnormality can cause major symptoms, sooner or later this abnormality, whatever it is, will be massaged, injected, put in a cast, corrected, or excised by a variety of practitioners. You will be treated sincerely and optimistically, but without a clear notion of how much the treatments will help you. However, this is such an abstract idea that it must be illuminated with a simple practical example.

I have a small wart at the base of my left thumb. I may believe that this wart is responsible for pains in my left arm and also for my headaches and my constant exhaustion, and I may be persuaded that amputating my left thumb will cure me. This sequence is clearly absurd. Most people are familiar with warts. They know them to be painless, and they will not undergo an amputation in hopes of eliminating the symptoms listed. However, it is easy to believe that small fibroids cause many symptoms: To most

TABLE 10.2   Gynecological Causes of Chronic Pelvic Pain

1. Endometriosis
2. Adenomyosis
3. Adhesions
4. Infections of the fallopian tubes
5. Residual ovary syndrome
6. Pelvic congestion syndrome
7. Varicosities of the pelvic veins
8. Other, less likely causes

people, fibroids are mysterious internal tumors that might cause any number of serious problems. Chapter 6 discusses fibroids and explains how common and harmless these tumors often (but not always) are. If you and your gynecologist believe that small (or medium-sized) fibroids can cause CPP, you will probably undergo hysterectomy; the uncertain outcome of this operation will be discussed in Chapter 11.

"It's All in Your Head"

And now we come to the use and meaning of that unfortunate phrase: "It's all in your head." I am astonished and dismayed to hear physicians use such language, but apparently they still do. I am convinced that women with CPP report their sensations and complaints accurately; none of their symptoms are imagined or pretended. The young gynecologists I have taught and worked with do not question the reality of the symptoms they hear about. The pains are real but in some women may be as baffling to understand as pain felt in amputated limbs. This condition, commonly called **phantom pain**, may be due to minor pain signals generated from nerves in the stump but magnified in the spinal cord, probably under the influence of higher centers in the brain, and felt in an arm or leg that was amputated. It is possible that something similar occurs in at least some women with CPP, and in this sense, CPP may be a physical disease, a neuropathy: an abnormality in the conduction and interpretation of pain signals.

But there is another important facet of pain perception: that anxiety and depression are likely to increase the depth and severity of many complaints. Anxiety and depression may be caused by months of unexplained suffering, but they may also be old problems that now contribute to the appearance of stubborn and severe symptoms. These two possibilities may be intertwined, impossible to separate out. In this sense, at least in some women, CPP may have an emotional component. Such notions are strongly supported by research conducted by Andrea J. Rapkin at the University of California in Los Angeles, discussed later in this chapter. Books written by Judith Lewis Herman offer further, equally persuasive evidence that psychological problems lead to anxiety and depression; her books are included as recommended reading in "References, Resources, and Recommended Reading" at the end of the book.

The Causes of Chronic Pelvic Pain

Experts believe that many gynecologic and other diseases may cause CPP; professional literature suggests over fifty possible causes. The tables and lists that follow include all common causes of CPP, but the lists and tables are also abbreviated and incomplete. You will shortly read about many conditions that have been accused of some involvement with pelvic pain. A little skepticism here will eliminate many unhelpful and dubious diagnoses that confuse so many women with CPP—although the confusions are mostly the consequence of the poor understanding physicians have of the causes of chronic pain, and the poor explanations usually given to patients. For instance, to use another example, a womb that is beginning to prolapse (fall out) has no direct way of causing constant pelvic pain, severe headaches, and lethargy. One of the problems with eliminating harmless coincidental conditions is that patients desperate for relief resort to surgery that fails to improve their symptoms.

Of course, patients are not in a strong position to argue with their doctors about their diagnoses or treatments. In the paragraphs that follow, I will discuss *likely* causes of severe CPP as well as other possible causes, including certain diagnoses of which I am skeptical. More important: If you have received treatments for three or four different diagnoses but have not experienced much (or any) improvement and your complaints continue to cause serious distress, perhaps you, too, should develop a measure of suspicion. If these lines apply to you, I'd recommend that you read the section that deals with chronic pain states slowly and carefully.

I have listed below most of the likely and some of the less likely causes of CPP. Gynecological causes, many of which are discussed throughout in this book, are listed first, followed by nongynecological causes.

Gynecological Diseases Causing CPP

1. **Endometriosis** may cause menstrual pains, infertility, and painful intercourse as well as abdominal and pelvic pains without a distinct pattern. A careful pelvic examination and expert ultrasound scans may be suggestive, but laparoscopy is the usual way of making (or excluding) this diagnosis. Recent research suggests that much undiagnosed CPP—in other words, CPP for which there is no honest explanation even after laparoscopy—may nevertheless be due to endometriosis. Some experts even recommend that women whose CPP has no obvious cause should be treated for endometriosis without the usual "workup"—in other words, without laparoscopy—partly to save surgical costs, but even more because laparoscopy is less than 100-percent reliable in diagnosing endometriosis. Endometriosis is discussed in great detail in Chapter 7.

2. **Adenomyosis** is a common cause of pelvic pain, although the pain is rarely severe. This disease is often painless, but if it causes too much pain and bleeding, hysterectomy will cure all symptoms. Adenomyosis is discussed after endometriosis in Chapter 7.

3. **Adhesions** are stringy, filament-like bands that glue organs to each other, much as if well-chewed gum were worked into the tightly packed mechanism of an old clock. Adhesions are best thought of as scar tissue usually found after tubal infections and pelvic surgery, such as surgery designed to promote fertility or surgery necessitated by a ruptured appendix. Old-fashioned myomectomies were notorious for causing dense, fibrous adhesions; laser-assisted myomectomies may be better in this regard. Adhesions do not imply an active, ongoing disease—instead, they are evidence of previous disease, like pockmarks signifying the occurrence of smallpox years before. Unfortunately, there are confusing disagreements about whether adhesions cause pain or not.

Most surgeons are skeptical of the notion that adhesions cause pain. This is a clinical opinion, based on the fact that many patients have severe adhesions but no symptoms at all. Ovarian cancer, a disease that causes pro-

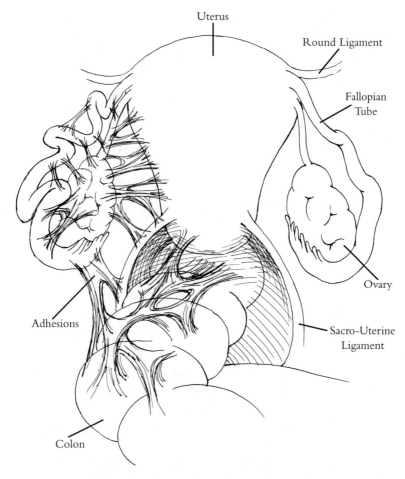

FIGURE 10.1   Adhesions (posterior view of internal organs)

found changes, including adhesions, in the pelvis, is a killer precisely because it is so insidious and symptom-free for months before complaints finally appear. (Do not be overly concerned about ovarian cancer if you
have CPP: After well over thirty years of looking after women with CPP, I
have yet to see a single woman who consulted me about CPP but was
found to have ovarian cancer instead). Specialists often find adhesions in
infertile women, who were free of pain and healthy all their lives and in
whom there was no suspicion of previous tubal infections. The extensive

tubal scarring and adhesions found in these women were most likely the consequence of a smoldering, chronic infection of the fallopian tubes with organisms called *Chlamydia*. These examples highlight an unfortunate fact: There may be much serious pelvic disease without any symptoms.

With CPP, we are considering the opposite side of the coin: women with serious complaints, but no definite disease to explain them. Andrea J. Rapkin, a professor of OB/GYN at UCLA, is one of the most thoughtful students of CPP in the United States. She compared CPP patients at her hospital to infertility patients and showed that adhesions are an unlikely cause of pain. Two other gynecologists, Arnold J. Kresch of the United States and the Canadian Anna Bodmer, compared CPP patients to well women undergoing tubal ligations and concluded that adhesions were a cause of pain. As often happens, and much to the dismay of all concerned, expert opinions clash, and definite proof is difficult to come by.[1]

Adhesiolysis, as the operation of dividing adhesions is called, fell into disrepute years ago. Major textbooks of abdominal surgery rarely have a chapter discussing this procedure. However, laparoscopic laser adhesiolysis is currently under investigation as a possible solution for at least some cases of CPP, and many gynecologists are optimistic that this operation will help sufferers. Adhesiolysis is discussed in Chapter 11.

4. **Infections** of the womb and fallopian tubes: acute and chronic salpingitis and pelvic abscesses; also called chronic pelvic inflammatory disease, or PID. Severe cases of these infections are relatively easy to diagnose, because fever, marked lower abdominal pain, and abnormalities of routine blood tests will be noted. Abscesses are slow to heal and may cause chronic pain. If the infection is not severe, blood tests may be normal, but pelvic examinations and ultrasound scans (sonograms) will suggest this diagnosis. Unfortunately, most women with CPP have taken courses of most avail-

---

[1]Rapkin, Kresch, and Bodmer were all correct with their conclusions. Compared to infertility patients, who usually have many adhesions and not much pain, CPP patients appear to be relatively adhesion free and pain prone, thereby weakening the causal connection between adhesions and pain. Compared to patients undergoing tubal ligations, who usually have no adhesions and have not had pelvic pain, CPP patients are prone to both, supporting the connection between adhesions and pain. Such complex thinking is difficult for most of us without a background in formal logic or statistics, but an easy problem for statisticians. The bottom line is that we are not sure how much pain may be attributed to adhesions.

able antibiotics without relief, and for this reason, I cannot regard PID as a reliable diagnosis. Since it is essential to find out what disease may be responsible for the pain, sooner or later laparoscopy is required to get accurate information; such studies have found few cases of chronic pelvic infections among women with CPP. This topic is further discussed in Chapter 13.

5. Pain after hysterectomy may be due to the **residual ovary syndrome**, a rare but well-recognized cause of CPP. The hysterectomy was typically performed to cure endometriosis or chronic salpingitis, and it was difficult because of adhesions. An ovary (or a fragment of an ovary) inadvertently remained behind, caught in adhesions, and continued to ovulate. Adhesions interfere with this process, causing pain. To make the diagnosis, the operative note and the pathologist's report from the hysterectomy should be reviewed. Blood tests used to identify the menopausal state (FSH, LH) and scans looking for ovarian tissue may be useful because they may show the existence of functioning ovarian tissue after these organs were thought to have been removed.

If ovulation is inhibited by medications such as BCPs or GnRH agonists, described in Chapter 8, the pains due to this syndrome should decrease. If surgery is undertaken to cure this condition, it is essential to find an experienced surgeon to do the operation. The residual ovary is not cancerous, but the precise dissection it requires is best done by a surgeon thoroughly versed in gynecological cancer surgery.

6. The **pelvic congestion syndrome** is an older theory, first proposed by Howard C. Taylor Jr., who had an exceptionally distinguished career in American gynecology. After World War II, Ivy League schools of medicine were preeminent, not yet rivaled by schools that were to arise later in the South and in California. Dr. Taylor was chairman of the Department of Obstetrics and Gynecology first at New York University, then at Columbia University College of Physicians and Surgeons. His colleagues remember him as a patrician figure and a careful and compassionate physician.

Howard Taylor was the first gynecologist to begin an organized, multidisciplinary effort to understand women with CPP. The clinic he opened at Columbia University's College of Physician and Surgeons was the first in the world to address this problem scientifically. Taylor was convinced that abnormalities of the pelvic vessels were an essential part of pelvic pain. He proposed that the pains were due to what he called the **pelvic congestion-**

fibrosis syndrome. This notion dates back to the ideas of European and American gynecologists of the nineteenth century, but Taylor hoped to demonstrate the disease in a way acceptable in the second half of the twentieth century.

For hundreds of years, women and their physicians have noted the presence of pains that were difficult to explain deep in the female pelvis. Previous generations of gynecologists put much ingenuity into designing names for the condition. There were names in English *(broad ligament neuritis)* and French *(plexalgie hypogastrique),* and some combined Greek and Latin *(pelipathia vegetativa).* One German synonym for chronic pelvic pain was translatable as "the disease with twenty names." Most diseases carry names instantly recognizable regardless of language barriers. Of course, inventing names is easily done, whereas understanding diseases and relieving symptoms is another, infinitely more important matter. The imprecise language of CPP diagnoses may also be contrasted with terms used when discussing illnesses such as appendicitis or lung cancer. There are no questions about names or arguments about the exact nature of these conditions, confusions characteristic of CPP.

The setting in which Howard Taylor began his research was rife with theories but poor in facts and even poorer with successful treatments. In line with then-current medical thinking, Taylor began by looking for a physical cause for the pain. He already knew from the work of the American physiologist Joseph Eldridge Markee that menstruation was a consequence of the sudden spasm of small arteries in the womb. Pregnancy is impossible without a massive dilatation of arteries and veins. The vascular flush of orgasm was just an assumption until it was demonstrated, many years after Taylor's work, by Masters and Johnson (of *Human Sexuality* fame) in St. Louis. Taylor surmised that the vessels might be involved and began to investigate their possible role in causing CPP.

Taylor had an engineer devise an ingenious instrument with which he could measure vaginal blood flow and showed that stressful questions sharply increased this flow in women. He also noted that many of his patients were women who had difficulties with orgasm. Engorged vessels were thought to be capable of causing severe (if transient) testicular pain in men. This pain was colloquially known as "blue balls" and was assumed to be the consequence of continued sexual excitement without orgasm. Taylor thought that something similar could be happening to women with CPP.

The theory he developed was that continued congestion of the pelvis, due to sexual excitement but unrelieved by orgasm, caused pelvic fibrosis, which in turn caused chronic pain. This was called the congestion-fibrosis syndrome, a theory that became popular for a decade or two. Five or six publications appeared in prestigious professional journals, but there were no photographs or drawings of the varicosities. Experienced surgeons reported that they rarely if ever saw the changes described by Taylor. Most damaging to the theory was the fact that after hysterectomy for CPP, examination of tissues removed showed neither congestion nor fibrosis.

Of course, during surgery patients are often in a tilted, head-down position to discourage the formation of clots in distended veins. Gravity makes the blood in pelvic veins flow toward the heart, collapsing them. The absence of visible varicosities during surgery could be explained away by the tilted position, but the absence of fibrosis, which should have been identifiable in hysterectomy specimens, was a more difficult objection.

Medical philosophy also changed. Even the opinions of respected professors were no longer accepted without questioning. Scientific proof was sought, and in this case, during Taylor's time, there was none. The theory gradually went into disfavor, to be resurrected decades later by Richard Beard in London.

Howard Taylor was struck by something unusual about his patients: They were often desperate with so many symptoms that life itself seemed to be one long list of dissatisfactions. Nervousness and anxiety, sexual difficulties, and exhaustion were the most frequently mentioned complaints. With Lothar Gidro-Frank, a Columbia University psychiatrist, Taylor investigated the psychiatric profiles of CPP sufferers and found that many had psychological problems.

Subsequently, much more sophisticated investigations using questionnaires such as the Minnesota Multiphasic Personality Inventory (MMPI) and others similar to it came to conflicting conclusions. Some showed that emotional difficulties were as frequent among women with pelvic pain as they were in the general population, whereas others claimed that women with pelvic pain were psychologically in worse shape than women without pains. However, it remained possible (and, to other researchers, likely) that the problems were the result and not the cause of the pain. Today, nearly fifty years later, this quandary remains.

7. **Pelvic varicosities**. During the 1970s, building on the work of American and Finnish researchers, Professor Richard Beard at St. Mary's Medical School in London reported an intriguing finding in women with CPP. An outpatient x-ray procedure, during which a dye was painlessly injected into the muscular wall at the top of the womb, showed dilated, varicose veins draining the upper uterus and the ovaries in many pelvic pain sufferers, while such veins were rarely observed in other patients without pain. The causes of the venous engorgement are unknown. Interestingly, during pregnancy the pelvic veins show an even greater degree of dilatation. Of course, during pregnancy lower abdominal aches and pains are exceedingly frequent. Rightly or wrongly, such pains are always attributed to other causes, not the veins.

Beard's work is convincing, although, as with adhesions, there may be large and easily visible varicosities, but no pain. The apparatus and procedure are simple but have not caught on in the United States. Color-enhanced ultrasound is another way of identifying engorged vessels. Work done at Duke University in North Carolina some years ago did not support Beard's observations, although this was more of a clinical opinion than a carefully designed study, such as Beard's was. In informal discussions, American experts are skeptical of the value of Beard's work with **uterine venograms** or **phlebograms**, synonymous technical terms for the procedure he used. Surgical removal of the veins may be difficult or impossible without major surgery; a few cases of embolization I have read about, a procedure discussed elsewhere in this book, were not successful. However, Beard has reported on the successful use of hysterectomy in alleviating pelvic pain in small groups of women. This work will be discussed in the next chapter.

At the 1991 meeting of the American Association of Gynecological Laparoscopists that I attended, pelvic pain was one of many topics discussed, but veins were not on the agenda. Subsequent meetings rarely mentioned varicosities. Originally an American notion, pelvic vein varicosities as a cause of CPP has been pursued mostly in the United Kingdom. Meanwhile, Beard's team at St. Mary's Hospital is looking at two other ideas. One is to consider medical ways of shrinking the veins, discussed with other treatments in Chapter 11. Beard and his team have also investigated the possibility that pelvic pain may be a disease that is psychosomatically determined. In an interview some years ago, Beard noted that many of his CPP patients had psychological problems that seemed to originate well before the pains appeared. Most of their patients are currently treated with medications and psychological treatments. This does not mean that the symptoms are merely "in the patient's head." The pain is real, but the underlying pathology is difficult to find. After years of suffering, the women need sympathy and reassurance as well as expert medical advice. The veins remain a tantalizing possibility, a single piece of a jigsaw puzzle that looks familiar but seems to belong in a corner where the pieces are beginning to fit together very slowly indeed.

8. I must also mention a number of other possibilities, although I am skeptical that these are genuine causes of CPP.

Ovarian cysts are painless unless they twist, which causes sudden, acute pain, not CPP. Rupture (except for rare instances of ruptured endometriotic or dermoid cysts) usually causes a little pain or none at all and is an unlikely cause of months or years of pain. Nevertheless, women are often told that this is the cause of their symptoms by gynecologists who have not listened to their patients and who are too focused on the present attack of pain. Ruptured or twisted endometriotic and dermoid cysts produce an abrupt emergency. These events, discussed in Chapters 7 and 14, are not easy to misdiagnose.

Fibroids, particularly if they are not large (in other words, smaller than an inch or two in diameter) are almost always painless. Even huge fibroids are usually (and amazingly) pain free. However, there are two processes that cause pain: torsion and degeneration. Torsion (twisting) of a fibroid hanging on a pedicle (stalk) may cause pain in a fibroid of any size; this pain is usually acute, but cannot last months. Degeneration, caused by an insufficient supply of blood, usually occurs in fibroids larger than two or three inches in diameter. This process, described in Chapter 6, may cause chronic pain. There may also be a steady ache or feelings of pelvic pressure from large fibroids. Ultrasound and other scans will identify degeneration, a change that occurs invisibly in the central area of the tumor, and laparoscopy will readily identify torsion, a sudden event. An extensive review of fibroids and their treatment is given in Chapters 6, 8, and 9.

Difficult deliveries may damage ligaments that support the womb in the pelvis, and an older theory holds that this may cause CPP. The damage is usually described as **broad ligament lacerations**. This condition was originally described in 1955 by two senior figures in American gynecology, Professors Willard Allen and William Masters (of Masters and Johnson fame) from Washington University in St. Louis. However, experienced surgeons see the characteristic lacerations so rarely that this condition has almost entirely lost favor as a possible cause of CPP. Broad ligament lacerations need laparoscopy for diagnosis and surgery, including hysterectomy, for treatment, but experts accept this diagnosis only rarely and reluctantly. Repair of the lacerations or hysterectomy is usually recommended. However, we have no carefully designed studies to tell us if these operations help.

Retroversion and **prolapse**, defined elsewhere, are typically pain free and should not be accused of causing the ravages of CPP. Prolapse may cause a pelvic ache or backache, sometimes helped with a **pessary**, a rubber or plastic device used to hold the uterus in place. **Retroversion** by itself is usually painless and harmless: Many older women have this. However, diseases that caused certain cases of retroversion, namely endometriosis and chronic salpingitis, must be identified because these may cause pain. Doctors' unwillingness to accept retroversion and prolapse as causes of pain may be labeled unsympathetic by women anxious to find a cause for their pains. Accepting this notion may seem more sympathetic but has led to millions of uterine suspension operations, now generally abandoned except, perhaps, for indications such as endometriosis.

Ovulatory pains (mittelschmerz) and **menstrual pains** (dysmenorrhea) may be confused with CPP. Ovulation occurs fourteen days before the next menstruation; recurring pains at this time may be caused by ovulation. Such pain rarely lasts longer than a few hours, or at most a day. Menstrual pains are felt in the midline and appear with menstruation—you don't need a male gynecologist to explain this to you. Keeping a calendar that shows periods and pain patterns helps to distinguish these two conditions from CPP, which usually has no correlation with menstrual cycles. Menstrual pains are usually relieved by antiprostaglandin medications, and even more consistently by BCPs that prevent ovulation.

Patients with **PMS** often have severe menstrual pains; much less often they have CPP as well. This is a complicated and unfortunate situation, and one for which some women have had hysterectomies performed, also excising both ovaries. If you have both conditions, each must be investigated and treated separately.

Intrauterine contraceptive devices (**IUCDs**) may cause painful periods but rarely cause CPP. On rare occasions, an IUCD may cause a sudden infection of the womb, which then spreads to the fallopian tubes, but this is an acute event. A chronic low-grade infection is a remote possibility, but under these circumstances, antibiotics are given and the IUCD is removed, usually with rapid relief.

If you consider all the above possible gynecological causes, I hope you will agree that it would not be easy to chart a course of investigations to fit all women with CPP. The gynecologist's first job may be to make sure that gynecological investigations and treatments are not scheduled for women whose problems originate from causes that are not gynecological. The irritable bowel syndrome (IBS) is, according to some experts, perhaps the most prominent of these problems.

Samuel Smith is a gynecological endocrinologist and director of the OB/GYN Department at Harbor Hospital Center in Baltimore. When I interviewed him in July 2000, Professor Smith, whose work includes looking after women with CPP, agreed that much pelvic and lower abdominal pain originates from gastrointestinal causes. IBS and particularly the constipation associated with IBS are the most important problems mistaken for CPP. Dr. Smith agreed that gynecological investigations such as laparoscopy and treatments with menopause-inducing drugs detailed in Chapter 11 are best timed *after* diseases of other systems have been excluded, but *before* hysterectomy begins to be discussed. And now let us concentrate on non-gynecological causes of CPP.

Non-Gynecological Causes of CPP

1. **Gastrointestinal diseases:** The **irritable bowel syndrome** (**IBS**) causes abdominal pain, intermittent attacks of diarrhea alternating with constipation, and gaseous distension with flatulence. Treatment is the domain of internists, gastroenterologists, or surgeons and consists of reeducating the bowel with a mixture of medications, laxatives, and dietary changes including high-fiber foods. The regimen is designed to eliminate cycles of diarrhea and constipation and is often successful.

Similar but worse symptoms, including bloody diarrhea, fever, and weight loss may be caused by **inflammatory bowel disease** (**IBD**).

TABLE 10.3   Non-Gynecological Causes of Chronic Pelvic Pain

1. Gastrointestinal causes of CPP:
    Irritable bowel syndrome
    Inflammatory bowel disease
    Lactose intolerance
2. Urological causes of CPP:
    Chronic interstitial cystitis
3. Orthopedic causes of CPP:
    Trigger points
4. Other causes of CPP:
    Chronic pain states
    Pain processing disorders
    Neuropathic pain

Other names for certain types of IBD are regional enteritis, ulcerative colitis, and Crohn's disease. These conditions are usually diagnosed by surgeons, gastroenterologists, or internists by means of special x-rays, and sigmoidoscopy or colonoscopy, the direct inspection of the inner surfaces of the colon. Medical treatment with sulfa drugs, anti-inflammatory agents, steroids, and other medications also helps certain cases. If the disease is severe, colectomy (excision of parts of the colon) may be necessary.

The symptoms of **lactose intolerance** consist of abdominal cramps, a bloated feeling, flatulence, and possibly diarrhea; it is caused by the absence from digestive juices of the enzyme *lactase,* essential for the digestion of lactose in milk and milk products. Some experts believe that severe lactose intolerance may cause CPP.

Ulcers (peptic, gastric, duodenal) and gallbladder disease are, as a rule, not difficult to diagnose and to treat. The pain is mostly in the upper abdomen and may follow specific meals or foods. It is relieved by appropriate medications. **Diverticulitis** is another cause of abdominal pain. In this disease, small pouches, which tend to get infected, bulge out of the colon. This disease usually occurs in men and women over the age of forty and is easy to diagnose with x-rays or a procedure called **sigmoidoscopy** (or colonoscopy).

2. **Urinary tract diseases: Chronic interstitial cystitis** (**IC** or **chronic IC**), is a disease of the walls of the bladder, and consists of lower abdominal and pelvic pains and a sharply increased, almost constant need to urinate. Many women with IC find intercourse painful; even more

claim that it took years of unsuccessful visits, often to supposedly expert practitioners, before the correct diagnosis was made. Early cases are difficult to diagnose, needing cystoscopy (looking into the bladder, usually under anesthesia) and biopsies of the bladder walls. The disease often shrinks the bladder to a smaller capacity; a simple test may tell you whether you might have such damage from more advanced IC. Drink six or eight glasses of water, wait until your bladder feels full, then empty your bladder and measure the volume of urine you have passed in a disposable measuring cup. Normal bladder capacity is 10–12 ounces. If you felt full and had an urgent need to empty your bladder with less than 6–8 ounces of urine in it, you need a competent urologist to examine you.

The Interstitial Cystitis Association of America (see the Resources section) will gladly provide more information on this condition, which is not diagnosed nearly as often as it occurs. Men suffer from IC very rarely.

The **urethral syndrome**. Urinary frequency and pain on urination are the hallmarks of the urethral syndrome. The urethra carries urine from the bladder toward the vagina; most of its length is located in the front wall of the vagina, terminating an inch below the clitoris. In this condition, direct but gentle pressure on the urethra, through the front wall of the vagina, is painful. The urethral syndrome is diagnosed by urologists; treatment consists of antibiotics and mechanical dilatation of the urethra.

Urinary tract infections and **stones** in the kidneys, ureters, or the bladder can cause severe flank, lower abdominal, and pelvic pains. Microscopic examination of the urine, cultures, and x-ray or ultrasound investigations are reasonably accurate ways to diagnose these conditions, which are rarely confused with CPP. Infections are treated with antibiotics; stones may be passed spontaneously or be excised. Modern equipment that uses sound waves to break up stones is beginning to be used. The fragments are then passed in urine, obviating the need for surgery. However, these conditions are rare causes of CPP.

3. **Orthopedic causes**: Modern x-ray investigations will show orthopedic diseases such as spinal infections, fractures, benign tumors, and cancerous deposits readily, but these are rare causes of pelvic pain. Much more often, degenerative diseases such as osteoarthritis will be found, but experts are reluctant to accept these as causes of pelvic pain. Many orthopedists, chiropractors, and physiotherapists regard severe chronic backaches as intractable, probably the way many gynecologists regard CPP. Herniated

intervertebral ("slipped") discs may be thought to cause CPP, but in my experience, orthopedists have rarely helped women with their pains.

4. **Trigger points**: Myofascial pain and pain originating from "trigger points" in muscles can cause pelvic pain. John C. Slocumb, a gynecologist from Denver, is the main proponent of this theory, according to which hypersensitive trigger points in myofascial planes cause the pain by irritating nerves. Slocumb believes that 74 percent of women with CPP suffer from pains that are myofascial in origin. In Slocumb's hands, the diagnosis is made by finding hypersensitive trigger points in myofascial planes, consisting of the skin of the abdominal wall and tissue along the cervix, the vagina, and the back. Injecting these points with an anesthetic solution produces relief. Other experts believe that myofascial pain occurs mostly after surgery, with an abdominal scar as the source of the pain. Since most gynecologists are not experts at diagnosing or treating this condition, if the above picture sounds familiar, you must consult with an up-to-date physiotherapist or pain clinic. According to Slocumb, treatment consists of the injections noted, with antidepressants, group psychotherapy, and acupuncture. Other experts regard trigger points as a poorly defined and oversold notion.

Chronic pain states, pain processing disorders, and **neuropathic pain**. There is substantial overlap in these diagnoses. Neuropathic pain (pain caused by malfunctioning spinal nerve centers) may be one of many mechanisms that ultimately leads to chronic pain states. Another possibility is that once habituated to pain, noxious patterns of pain are embedded somewhere in the brain itself. When I interviewed him in August 2000, Clifford Gevirtz, associate professor of anesthesiology at New York's Mt. Sinai Hospital, related information gynecologists (and indeed most physicians) don't usually know: After months or years of unremitting pain, even a spinal block may not provide relief. Fortunately, this is a very rare event, but there are few options left now: complex neurosurgical interventions or major tranquilizers such as Haldol. In the years to come, these ideas will be clarified by neuroscientists; more important, I hope to see better treatment choices for women. At present, such ideas are familiar to researchers, up-to-date neurologists, and staff working in pain clinics, but they are virtually unknown to the rest of the medical world.

Miscellaneous other possibilities include medical diseases such as advanced syphilis, sickle cell disease, and narrowed arteries supplying blood to bowel: rare but distinct causes of chronic abdominal pain. In the hands of competent internists, they should not be confused with CPP. Chronic appendicitis, a popular diagnosis around the turn of the century, occurs rarely and is an unlikely cause of CPP.

Pelvic Pain and Post-Traumatic Stress Syndrome

Western thinking divides symptoms into physical and mental categories, a dualism that causes difficulties. It is counterproductive and inaccurate to imagine that most symptoms are due to a physical disease, whereas a few, whose exact cause is obscure, are "mental" in origin. The two are often intertwined: The woman who loses her breast to cancer gets depressed; the man whose business fails gets an ulcer. This artificial division has been broken down with a new diagnosis: the **post-traumatic stress disorder (PTSD)**. PTSD was originally described in men but also occurs in women who have experienced physical or sexual abuse as infants or children.

PTSD was first diagnosed in the mid- to late 1970s, when the term was coined for Vietnam veterans who suffered from a well-defined group of symptoms, including sleeplessness, nightmares, a jumpy, hyper-alert manner, and difficulties with concentration and relationships. The symptoms are thought to be the consequence of prolonged exposure to the enormous violence of the conflict in Vietnam. With the diagnosis of PTSD, psychologically unbearable events came to be accepted as the cause of symptoms appearing much later in large numbers of physically healthy young men. The symptoms all involve feelings, psychological states of mind; their causes may be subjective and open to various explanations. For Vietnam veterans, PTSD has become an acceptable diagnosis to explain symptoms without insisting on finding a "physical" disease. Many experts think that something similar may be causing the sufferings of at least some women with CPP in whom a physical disease cannot be found. Interestingly, women develop PTSD more often than men do, even though they were combatants in Vietnam much less often than men were.

The multiple complaints often seen with CPP are, of course, different from the symptoms of Vietnam veterans. But the headaches and lethargy, the loss of the joy of life, and the preoccupation with bodily symptoms that are so frequent and so debilitating among women with CPP have never had a satisfactory explanation. Significantly, women with arthritis or other equally severe illnesses rarely develop such a profusion of these symptoms.

The psychologists and social workers of the Pelvic Pain Clinic noticed that women with CPP often had experienced physical violence and sexual abuse when they were young. One reasonable explanation of their despairing effect may be that these symptoms are a consequence of physical or sexual abuse constituting a delayed reaction to unbearable stresses occurring years before. Much of the work in PTSD originates from women, making it more difficult to dismiss the hypothesis on ideological grounds. This concept is only too familiar to social workers and women involved in counseling the victims of abuse: Terrible experiences in childhood may wreck your ability to enjoy a productive and happy adulthood.

Judith Lewis Herman is an associate clinical professor of psychiatry at Harvard Medical School and director of the Women's Mental Health Collective in Somerville, Massachusetts. She is also the author of *Father-Daughter Incest* (Harvard University Press, 2000) and, later, of *Trauma and Recovery* (Basic Books, 1997). Dr. Herman has written eloquently and extensively on the subject of the lifelong anguish often experienced by survivors of incest. Her books document how frequently young girls and adolescents become the victims of the uncontrolled sex drives and violence of their fathers, stepfathers, and other male relatives. In an interview, Dr. Herman reiterated that incest and other forms of sexual assault are very frequent. She emphasized the strong probability that such exceptional stresses cause long-lasting damage. Among symptoms frequently observed are anxiety, depression, and the tendency to develop multiple health complaints that are difficult to explain.

Other compelling ideas come from Andrea J. Rapkin, whose work on adhesions has been mentioned already. Dr. Rapkin believes that physical violence in early childhood is an even stronger influence than incest in leading to the development of CPP. She studied a group of women with CPP and found that a very high proportion (nearly 40 percent) suffered from physical trauma when young. Twenty percent were sexually assaulted while children. Thinking about PTSD and the work of Drs. Herman and Rapkin, in 1992 I interviewed two women whose work gave them intimate insights into the world of the physically or sexually abused woman.

Since the inception of the Rape Intervention Program at St. Luke's Hospital Center–Woman's Hospital, social worker Susan Xenarios has been in charge of the program and therapist Louise Kindley has been working with women who have survived sexual assault and related experiences. I have known these women since the late 1970s, when I was the gynecologist among a group of hospital employees who started the program. Susan Xenarios and Louise Kindley are not women who go along with old-fashioned patriarchal ideas without an immediate and articulate protest. They, too, have noticed that abuse, whether physical or sexual, scars the victim for life, leaving her worried about bodily functions, hypersensitive to feelings she cannot account for, and prone to develop complaints for which there is no easy explanation. They also remind me how painful these memories may be, how some women begin to recollect memories of incestuous attacks inflicted during formative years only after hours of gentle, delicately probing conversations. One example they gave was that of a young woman who suffered from what she thought were sinus headaches, feeling that her sinuses and head were about to explode. Through therapy, she realized that oral sex was repeatedly forced on her during her infancy, explaining (as much as such feelings can be explained) her feelings years later.

The events some women have survived may have been so traumatic that the memories have been completely repressed. It is not only the survivors of such attacks who find it difficult to discuss these betrayals. Even seasoned mental health professionals are often ill at ease discussing incest; I know I must prepare myself (and my patient) carefully before venturing into these difficult areas. Women caring for victims of sexual assault have recognized that the aftereffects of rape, in particular, may be felt for decades. The media have recently also reported a number of instances in which victims of incest have repressed all memory of their sufferings for years, when therapy or some unpredictable event made the memories surface—although the opposite claim, that recovered memories are often false, has also been voiced.

In pediatric circles, it is one of the saddest axioms that incest is a frequent crime, but the least-reported one, against children. Symptoms such as depression, lack of sexual desire, a preoccupation with disease, lethargy, and CPP may all be a delayed reaction to repeated physical or sexual assaults many years before.

A bright five-year-old stands out in my memory. She complained of a vaginal discharge, but when I examined her, everything seemed normal. Her mother brought her back four days later because the discharge was worse. The little girl kept insisting that nothing unusual happened during the recent week she had spent with an aunt and an uncle. I was reluctant to upset her with a second examination, but she seemed more distressed than before. Sad to say, this time I found the unmistakable eruption of genital herpes, and the whole story fell into place.

The frequency of sexual attacks is shockingly high. It would be very naive to believe that all pelvic pain follows this pattern, and I have never advised anyone directly that a long-forgotten sexual attack was the "real" cause of their symptoms: Such language would be unacceptable. Women with pelvic pain of obscure cause need a careful approach that considers the whole person, not statements that may be unfounded or likely to anger or insult them. At the same time, particularly when there are multiple debilitating symptoms of obscure cause, the possibility of having survived painful events must be considered.

CPP of Obscure Cause— a Psychological View

Women with CPP are often indignant or furious with concepts involving psychological terms. Most people consider that physical disease is the only legitimate cause of pain; for them, the suggestion of psychosomatic factors or concepts is often regarded as evasive and insulting. Feminists point out that women receive what they consider put-downs in psychological terms much more often than men.

Elaine Showalter, a Princeton professor of English, has written with great understanding about the illnesses of women around the turn of the last century. Showalter sees the "madness" of these women as the "desperate communication of the powerless." Phyllis Chesler's book *Women and Madness* (Doubleday, 1972) is perhaps the most emphatic account detailing profound feminist objections to sexism in psychiatric thinking.

The language used by psychiatrists tends to be disagreeable, objectionable, and perhaps offensive to some women. Because the stigma of mental disease is so strong, anger makes sense as a response to diagnoses expressed in odious language. Even if psychiatric labels are avoided, psychological considerations remain unpalatable to many. I have tried various ways of discussing these ideas with women who appeared deeply and unmistakably depressed. The message was intended to be sympathetic, but too often it was received as a harshly critical accusation that was demeaning to them. One legitimate reaction from patients has been that if they are psychologically affected, this is due to years of suffering and confused diagnoses. This view is backed by solid research. The Belgian gynecologist Professor Marcel Joseph Renaer, who coined the abbreviation CPP-WOP, meaning chronic pelvic pain without obvious cause, has shown that prolonged pelvic pain has profound and adverse psychological consequences on women.

Sadly, too often women with CPP are caught between poorly diagnosed physical diseases, for which there seem to be no effective treatments, and difficult symptoms that only the psychiatric community is willing to take seriously. Psychological diagnoses are likely to be applied to women more often than to men. But choosing a symptom to be presented for psychological analysis (either by the patient or the gynecologist) is determined by our attitudes concerning mental health, and these have a sexist bias. I am often tempted to define the tendency to kill, maim, rape, or assault other people as a mental disease, a notion not unheard of among criminal lawyers. If we did so, a different picture would emerge. Men would be shuffling interminably through psychiatric rather than penal systems, feeling depressed and victimized.

During the interview with Louise Kindley and Susan Xenarios, they repeatedly used a phrase that rings true: "body memory." The phrase reminds me of recent theories of chronic pain and the existence of a condition called the chronic pain state.

Chronic Pain States

Chronic pain differs from acute pain, and is, unfortunately, poorly understood. In acute pain, there is a disease, discernible as tissue damage, usually identifiable under a microscope. With treatment, or perhaps on its own, the damage heals. Within weeks, the pain leaves, and the illness is over. In chronic pain, the original disease is often less distinct and the microscope may not provide a diagnosis, but the pain stands out ever after with stark reality. There is some evidence that the difference is caused by a change in the nervous system, which becomes overexcited and too ready to send pain reports to higher centers in the brain, often in response to events that cause minimal distress at most in other people. The patient has no control over the pain, but there is no question that CPP patients feel all the pain they report. None of it is invented, explaining the anger these women feel when it is implied that their symptoms are imaginary.

Theories that involve the nervous system go by a variety of names: pain processing disorder and neuropathy are current favorites. There is an eternal debate between doctors who are paralyzed by their failure to understand what might be causing pain and patients who categorically state that the pains are severe enough to drive them crazy; fibromyalgia and CPP are two such diseases. Neuropathy is not just a fancy name for a mysterious condition; there is experimental evidence that it exists, and treatments are beginning to be developed for it.

Chronic pain is different from acute pain in one other important respect. After a few months of pain, it no longer matters what the original disease was. When CPP occurs, in some extreme cases it may no longer be appropriate to regard the condition as purely gynecological. Now the disease is chronic pelvic pain, which may respond better to treatments with antidepressants, acupuncture, new medications, and psychological treatments than it does to pain medications or to gynecological surgery.

When should the diagnosis of a chronic pain state be made? This is not as simple as diagnosing a broken bone with an x-ray. More pronounced cases are easier to identify confidently; less severe cases remain arguable. The more a woman's story resembles the following clinical picture, the likelier it is that she is suffering from a chronic pain state:

- Multiple symptoms are being investigated and multiple diagnoses are being made. The patient with pains all over her body, palpitations, dizzy spells, extreme lethargy, depression, and frequent crying spells is probably suffering from a chronic pain state. The woman who is disabled by pain and who is told that her symptoms are due to tubal infections, ovarian cysts, fibroids, PMS, and food allergies, but whose diagnoses cannot be verified, may also be suffering from a chronic pain state.

- Symptoms, diagnoses, and treatments are beginning to take over the patient's (and perhaps her family's) existence. When meals and nonmedical appointments are being missed because of the pain and sexual matters and friendships are neglected, the woman and the gynecologist should begin to think in terms of chronic pain states.

- The response to all treatments is disappointing. No treatment is ever guaranteed, but the lack of response to all imaginable treatments is a strong hint to consider the possibility that a chronic pain state may be the cause of all symptoms.

John Bonica, an anesthesiologist from Seattle who died recently, developed an interest in chronic pain almost fifty years ago. Bonica was the senior editor and one of the main contributors of a compendium of over 2,000 pages called *The Management of Pain* (Lea and Febiger, 1991). The book covers pain caused by cancer. There are also sections on the pain felt by amputees in phantom limbs and on headaches, backaches, temporomandibular joint pains, chest and abdominal pains, and pelvic pains. Bonica estimated that the annual cost of chronic pain states is in excess of $60–80 billion a year; much of this vast sum is currently spent unwisely, on old-fashioned and ineffective treatments.

The existence of chronic pain states is unappreciated by many physicians. Pain clinics have proliferated, and they have proven their worth in terms of pain relief and the successful return of sufferers to work. However, public acceptance has been slow. One reason for this may be that these clinics require the continued active participation of the patient for success, a far cry from most medical and surgical treatments. Also, pain clinics are expensive. Pain clinics are discussed in Chapter 11.

You may be interested in learning what happened to the two women whose stories opened this chapter. The first, whose pains were always thought to be due to infections, had laparoscopy and was found to have endometriosis. With conventional treatment, she improved. The second got her hysterectomy at another hospital but fared less well. Within a year, she was back to see me with all her usual symptoms. I encouraged her to enroll in our pain clinic, but to no avail. I knew enough about her background to know that I had to worry about the consequences of both physical and sexual abuse during her teens. When I last saw her, some years ago, she was busy visiting clinic after clinic, each focused on one bodily system and each unsuccessful. I understand her reluctance to delve into her painful past. However, I fear that her life is being ruined by her ill health, and it saddens me that I could not help her more.

Not all cases of CPP are as extreme as the case of the second woman, and only a few sufferers need such extensive care. The cause of pelvic pain may be difficult to pinpoint. In many, the symptoms come and go. The cause of the pain may be a gynecological disease such as endometriosis, or it may be a non-gynecological disease. Maddeningly, all manner of diagnoses may be made, but relief may never arrive. As more and more symptoms interfere with a happy and productive life, it becomes time to consider such diagnoses as the chronic pain state. However, too many gynecologists shy away from unfamiliar diagnoses and complicated treatments, and many women pay a high price for their insistence on a gynecological solution: hysterectomy with an uncertain chance of success.

· · · II · · ·

Chronic Pelvic Pain: Treatments

Of all the chapters in this book, the two dealing with CPP required the most extensive rethinking and rewriting for this second edition, a consequence of our better understanding of this problem. As recently as ten years ago, our notions of CPP were primitive; today we have much better treatments for women suffering from this distressing problem. These words, unfortunately, do not mean that women suffering from CPP can now obtain immediate and lasting relief. Persistence and intelligence are still needed to make sense of the universe of possible causes and treatments, but at long last, light is beginning to show at the end of the tunnel.

In this chapter, I will outline a number of medical treatments effective in relieving CPP. Some are uncomplicated and may be prescribed by any physician; others need much gynecological expertise, even a gynecological endocrinologist. Treatments may be provided by an internist, an expert urologist, possibly other specialists. Surgery, including hysterectomy, will be discussed last. The effect of surgery on CPP is a complicated story; because of its obvious importance, it will be considered in detail. The treatments I describe will bring substantial relief to at least half of all women suffering from CPP, but they will not cure everyone.

One mysterious aspect of CPP consists of the amazingly large numbers of treatments proposed to women with CPP. During the 1950s, one prestigious British gynecologist still recommended painting the endometrial lining with silver nitrate, the mildly cauterizing chemical in old-fashioned styptic pencils, which were used to stop bleeding from inadvertent shaving nicks, as an effective treatment for pelvic pain. Such notions do not die easily, and this British idea was resurrected in an aggressive modern form. At the Twentieth Annual Meeting of the American Association of Gynecological Laparoscopists, held in Las Vegas in late 1991, one panelist delivered a paper that claimed that a thick endometrial lining caused both PMS and CPP. The proposed treatment was surgical ablation (destruction) of this seemingly innocent layer of tissue; the panelist reported excellent results from the operation. The theory behind ablation was that the endometrium may produce chemicals that caused extensive symptoms. In common with silver nitrate and many other treatments, ablation was soon forgotten as a treatment for CPP, and has never resurfaced.

More recently, a group of researchers led by a prestigious gynecologist, whose research interests have included the effects of hysterectomy as well as the use of menopause-inducing drugs for women with CPP, reported another unusual treatment. Their treatment of CPP consisted of magnets applied to abdominal trigger points; the magnets were found to provide significant relief. This study was presented at the Forty-Eighth Annual Clinical Meeting of the American College of Obstetricians and Gynecologists, held in San Francisco in May 2000. The trial involved fourteen patients only, raising statistical problems academic physicians take very seriously, but otherwise it was a properly designed study that showed good results.

An unusually large number of extraordinary diagnoses and treatments have been proposed for women with CPP. There may be many causes, but the availability of all these treatments implies that none works well for every patient. This chapter will describe treatments that almost all mainstream practitioners can undertake and will go on to note other important ideas. However, it will not mention or comment on myriad other treatments that originate from a few enthusiastic supporters but have no national recognition.

You may be able to cope with your symptoms through the help of various systems of healing, from acupuncture through meditation, ginseng, or

St. John's wort, or pain medications, Tai-Chi exercises, massage, or a variety of diets. These and other similar approaches are fine. If your treatment is working, there is no need to worry about the exact diagnosis. However, if severe symptoms recur and your illness has taken over your life, another possibility must be considered. You may have developed a newly recognized condition described in Chapter 10, called the chronic pain state. This is neither cancerous nor life-threatening, but it menaces the quality of the remainder of your life. If you continue to suffer from CPP, you may need the services of a pain clinic. These clinics are a new and innovative branch of medicine and have developed a wide range of treatments to help those whom more traditional medical approaches have not helped.

Chronic pain clinics offer effective treatments, but these include a novel feature: You are not a passive recipient of treatments but an important part of the team taking care of you. By definition, severe cases of CPP and other chronic pain states represent the failure of all previous treatments. Depending on the knowledge and skills possessed by your doctors, your diagnosis, your temperament, and support systems (and, unfortunately, your medical insurance coverage), certain treatments remain to be used; some are excellent at solving even intractable pain problems.

Medical Treatments

Pain medications are usually tried first, but for reasons that are not clear, their effectiveness is unpredictable. In Chapter 10, I mentioned the Seattle anesthesiologist John Bonica, a pioneering physician who died recently. He and his colleagues in **algology**, the branch of medicine that deals with pain, established the first chronic pain clinic in Seattle. Early in his career, Bonica highlighted a humbling fact: Conventional pain medications may not relieve chronic pain. The reason may be as simple as nervous tissue getting used to pain-relieving drugs and requiring ever-higher doses to be effective. Unfortunately, many physicians have been slow to appreciate this and continue to treat sufferers with a variety of pain medications even when they are clearly not helpful.

A few women get all the help they need from the intermittent use of pain medications, but more often these are effective only temporarily. Any medication, from simple analgesics (mild pain-relieving medications) such as Tylenol, Aleve, Motrin, and others to more potent narcotics such as codeine-containing compounds and drugs such as Dilaudid may be tried. Potent medications currently in vogue include long-acting drugs such as MS Contin, a drug similar to morphine, and Oxycontin, derived from codeine. There are adverse outcomes to this approach: These medications may not work, they may cause constipation or drowsiness, and there is a small but distinct risk of addiction. You and the physician who issues your prescriptions must discuss these problems honestly.

Antibiotics, often combined with analgesics or narcotics, must be mentioned even though they are valuable only if the pain is due to an infection. The often difficult diagnosis of PID is discussed in Chapters 10 and 13. Most women with CPP have consumed successive courses of every available antibiotic without much effect, except for a complication: the yeast infections *(monilial vaginitis)* that follow the use of antibiotics. These drugs eradicate the bacteria that normally inhabit the vagina, including bacteria that maintain the normal acidity and normal bacterial contents of the vagina, allowing the overgrowth of yeast organisms. If you are prone to yeast infections and you are given antibiotics, be sure that you use one of the many standard antifungal creams or suppositories as long as you are taking antibiotics, and ideally for a few days longer. Another approach is the use of Diflucan, a single swallowed tablet. Also, be tested for diabetes, another frequent cause of yeast, or fungal, vaginitis.

Birth Control Pills (BCPs) are excellent for mittelschmerz, which is ovulatory, or midcycle pain, and for menstrual pains. If you have noticed an accentuation of your symptoms during your midcycle, premenstrually and menstrually, BCPs are worth trying. It might be best to take one of the monophasic BCPs continuously first, taking a hormone-containing tablet every single day for three months, although most gynecologists are more familiar with the customary cyclic use: three weeks on, one week off. BCPs are discussed in full in Chapter 8. Most women I have seen with CPP did not respond well to treatment with BCPs, but this may be because those who were helped no longer had any need to enroll in a CPP clinic. Relief during BCP use may indicate that the CPP is due to endometriosis, in which case even better pain relief may be had: the GnRH agonists.

Since the mid-1990s, good results have been reported using the **GnRH agonists,** mentioned in Chapter 8 as treatments for fibroids and for endometriosis. The success of these drugs may depend on their beneficial effects on endometriosis; you may recall that this disease, visible in the pelvis, or invisible in deeper pelvic tissues, is a common cause of CPP. The GnRH agonists also produce menopausal hibernation in most pelvic tissues, shrinking muscles as well blood vessels including varicosities—pelvic congestion with dilated veins is another possible cause of CPP. Thus, GnRH agonists may help with two recognized causes of CPP.

GnRH agonists can be used up to six months; if extended beyond six months, the prolonged hypo-estrogenic state induced may cause osteoporosis. However, if there is sufficient pain relief, the GnRH agonists can be prescribed for longer than six months, provided that "add-back" estrogen and progesterone are also prescribed. These drugs are used for women with CPP exactly as they are used for women with endometriosis; details are found in Chapter 8. More important, according to Samuel Smith, an associate professor of gynecology and obstetrics at Johns Hopkins and University of Maryland Medical Schools in Baltimore, these medications have given good results in over 50 percent of women to whom they were given.

Antidepressants help women with other chronic pain states such as chronic backaches and have proved effective even for women with severe CPP. An experienced team, from Washington University in Seattle, found antidepressants very potent in relieving CPP, and these drugs are in steady use in pain clinics. Tricyclic antidepressants may be useful for anyone with prolonged and severe pain regardless of the cause; these antidepressants are preferred to medications such as Prozac. The main obstacle to the use of antidepressants is patients' reluctance to accept them. This applies to men with chronic backaches as well as to women with CPP and derives at least in part from the stigma of mental disease.

There may be other reasons for not using these medications, but I suspect that had antidepressants been first marketed as neurotransmitter modifiers (an equally accurate if obscure name), it would likely be much easier to persuade patients to use them. You may be less resistant to using antidepressants if your gynecologist does not dwell on complicated psychological theories about the cause of the pain. Instead, the medications should be tried as an experiment that should last at least six to eight weeks. I must emphasize again that if you suffer from CPP, you are not imagining anything, nor are you responsible for your symptoms; you are responsible only for making sure that you get the best care available.

Tranquilizers and **sedatives** have not provided much help after the initial relief any new medication usually brings. They deserve mention because some physicians who lack insight into the problems faced by women with CPP may prescribe them.

Myofascial pain: There are some newer treatments underway as well. John C. Slocumb, a gynecologist from Denver and one of a handful of American researchers with new ideas about CPP, has introduced a new therapy. This consists of an array of methods, including trigger point blocks (injections with anesthetic agents), pain medications, antidepressants and medications prescribed to help with anxiety, and various forms of psychological and hormonal therapies. Slocumb's results are reportedly excellent: Half his patients are pain free and almost 90 percent improve after treatment. Other experts agree with the concept of myofascial pain but believe that it is seen mostly in women who have abdominal scars from previous surgery. Many women with CPP are operated on sooner or later; the pain may precede or follow surgery; it may be difficult to distinguish cause from effect.

Pelvic congestion, pelvic varicosities: A British center with a special interest in CPP may have other drugs or combinations of treatments for women with this problem. Richard Beard and his team at St. Mary's Medical School in London have had a strong interest in the treatment of pelvic pain since the 1970s. Following Taylor's work mentioned in Chapter 10, Beard and his colleagues believe that varicosities of pelvic veins are responsible for CPP in many women. The varicosities are thought to be similar to the large, distended varicose veins that may be seen in leg veins, which may be painful. It may be possible to shrink the varicosities medically, and Beard's team is conducting clinical research in this field. Drugs under investigation include Provera (discussed in Chapter 8) and ergot preparations.

Every American gynecologist prescribes Provera, but they are not familiar with this use and may not want to prescribe it for CPP, particularly because the doses required (20–40 mgms a day) are higher than customarily written in the United States. Ergot preparations have also been researched for women with CPP. These chemicals contract muscles in vessel walls, reducing the flow of blood through arteries and veins. They are familiar to women suffering from migrainous headaches, caused by a transient but marked dilatation of vessels in the brain. Ergot is also used to control bleeding from the uterus after deliveries. However, ergot preparations are limited by their toxicity. Overdoses may be fatal, and too much ergot, or even standard doses used for too long, may cause widespread damage to arteries. Gangrene of the fingers, toes, and even limbs has been described, though not in recent decades. Ergot preparations have been used from medieval times in an effort to produce abortions. Physicians also became familiar with ergot poisoning, which was more often accidental, the consequence of eating rye contaminated by an ergot-producing fungal growth. The illness was known by the colorful name of St. Joseph's fire, supposedly because affected extremities felt as if they were on fire. A visit to St. Joseph's shrine often produced a cure, probably by removing the sufferer from the diet of contaminated rye.

Surgical Treatments

There are several possible surgical treatments for CPP.

Laparoscopy, surgery during which organs in the abdomen and pelvis are inspected through a small incision just below the navel, is an excellent way of identifying disease (or normal, healthy tissues) in various organs. Laparoscopy has had extensive use in CPP and is particularly reassuring to women wondering about the state of health of their internal organs. Without laparoscopy, your gynecologist is just guessing at the diagnosis, not a good approach for potentially serious complaints, and certainly not for dealing with CPP. However, laparoscopy, while certainly mainstream American gynecology, has its opponents. Some gynecologists recommend that laparoscopy should be dispensed with, arguing that endometriosis may not be properly identified at laparoscopy: an expensive (and minimally risky) way to obtain misleading information. Their contention is that GnRH agonist medications should be tried without laparoscopy. This is a therapeutic trial: an elaborate way of saying, "Let's see what these drugs will do for this patient."

Surgery can cut nerves that carry pain signals from the uterus to the spinal cord and on to the brain, an idea attractive in its simplicity. Such operations are excellent for menstrual cramps, but such drastic measures are rarely necessary. CPP is rarely helped by the interruption of bundles of nerves that are thought to carry pain messages. However, these operations are still recommended for women with CPP. For this reason, you must understand what they are, and what they can (and cannot) do for you.

Any one of a number of operations should work to ease painful menstrual periods. The easiest fibers to interrupt are located in the **uterosacral (US) ligaments,** located just above and behind the cervix. The surgery may be done vaginally, in which case the operation is called **Doyle's procedure**. Doyle was, you may recall, one of the earliest American critics of unnecessary hysterectomies. It can also be done by means of old-fashioned abdominal surgery. If done the modern way, laparoscopically, it is called **LUNA**, an abbreviation for **laparoscopic uterine nerve ablation**. Except for surgery for some women with endometriosis, specifically those with exceptionally severe menstrual pains, I am not enthusiastic about either of these operations, mostly because there are easier ways to help painful periods. The LUNA procedure may, on rare occasions, damage the ureters, two ducts that carry urine from the kidneys to the bladder. Whenever this occurs, elaborate surgery is required to repair the damage. Recurrences of menstrual pains within a year of LUNA procedures are also common—the final reason that these operations have been largely abandoned.

Nerve blocks: Injecting the US ligaments with drugs derived from cocaine used to be another choice. This method dates back to Freud's discovery of the anesthetic properties of cocaine toward the end of the nineteenth century. The technique is the same as a paracervical nerve block, used for abortions performed under local anesthesia. It is only minimally painful. Since the effects of cocaine, like the effects of dental nerve blocks, wear off, alcohol or dilute solutions of a potent poison (phenol) can be used instead of local anesthetics to destroy nerve fibers permanently. However, there are no detailed studies of the effects of these injections, and they are not in current use.

Presacral neurectomy is a more extensive operation that interrupts pelvic nerves behind the peritoneum, in front of the spinal cord. It works better (and longer) than the LUNA procedure, but it may damage the nerves needed for emptying the bladder, and it may cause constipation. Presacral neurectomy is usually performed through a lower abdominal incision, although experts have performed it laparoscopically. According to sources at Blue Cross/Blue Shield, this operation has been so extensively abused that most often their plans do not pay for it. The operation may have a role during surgery for severe endometriosis, and it does help painful periods. It can, perhaps, be tried if your pains are felt in the middle of your pelvis only: pain that gynecologists call "midline pain." However, it has not helped my chronic pelvic pain patients and cannot, as a rule, be recommended as a solution.

I recall one woman who came to me, expressly asking for presacral neurectomy. After a lengthy discussion, she departed, clearly not happy with my ideas. She called in triumph about a month later to tell me that she had the surgery done elsewhere and was at long last pain free. I congratulated her, thanked her for calling me, and wished her well. Two or three months later, she called again, to tell me that her pains were back, virtually unchanged. This time I persuaded her to try nonsurgical treatments, which gave her relief that was less complete but lasted longer.

Adhesiolysis: John F. Steege, a gynecologist at Duke University Medical Center in Durham, North Carolina, has reported his experiences in using **laser adhesiolysis** to relieve CPP in thirty patients. One of the difficulties of evaluating adhesiolysis is that the adhesions reappear within a month or two of the procedure. During the surgery, Steege took particular care to prevent the reformation of adhesions by covering surgical sites with a material called Interceed, which may prevent recurrences. Steege and his coworker, the psychologist Anna L. Stout, concluded that (based on their patients' extensive symptoms) ten women had a chronic pain syndrome. The twenty women who did not have this condition obtained significantly more relief from the surgery than did the ten who were thought to have it. Painful intercourse was particularly difficult to help, and most patients reported no change in this annoying complaint. Some improved, but a few got worse, a troublesome and incomprehensible outcome after surgery. Overall, the ten women with extensive symptoms did very poorly. Most improved temporarily but relapsed within months of the operation. Although the reformation of adhesions remains a possibility, reoperating every few months can hardly be recommended. Since medications such as Pirfenidone, used in Europe to prevent the formation of fibrous tissue cells, are not available in the United States, state-of-the-art surgery was not the answer for these women.

Stout and Steege concluded that patients with chronic pain syndromes had less to gain from surgery and expressed a preference for nonsurgical treatments. Most gynecologists wish that the solution to the problems faced by women with CPP were as simple as operating and dividing adhesions. The fact that this procedure has not, in over a century of surgery, emerged as a remedy is, I think, telling in itself. However, meticulously performed adhesiolysis, using techniques similar to Steege's, may prove useful, at least for patients not suffering from chronic pain states.

Views similar to those of Steege and Stout are heard increasingly often from gynecologists with laparoscopic laser skills, and any surgery that might offer lasting help should be welcomed. It is hoped that laser adhesiolysis will help at least some women with CPP and that it will eventually become recognized as effective surgery. Severe adhesions involving the bowel are thought to be definite cause of pain at least by some gynecologists. Meanwhile, perhaps we should still regard laser adhesiolysis as an experimental idea, and women should exercise caution before undergoing adhesiolysis to relieve pain. In competent hands, adhesiolysis is a reasonably safe operation; complications have been rare—but occasionally they have been catastrophic. If you have not had laparoscopy and this operation is scheduled, it would make sense to have the laparoscopy performed by an expert surgeon skilled at adhesiolysis.

Chronic Pelvic Pain and Hysterectomy

Finally, there is the possibility of **hysterectomy.** Among Steege's thirty patients, ten were thought to have a chronic pain syndrome. Not fewer than eight of these ten women had already undergone hysterectomy to relieve their CPP. This finding emphasizes something well known to gynecologists: Hysterectomy cannot be relied upon to relieve CPP. Nevertheless, as mentioned earlier, large numbers of hysterectomies are performed annually in the United States in the often desperate search for the relief of pelvic pain.

It is very difficult to know how much pain relief may be gained from hysterectomy. Opinions based on the experiences of any gynecologist are subjective and vary enormously. If dissatisfied women leave the gynecologist without complaining, he or she is left with grateful patients, and the operation is believed to be successful. If patients worsen after the surgery and begin to complain about their predicament, surgical enthusiasm will wither rapidly. Perhaps the strongest argument against hysterectomy is something all experts have noticed: the tendency of the pain to return months or even years after the operation. An argument in favor of hysterectomy consists of the fact that a number of recent studies cautiously claim that for some women at least, hysterectomy will relieve pain.

Remarkably, there are few studies of the effects of hysterectomy on women with CPP. Contrary to most expert opinion of previous years, the authors of the first study, Drs. Thomas G. Stovall, Frank W. Ling, and Donald A. Crawford of the University of Tennessee found that hysterectomy is reasonably successful in relieving CPP. Appearing in the April 1990 issue of *Obstetrics and Gynecology,* their article reported the results of hysterectomies on 99 women who had their surgery at Baptist Memorial Hospital in Memphis. These 99 operations were collected from a total of 500 performed during the five years from 1982 through 1987, a considerable experience. The age range of the women ranged from 20 to 51, with an average of 34 years. I was astonished when I read this paper. In various Midwestern and Northeastern academic hospitals that I am familiar with, not to mention British teaching hospitals (with the exception of Beard's hospital, St. Mary's in London), it was virtually unheard of to undertake even one hysterectomy for the relief of pelvic pain. It also seemed absurd to perform such an operation on a twenty-year-old woman, although such a judgment cannot be offered in the absence of clinical details that might have made for a more convincing case for the hysterectomy.

The authors reported that among the 99 women whose charts were available for at least a full year after surgery, 77 were free of pain after hysterectomy. Unfortunately, 22 had persistent pain, and 5 of the 22 were in significantly more pain than they had before surgery. To my disappointment, the paper shed no light at all on the cause of the pain or why almost one-fourth of the patients did not improve or actually got worse. Most important, endometriosis was not mentioned as one of the abnormalities identified in the specimens removed, sharply undercutting the claim that endometriosis is the secret cause of much CPP.

If this were the entire picture, at least one could offer women with CPP a simple statement: With hysterectomy, there is a 75-percent chance of improvement and a 25-percent chance of no change, or even the very small but inexplicable possibility of deterioration. Unfortunately, it is difficult to be sure of the reliability of this study. The authors did not interview any of the women; they merely reviewed their charts. Such appraisals are not as accurate as questioning patients, for instance, to find out if they developed other possibly severe symptoms after surgery. An even more troublesome consideration is that of 500 women, only 99 qualified to be included in the study. One reason for excluding women was that their medical course could not be followed from chart reviews for at least one year after surgery. Suppose that there were women whose pains got so much worse after surgery that they left the clinic in disgust, never to return. They were now excluded from the study because they were not helped. Had they been identified and included in the study, a reevaluation of the authors' conclusions would have been in order, very likely diminishing the value of hysterectomy. However, this paper, while seriously flawed, drew attention to the fact that contrary to expert gynecological opinions, hysterectomy was apparently successful in relieving CPP in at least some women. Further, the study confirmed that hysterectomy made CPP worse in a smaller but appreciable number of other women.

In recent years, some experts have become less harsh with views against hysterectomy. For instance, Richard Beard, in London, who previously did not advocate hysterectomy, has reported (with six coauthors) on a small number of such operations with good results. Beard believes that the pain may originate in dilated and congested pelvic veins, a notion already discussed. Since these veins drain blood from the womb as well as from the ovaries, Beard removed these organs from 36 women, who were between 27 and 46 years old, with an average age of 35.3 years. Five of his patients had no children, and 31 had at least 2 children. All the women were given hormone replacements after surgery; all were reexamined periodically, including an examination a year after the surgery. The results were unexpectedly good: 24 were completely relieved of their CPP, 11 were substantially relieved, and 1 improved "somewhat." None were unchanged, and none deteriorated. After hysterectomy, the frequency of intercourse increased significantly, from an average of once per month to eight times a month. Postcoital ache, previously a frequent occurrence in all, disappeared in 29 women, improved in 4, and was not recorded in 3.

Interviewed in London in late 1992, Professor Beard discussed his CPP research. His group found that about 60 percent of women with CPP had a traumatic childhood. Many were orphaned at an early age and had formed troublesome relationships with parents and stepparents. Others developed CPP after childbirth or a gynecological illness. Many had small ovarian cysts. Beard's treatments and ideas combine physical with psychosomatic causes.

Reasoning that hysterectomy may not be essential to remove the distended veins, Beard started another project. Instead of hysterectomy, his patients underwent the laparoscopic removal of their ovaries and tubes. This operation excises most of the tissues that contain the veins, which, unfortunately, are difficult to remove without such drastic surgery. Again, his patients improved. The premature menopause that resulted was treated with hormones, a subject discussed in Chapter 14. Pregnancy was still achievable through elaborate and expensive means, using donated ova and assisted reproductive (in vitro fertilization) technology.

Other articles, appearing during the mid–1990s, indicated that hysterectomy was, again contrary to expert opinion, successful in relieving CPP. Karen J. Carlson, reporting in 1994 on over 400 hysterectomies performed in Maine, found that there was substantial pain relief after surgery. However, this study included CPP patients lumped together with women whose pains were caused by fibroids and other diseases. This is not as clear-cut an answer as I'd like to have—but at least the paper noted that few women reported new gynecological problems after hysterectomy. More important, in 1995 Susan D. Hillis, Ph.D., and her associates reported on over 300 hysterectomies performed on women with CPP. Their conclusion was that almost three-fourths of these women experienced complete resolution of the pain, about 20 percent had partial relief, and only 5 percent were unchanged or got worse. Women under thirty years of age, uninsured women (or those on welfare), and women whose tissues, after surgery, showed no disease were the most likely to report continued pain.

It is amazing that we cannot answer an apparently simple question clearly and definitively: Might hysterectomy help women who have CPP? One authoritative monograph, *Chronic Pelvic Pain: An Integrated Approach,* written by five prominent experts, sponsored by responsible independent organizations, and published as recently as January 2000, does not even mention hysterectomy as a choice. On the contrary, guidelines issued by the American College of Obstetricians and Gynecologists (ACOG Technical Bulletin No. 223, May 1996) outline very specifically under what circumstances hysterectomy should be performed. There are good reasons for such disagreements, and they have to do with the precise and elaborate statistical studies that gynecologists require for definitive answers. Without these statistics (and I regret to add that they are so demanding and complex that they might never become available) what we have are "expert opinions"—opinions overly dependent on the personal experiences of the experts.

These are all thought-provoking and troublesome studies to ponder. I am disturbed by these operations that seem to work for some, or for many, but fail at least a few others and make a few patients worse. However, I find it easier to remain open to what may be helpful new information than to reject studies because they clash with my experiences and convictions. According to the articles I cited, some CPP patients may be helped by hysterectomy with or without the removal of their ovaries. It also appears likely that if no disease is identified and the woman comes from a disadvantaged group, with poor education, poor medical insurance, and no job, her surgery is much more likely to fail. At the time these words are written, in late 2000, this remains an open and controversial issue, with only the information cited to help you decide.

The usual response to reports such as those described is to repeat the studies. This, of course, means more hysterectomies. However, the objective is not to cling to our prejudices but to get the facts as clear as possible and to try to help people in pain. I am not eager to perform hysterectomies solely to relieve pain but cannot dispute that on occasion it has helped. I can recall doing a hysterectomy for pelvic pain only once during the last twenty years. This patient was Irene, a hospital employee who was in my care three or four years before we agreed on hysterectomy. Irene was in her late thirties and had already had four or five operations for pain—not an unusual story. Some of these were to remove ovarian cysts, but there was also an adhesiolysis and an appendectomy. To correct a retroverted ("tipped back") uterus, she also underwent a so-called suspension procedure, all to no avail. By the time she became my patient, she had also been using BCPs to inhibit the formation of ovarian cysts, antibiotics against infections, and other treatments without relief. Now she had another medium-sized ovarian cyst, small fibroids, and irregular bleeding. In addition, her pains were getting worse again. From previous surgical notes, I knew that Irene had many adhesions, and I thought she probably had, in effect, a residual ovary syndrome. (This condition is mentioned earlier, in Chapter 10; this usually develops after hysterectomy, when the ovary is buried deep in adhesions and tends to form cysts instead of ovulating cleanly into an adhesion-free peritoneal cavity.) Irene's adhesions had probably recurred, and she was anxious to have a hysterectomy. I thought that this was not an unreasonable plan and agreed to go ahead, as long as she understood that I could not guarantee that she would be pain free afterward.

Irene obtained a second opinion from a gynecologist with a national reputation, who agreed with the operation. Pelvic pain was not regarded as a reason for hysterectomy at the hospital where the surgery was to be performed. I gave the pathologist a list of all the operations Irene had had, explaining that the recurring cysts, the pain, the adhesions, and the fibroids were all indications for operating.

Because of the adhesions, Irene had a difficult hysterectomy, in the course of which I removed one badly scarred ovary and left the other where I thought it would not become entangled in the adhesions she was likely to develop. The pathologist called me two days later because of an unexpected finding: High in the cervical canal there was an area of marked precancerous change. This was an instance of misleading, "false-negative" Pap smears, taken not only in my office but also in the office of the gynecologist who provided the second opinion consultation. The growth had escaped detection because none of the Pap smears picked up any cells from the precancerous area. Irene was not entirely free of pain after this operation, but she certainly improved. Cancers high in the cervical canal are often detected late and therefore have a poor outcome; the hysterectomy probably saved her life. However, this was a lucky coincidence, one that has no bearing on hysterectomy for CPP.

Chronic Pain Clinics

Medical science has not been very successful with chronic pain, as witnessed by women and men with chronic headaches, backaches, or pain due to metastatic cancer, or from arthritis, temporo-mandibular joint pains, and pain in countless other sites from which it will not budge. There has always been an impasse between patients in severe, unremitting pain and a profession generally not too good at helping them. The recognition of chronic pain states has changed this situation. This corner of medicine owes its existence to John J. Bonica, a visionary physician who pioneered the introduction of multidisciplinary pain clinics. Pain clinics place less emphasis on the diagnosis and concentrate more on pain relief, regardless of its cause. They treat chronic pain with a variety of methods, most of them nonsurgical.

However, the patient is no longer a passive recipient of treatments. Instead, he or she is actively involved in the process of obtaining pain relief.

Pain clinics are usually the last resort for women for whom all other approaches have failed. They offer treatments that may give substantial pain relief to some without much patient participation; for others, they will find at least partial relief after involving patients in their own care. There is, however, a major financial difficulty to be faced: Almost all forms of medical care in the United States are expensive, and pain clinics are not excepted. The emergence of HMO-financed care, with its emphasis on limiting costs, has placed pain clinics out of the reach of many. If your medical insurance is good, you may be referred to a pain clinic without trouble. However, if you belong to some form of "managed care"—another euphemism for cutting costs—you may find substantial resistance from "gatekeepers" (physicians, nurses, or administrators charged with limiting access to expensive modes of care) to such an idea. There is evidence that pain clinics save money by providing effective care that speeds recovery; nevertheless it occurs commonly that the problems faced by people with pain-related illnesses are minimized or disregarded.

Pain clinics are usually directed by an anesthesiologist or a neurologist; others may be led by physicians trained in rehabilitation medicine. They have access to consultants in other fields: internists, orthopedists, psychologists or psychiatrists, gynecologists, neurosurgeons, and other specialists as required. Most of their work is for patients who come to the clinic by appointment; there is the occasional emergency; and some patients are admitted to a hospital or other facility as inpatients. Most important, while pain clinics differ from each other in the way they are organized, virtually all of them offer care described as interdisciplinary or multimodal: Care is individualized and coordinated, using the knowledge and skills of various specialists.

Chronic Pain Clinics—Treatments

Medications

A number of drugs have already been noted: analgesics and narcotics used to relieve pain, certain hormones, antidepressants, antibiotics, the GnRH agonists, and so on. Women registering in pain clinics have usually exhausted these without relief, which is why they have decided, as a last resort, to try pain clinics. Other medications are available from the neurologists, particularly gabapentin (Neurontin) and mexiletine.

Physical Treatments

Acupuncture. Although it originated in China, acupuncture has become a mainstream Western therapy. Acupuncture consists of the temporary insertion of sterile needles at strategically selected locations in the patient's body; it may provide sufficient pain relief to allow major surgery without general anesthesia. The precise mechanism whereby acupuncture works is unknown but is thought to involve the stimulation of pain fibers, distracting the nervous system from other, stronger signals originating in deeper organs. Other theories involve the release of neurotransmitters, including natural morphine-like compounds, caused by the needles. Of course, *precision* is a Western concept; Oriental explanations of acupuncture state that the needles restore a more balanced flow of energy along channels and meridians.

Acupuncture works well to relieve pain, and it is unusually safe as long as it does not distract attention from other, well-established medical procedures. I know of one young man who died because a tumor he developed was treated by means of acupuncture instead of surgery and chemotherapy.

Transcutaneous Electrical Nerve Stimulation, or **TENS**: TENS uses a small, battery-powered device to stimulate the patient's skin. To treat chronic backaches and CPP, the device is usually strapped to the patient's lower abdomen or over her lower back. TENS has given long-term relief to a few women with CPP, but there are no large-scale studies to attest to its effectiveness.

Trigger Point Injections. Trigger point injections consist of multiple injections of local anesthetics such as Lidocaine or Marcaine into sites identified by a physician's careful palpation of the patient's skin as trigger points. Other substances such as steroids or saline (saltwater) may also be injected into appropriate sites. These injections are thought to disrupt trigger points or to block the transmission of signals that register in the brain as pain.

Dr. Slocumb's treatment of CPP patients described in Chapter 10 uses trigger point injections combined with other treatments, apparently with excellent results.

Massage. For centuries, it has been known that gentle irritation of skin surfaces may relieve pain originating from deeper tissues or organs. The use of liniments to soothe aching muscles after strenuous exercise is an example of this principle. Massage is in frequent use in chronic pain clinics; its mechanism of action may depend on similar principles. A variety of specialized massage techniques may be used. The Alexander technique for backaches and Shiatsu are well-known examples of massage-based treatments. There are others, including osteopathic and chiropractic methods. All have enthusiastic and committed adherents, but it is difficult to know how effective these methods are. They are certainly safe; if they don't work or if the beneficial effects wear off, only time and money have been spent.

Superior Hypogastric Plexus Blocks. These high-technology injections are used as a last resort to obtain relief from severe pain. They consist of the injection of a local anesthetic agent into a nerve center deep in the abdomen. If there is good relief from intractable pain, alcohol or other substances such as phenol may be injected by anesthesiologists as permanent treatment. The injections have an uncertain duration of action. While immediate and dramatic pain relief may be obtained, complications such as persistent diarrhea may also result.

Other aggressive, expensive, and complex treatments include the injection of various medications (morphine-like drugs, local anesthetics, and other drugs) into the space surrounding the spinal cord. If successful, pumps containing a reservoir of medications can be implanted under the skin. The pump continuously delivers appropriate doses of medications that bathe and anesthetize nerves as they emerge from the spinal cord. Unfortunately, such treatments are unusually expensive—the cost of the first year of care is often above $10,000. You may argue that this is not a vast sum, or that the costs of months of work missed because of severe pain exceed this sum, or that not extending such care amounts to discrimination. There are other arguments, too; the problem is that you will not be arguing with doctors; the arguments will be between you and your physicians on one side and various employees of the organization that pays for your medical care on the other side—in other words, not an equal struggle.

Psychological Treatments

Pain clinics also use psychological treatments consisting of relaxation techniques, hypnosis, biofeedback, and behavior therapy. Other methods such as meditation, yoga, and cognitive therapy may also be employed.

Relaxation Therapy. Originally conceived as a treatment for anxiety states, relaxation therapy has been found to be useful in managing pain as well. Like other psychological treatments, relaxation therapy is best combined with physical treatments such as acupuncture and other psychological treatments. Relaxation therapy teaches techniques such as deep breathing exercises and guided imagery as distractions from the pain. This therapy requires no equipment and is usually well accepted by patients wary of conventional psychotherapy.

Hypnosis. Hypnosis has been accepted as a reliable treatment by both the American Medical Association (AMA) and the British Medical Association (BMA). It has been used increasingly in the management of chronic pain states. Not everyone is easy to hypnotize, but patients in whom a hypnotic trance can be induced may enjoy striking pain relief without having to worry about a wide range of complications.

Biofeedback. Biofeedback uses special equipment to familiarize patients with selected bodily functions such as tension in selected muscles, blood pressure, sweating, or the pulse rate. Changes in these functions are measured and the information is fed back as audible signals to patients, who are taught to recognize their responses to emotionally charged ideas. With practice, the correlation between emotions and symptoms becomes apparent, resulting in pain relief.

Behavior Therapy. Behavior therapy is not an easy concept to explain. Briefly, the therapist and the patient attempt to modify the patient's behavior and his or her environment to improve communications and diminish interpersonal stresses. Relatives, friends, support groups, and other influential parties may also be asked to participate in behavior therapy.

Some patients derive relief from one of the above therapies, applied by one trusted practitioner. Others find more permanent relief if a number of these therapies are applied in an organized program, almost always taking place in a center specializing in the treatment of chronic pain.

It is very difficult to know which of these treatments will provide the most pain relief for particular patients. After listening to women with CPP as well as experts on chronic pain and studying the methods outlined, I believe the best methods combine acupuncture, antidepressants, and at least one of the psychological methods outlined above.

Cancer and the Uterus

When cancers of the female genital organs are diagnosed, some combination of surgery, radiation, and hormonal or chemotherapy is usually unavoidable. However, this stark recommendation emphatically does not apply to a range of less serious conditions of the cervix or the endometrium usually described as "precancerous," "premalignant," or "preinvasive." Fortunately, the process of reaching an exact diagnosis is rarely complicated. The crucial step is to distinguish outright, "invasive" cancer—a term we'll discuss shortly—from its forerunners, which doctors call by any of the three adjectives just listed; the term "precursor" is also used. However, women must watch out for something that may be presented either openly, as an unbending view, or covertly, as a sly innuendo: that even if there is no cancer to be found in the uterus now, nor an immediate precursor, its appearance in the distant future must be prevented through hysterectomy. Except for women with a strong family history of breast and ovarian cancer, such statements are often exaggerated, adding to the toll of unnecessary hysterectomies.

Paula, whom I knew socially, was the thirty-five-year-old friend of one of my patients. She gave me a panicked call around 10 P.M. one evening some years ago. She was planning to have her tubes tied and had a new and well-recommended gynecologist take a Pap smear as part of her preoperative evaluation. The abnormal result led to colposcopy, a term we'll discuss shortly, in the course of which cervical biopsies were taken. These showed a condition of her cervix then called "moderate dysplasia." Her gynecologist exaggerated the seriousness of the situation, frightening Paula toward a hysterectomy. Paula became my patient and had a much simpler but equally effective treatment. Five minutes of cryosurgery, or freezing the cervix, cured her. She postponed the surgery on her tubes and had one more child; we never had to discuss hysterectomy again. Cryosurgery has been supplanted by better treatments, but the principle still applies: Short of invasive cancer, it is usually possible to resect or otherwise remove the most dangerous areas, leaving behind healthy tissues or tissues that can be expected to recover. Sad to say, Paula's was not an unusual story, but one heard with disheartening regularity.

Women have also been frightened by recent reports about the unreliability of Pap smears, which have helped diminish deaths due to cervical cancer. Like virtually all investigations, Pap tests have on occasion given anxiety-fueling misinformation. However, it is not difficult to protect yourself against reports that are overly alarming or misleadingly reassuring. Having vaginal infections that occasionally lead to abnormal Pap smears treated, getting additional Pap smears, and undergoing colposcopy (discussed later in this chapter) will almost always provide an accurate diagnosis. A number of modern versions of the traditional Pap smear have also appeared; in due course we'll discuss the advantages and disadvantages of these improvements.

Cervical cancer was lethal for generations of women in the past, but with reasonably good care, it is highly unlikely that you will ever develop this condition. Modern investigations have also simplified the early diagnosis of endometrial cancer. These two cancers may be prevented through the detection and treatment of precancerous conditions. Unfortunately, if you do not understand the ideas and language used by gynecologists and your questions are not answered satisfactorily, you may find that you are receiving second-rate care. This includes the possibility that hysterectomy will be recommended (and performed) for insufficient reasons. This almost happened to Paula and still happens whenever women are frightened by the calculated use of the word "cancer." Armed with basic information and an understanding of gynecological ideas and language, you will be able to ask for and receive safe and effective care.

There are four major female cancers: breast, cervical, endometrial, and ovarian. Diseases of the breast are beyond the purview of this book but are thoroughly presented in *Dr. Susan Love's Breast Book* by Love and Lindsey (Perseus Books, 2000). While the fallopian tubes and the vagina spontaneously turn cancerous very rarely, so-called "DES daughters" are at an increased risk of cancer of the vagina. DES (diethylstilbestrol) was the first estrogenic hormone to be synthesized; much later, it was used in an effort prevent miscarriages. This use continued until the 1960s, even after it was shown to be ineffective. To be fair to physicians, the notion that a medication taken by a pregnant woman might damage her baby was virtually unheard of during the fifties—there were fewer drugs, few of them toxic. Twenty years later, the dimensions of the DES disaster began to unfold. Even if your mother took DES while she was pregnant with you (and such cases occur less and less often as the generation of women who used DES for this purpose becomes menopausal), vaginal cancer remains an unlikely possibility. This tragedy usually followed the use of DES from the second through the fourth months of pregnancy and was typically estimated at about one vaginal cancer in each group of 1,000 DES daughters. The resulting cancers were treated with extensive surgery—excising the cancer, then possibly reconstructing the vagina. Reproductive difficulties in DES daughters—such as repeated miscarriages—have been a much more frequent consequence of the maternal use of DES. And in case you are curious: DES taken by pregnant women also damaged their male newborns, although cancer was not a consequence. Testicular damage and problems fathering children were the difficulties most often reported by urologists looking after such men.

Cancers of the breasts, the cervix, and the endometrium are now easier to diagnose at an early, more treatable stage; only ovarian cancer continues to defy efforts at early detection and effective treatment. In this chapter, diseases of the cervix and the endometrial lining of the womb are discussed; ovarian cancer will be discussed in Chapter 14.

Cancer of the Cervix

The cervix is so easy to find, to look at, and to biopsy that cancer in this site is better understood than cancer in any other organ. We know little about the causes of pancreatic or brain cancer; more is known about smoking and lung cancer or sunlight and melanomas. In contrast, there is abundant and precise information about why and how cervical cancer develops, how it may be prevented, and how best to treat it.

The villain of cervical cancer is the **human papillomavirus (HPV)**, the cause of genital or venereal warts as well as cervical cancer. The process that leads to cancer begins in women who became sexually active at an early age, with the papillomavirus finding an easy entry into the **mucosa**, the delicate skinlike covering of the cervix. The source of the virus is the skin covering the penis of an affected male, and the virus is picked up by women during intercourse without condoms. In teenage boys, who are often the silent carriers of the virus, the skin may look perfectly normal. Even years later, it may require using a magnifying glass (or a **colposcope**) on the skin of the penis to reveal the tiny bumps and telltale plaques that signal the presence of the virus. Such skin is surreptitiously shedding HPV, infecting cervical cells. Acquiring such an infection may also occur years later, but the sequence that ultimately leads to cervical cancer often seems to start in the relatively immature cervical cells of teenagers.

Years before cancer appears, the cells that make up the surface of the cervix begin to develop changes described as premalignant or precancerous. These go by a variety of names and abbreviations: dysplasia, low-grade and high-grade CIN (cervical intraepithelial neoplasia), carcinoma *in situ,* and SIL (squamous intraepithelial lesion) are all terms in recent or current use. More important, some of the earliest precancerous changes are mild and may disappear with simple medical measures such as the treatment of vaginal and cervical infections with antibiotics or the consistent use of condoms for six to nine months. These treatments rely on a balance between the damage caused by repeated exposure to the papillomavirus, and a normally functioning immune system, which destroys abnormal cells, hastening healing. Unfortunately, there is no guarantee that healing will be complete. Also, the more advanced the cervical disease, the less likely it is to retreat to a lesser grade of severity or to disappear. The recent epidemic of infections with HPV has made cancer specialists very cautious about undertaking unaggressive treatment plans. Faced with a potentially lethal process, few women (and even fewer gynecologists) will choose an option that calls for years of observation with colposcopies and biopsies without definitive, virtually guaranteed-to-succeed treatment.

Cervical cancer has been known for decades to be a venereal disease, one associated with intercourse at an early age and with multiple partners. Catholic nuns, for example, do not get cervical cancer; reportedly, only one nun ever developed cervical cancer, and she ultimately revealed that before becoming a nun, she was very promiscuous. This story might be apocryphal, but such ideas should not be discussed with women who have recently been found to have cervical cancer or its precursors. They are upset enough without the guilt and self-blame such information causes, and the theories add nothing to effective care. Instead, I regularly advise teenagers to use condoms not only to prevent pregnancy but also the common venereal diseases syphilis and gonorrhea. Infections with the viruses of HPV and HIV are the final and strongest argument in favor of the use of condoms. No one ever knows for sure who has had (or is still having) intercourse with whom. Intravenous drug use, homosexuality, bisexuality, and intercourse with more than one partner may be closely guarded secrets. Negative HIV tests in both partners combined with monogamy may eliminate these anxieties, but for many women, condoms are a must.

Older studies indicated that cancer is more likely to develop in women who are married to men whose previous wives developed cervical cancer. This implied an infectious agent, spread from men to women, although, of course, the virus also passes from women to men. More recently, certain strains within the large family of papillomaviruses have been implicated. Laboratory tests are available to identify which strain, if any, might be multiplying in a woman's cervical cells, but these tests have not achieved much acceptance among gynecologists. However, these strains appear to be able to damage the chromosomes of cervical cells more rapidly than previously thought possible. This bears a certain resemblance to the transmission of AIDS. In both cases, intimate contact, sexual or other, is required. Years after what may have been a brief relationship (or even a one-night affair), the virus may surface and cause the development of lethal diseases. Condoms may not offer perfect contraception or guaranteed protection against venereal diseases, including cervical cancer and AIDS, but they are simple and effective measures and are highly recommended.

As HPV infects the cervix, millions of viruses lodge in sheets of cervical cells, and the chromosomal material in these cells begins to undergo a drastic change. Layers of cells that used to grow in an orderly fashion now begin to grow abnormally and at an accelerated pace. Previously they adhered to each other; now they break away from each other. As long as these changes are confined to the surface of mucosal skin, the illness is localized and treatable in your gynecologist's office. This is true even for the most advanced form, which is often referred to as carcinoma *in situ:* a localized, noninvasive form of cancer. Perhaps it should be called "not-yet-invasive-cancer": If not treated, the cells begin to push against the **basement membrane**, a strong, leathery sheet of cells in the skin covering the cervix, and in due course they penetrate it. This event resembles a small group of rowdy hooligans breaking through a solid barrier, followed by a crowd, spreading out and causing mayhem.

Similarly, with the basement membrane penetrated, cancerous cells begin to stream into surrounding tissues. This crucial and potentially deadly event is signified by the word "invasive." The malignant cells have broken through; they have escaped from their original site and are now ranging further into new locations. They may be picked up by the lymphatic system, vessels that slowly sweep lymphatic fluid and cancerous cells toward nearby lymph glands. Some weeks or months later, these glands can no longer contain the spread of the cells, and as they allow the malignant cells to pass through, lymph glands further away are invaded. From the cervix, this process usually takes many months to become widespread, although in other sites (for instance, in the ovary) a much faster rate of spread occurs. The cancerous cells soon range so widely that it may no longer be possible to remove them all, even by cutting out large blocks of tissue such as the entire uterus. Such a cancer was initially operable, but it can no longer be excised completely. This explains the need for additional treatments such as chemotherapy, radiation, or one of the more experimental immunotherapies.

Cervical cancer has killed teenagers, for instance, young prostitutes from Miami, in whom the disease must have developed with unprecedented speed, probably the consequence of an infection with a virulent strain of the papillomavirus. Gynecologists do not support intermittent federal efforts to lengthen the recommended interval between Pap smears to save money. Once a year seems a reasonable minimum interval for this inexpensive test, but more frequent Pap smears are recommended if you began your sexual life at an early age and have had numerous partners.

Today we know that AIDS, because it ruins the immune system, also allows the accelerated development of cervical cancer. In some municipal clinics that serve large populations of indigent women, a high proportion of patients may test positive for HIV. Cervical cancer is frequent in such settings. The lessons from this are that using condoms regularly and getting Pap smears at least once a year (and perhaps more often) are essential. If the Pap shows abnormal cells, the source must be meticulously identified and treated.

To return to less extreme circumstances, you may want to look at the exact language in the report that gave you the news of the abnormal Pap smear. A number of terms are used; some are more ominous than others. If your smear is abnormal, you will come across words and phrases such as the ones shown in Table 12.1. However, unless the phrase "invasive cancer" is used, most likely you don't have cervical cancer.

TABLE 12.1   Pap Smear Reports

Language Used	Meaning
Normal	No abnormal cell identified.
Specimen unsatisfactory	Not enough cells or poorly preserved cells—best to repeat Pap smear.
Atypia of known significance Reactive or reparative changes Inflammatory chances Squamous metaplasia Atrophy Trichomonas, Monilia, bacteria, or other organisms noted	These descriptions indicate that the effects of infection, inflammation, repair process, or aging have been noted. Treatment may be required, but cancer is not suspected.
Atypia of undetermined significance (ASCUS)	Abnormal cells are present, but not abnormal enough to classify as inflammatory or precancerous. Treatment may be prescribed. Must be investigated by at least a repeat Pap smear in 3–4 months or by colposcopy.
Low-grade squamous cell lesion, HPV, koilocytosis, mild dysplasia, CIN 1 (Cervical Intraepithelial Neoplasia)	Abnormal cells are present and colposcopy with or without biopsy is recommended to confirm diagnosis. Cancer is unlikely. Treatment not absolutely essential because many of these abnormalities disappear spontaneously. Follow-up essential.
Cancer: squamous cell carcinoma or Adenocarcinoma	Colposcopy and biopsy are needed urgently.
Sperm	Recent intercourse, sperm identified.

Abnormal Pap smears are investigated by means of a group of procedures collectively called **colposcopy**. Colposcopy itself is pain free: A
speculum is inserted, the cervix is cleansed with vinegar and is then inspected with a colposcope, which enlarges the cervix eightfold or tenfold,
or more if needed. Vinegar (acetic acid) makes abnormal areas easy to identify, and these are next biopsied. A **biopsy** is a tiny sample of tissue, removed with sharp forceps. This may be pain free or somewhat painful, particularly if the instrument with which the biopsy is taken is not sharp.
Depending on how widespread the abnormal area appears, one, or two, or
three biopsies may be taken, each as small as a pea. It is rare that three biopsies are not enough and more must be taken.

The pain of having a biopsy taken may be lessened by taking a pain
medication such as Aleve, Motrin, Anaprox, or Tylenol with codeine half an
hour or an hour before the biopsy is taken. Not all gynecologists recommend this simple precaution routinely. If you are exceptionally sensitive to
pain, even a tranquilizer may be added or a nerve block given with a small-
gauge needle. For even more pain relief, intravenous drugs may be used.
However, these measures require more than the usual gynecological office
and staff, and they are rarely needed. The facilities are usually available, but
if you think you will need them, you may have to insist on getting them
well before your turn to undergo colposcopy arrives.

Another type of biopsy, called **endocervical curettage** (**ECC**), is often
added. This procedure, less painful than cervical biopsies, consists of gently
scraping (curetting) the cervical canal, most of which is invisible. Many
cancer specialists consider the ECC an essential safeguard against a basic
error in diagnosis and treatment: that is, treating a less serious lesion on the
outer, visible part of the cervix, unaware that a more serious, even cancerous condition may be lurking an inch higher. If your gynecologist does not
specifically discuss the ECC, you may mention casually that you know
about this test and ask for his or her reasons for omitting it. The ECC is
uncomfortable but rarely painful; most of my patients have found it easier
to tolerate than the cervical biopsies.

All the tissues obtained through biopsy are sent to a pathologist, who has
them stained and then examines thin slices, mounted on glass slides, under
a microscope. The report should be available to your gynecologist (and to
you) within a few days or a week. The delay depends mostly on where the
pathologist works, how the biopsies are sent, and how the reports are re-

turned. In order to prevent delays due to reports lost in the mail or otherwise mislaid, a good laboratory will call the gynecologist if cancer is identified.

The terms used in the pathologist's report are explained in Table 12.2:

Asking for a photocopy of Pap smear and biopsy reports is not routine, but there is no reason why the exact language of the report should not be available to you. I know one woman who left her gynecologist because his office staff did not have standing orders to give out all the information

TABLE 12.2   Cervical and ECC Biopsy Reports

NORMAL Cervical Biopsy	

Normal epithelium
Squamous metaplasia
Chronic cervicitis
Microglandular hyperplasia
	These reports are reassuring.
	  They indicate changes that are not
	  precancerous.
	Chronic cervicitis is a frequent change,
	  particularly after childbirths. Micro-
	  glandular hyperplasia is common in birth
	  control pill users.

ABNORMAL Cervical Biopsy	

Koilocytosis, HPV
Mild dysplasia, CIN I
Moderate, severe dysplasia
CIN II, III, carcinoma *in situ*
	These words and phrases indicate the
	  presence of increasingly worrisome
	  changes. They must be followed up or
	  treated. Continued care ("follow-up") is
	  needed even after treatment.

Microinvasive cancer	This is a very early cancer and must be
	  evaluated to determine how widely the
	  cancer has spread. Treatment needed may
	  be less extensive than for frankly invasive
	  cancer.

Invasive cancer: Squamous cancer or
  adenocarcinoma
	Diagnosis is established; proceed to staging
	  to determine treatment: surgery, radiation,
	  chemotherapy, or combinations of these.

ABNORMAL ECC (Endocervical Curettage)	

Koilocytosis, HPV
Dysplasia: mild, moderate, severe
CIN I, II, III, carcinoma *in situ*
	These descriptions may indicate abnormal
	  changes inside the certical canal that may
	  not be apparent by looking. A cone
	  biopsy may be needed.

Invasive cancer: squamous or
  adenocarcinoma
	Diagnosis established; proceed to staging and
	  treatment.

made available to them in the Pap smear report. In her case, this indicated the presence of yeast organisms called *actinomyces,* occasionally found in women using an intrauterine contraceptive device (IUCD). Such a report calls for a discussion of treatment options to prevent a major infection. It is important for you to get as much of the information as possible. As mentioned earlier, if you participate in your care and if you understand the language and principles used by gynecologists and pathologists, you will get better care.

Treatments

Cervical cancer is usually preventable. Once abnormalities appear, years may pass before cancer appears. Modern treatments have largely replaced older procedures such as conization of the cervix (the removal of a small, cone-shaped piece of the cervix) and prophylactic hysterectomy. The new treatments are usually less extensive and less expensive and are easier to accept. Amazingly, almost any treatment that eliminates the area in which abnormalities are developing is very likely to cure the illness, and this is true as long as cancer has not developed. The gynecologist's job is fairly easy: Make sure how severe the disease is, pinpoint all the sites involved, and arrange treatment.

Simple **electrocautery** was the oldest treatment, but it has been abandoned in the United States, because electrocautery burned away tissue, which could not be examined under a microscope by a pathologist. Electrocautery was superseded by conization, which allowed for careful microscopic examination, an important step in distinguishing cancer from less serious conditions.

Conization has also become largely obsolete. It is still used if there is some unusual feature that calls for it—for instance, ominous Pap reports from women whose colposcopy and biopsies are inconclusive. Disease high in the cervical canal, as shown by the ECC procedure, is another good reason for conization. Conization may, however, damage the cervix for future childbearing. If the accent is on preserving reproductive function, conization should be avoided as much as possible. If the accent is on making absolutely certain that there is no cancer, conizations will continue to be done. Large clinics whose patients do not always return for continued care are more apt to offer a procedure that not only diagnoses precisely but often cures the disease being investigated.

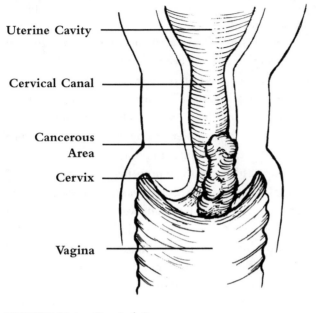

Uterine Cavity

Cervical Canal

Cancerous
Area

Cervix

Vagina

FIGURE 12.1   Cervical Cancer

Cryosurgery consists of freezing the cervix with a specially designed probe, cooled with liquid nitrogen. Freezing works because it destroys tissue just as much as heating it with electricity does. This is an outpatient procedure, minimally painful, relatively inexpensive, and successful about 90 percent of the time. If it does not work, another session of cryosurgery may solve the problem, and other treatments remain available. After frozen tissues thaw, cryosurgery is followed by about ten days of a profuse, watery discharge that is best managed with sanitary pads rather than tampons.

Laser surgery is substantially more expensive than other treatments, with roughly similar rates of cure. It is better for larger and multiple lesions and may cause less scarring than either conization or freezing the cervix (cryosurgery).

The latest innovation is the use of improved electrosurgical methods called **LEEP** (for **loop electric excision procedure**) or **LLEETZ** (for **large loop electric excision of the transformation zone**, the area in which most precancerous lesions appear). Early reports indicate that these procedures offer substantial improvements over previous methods. If there is no disease higher up in the cervical canal, as shown by a negative ECC, all the remaining work can be combined into one efficient office procedure, performed under local anesthesia.

Hysterectomy has a very limited place in the care of women with these lesions. If you have any condition short of cancer, lesser procedures should be curative. If invasive cancer is found, there is a chance that the disease is no longer confined to the cervix. Therefore, more extensive treatments are needed: radiation, a radical hysterectomy, chemotherapy, or combined treatments. In this case, simple hysterectomy (in contrast to radical hysterectomy) is not advised because results are poor.

There is one small group of patients for whom hysterectomy is appropriate. If the cervical biopsy diagnosis is **microinvasive cancer**, the cancer has broken through the basement membrane very recently, but in all likelihood it has not spread far. Microinvasion is defined as invasion less than 3 millimeters deep from the basement membrane. A conization procedure should now be performed to be sure that there is not deeper penetration in another, nearby patch of microinvasion. If there is not, simple hysterectomy is reasonable treatment, with excellent chances of a cure. Once cancer has spread deeper, lymph nodes may be involved, necessitating radical hysterectomy, radiation, or a combination of these.

Endometrial Cancer

Abnormal bleeding during the years just before or anytime after menopause is usually caused by diseases of the endometrial lining, such as **hyperplasia**. This term describes the appearance, under a microscope, of endometrial tissue obtained through biopsies or curettage. The changes may be caused by prolonged estrogenic stimulation without the balancing effect of progesterone. Bleeding may also be caused by **polyps**—fleshy, fingerlike growths that are almost always noncancerous; by hormone replacement therapy (HRT), discussed in Chapter 14; and by vaginal infections and atrophy. Abnormal bleeding, particularly after menopause, may call for investigations such as sonograms, but the most urgent need is for samples of the lining to be examined under the microscope, to exclude the possibility of cancer of the endometrium. Pap smears are virtually useless at diagnosing endometrial cancer, because the samples of cells taken for a Pap smear are from the lower cervix, whereas the cancer may be growing two or three inches higher up, inside the womb.

Complicated matters must be discussed when one of the endometrial hyperplasias are diagnosed. These conditions go by names such as **simple hyperplasia**, **cystic** or **Swiss cheese hyperplasia**, **glandular** or **adenomatous hyperplasia**, **atypical hyperplasia**, and, finally, **carcinoma *in situ*** of the endometrium. Our first difficulty is that there is much individual variation in the way pathologists use these terms, and occasionally there are disputes about the exact significance of the microscopic picture seen by two or more pathologists. There is also disagreement over whether simple and cystic hyperplasia are precancerous. If they are (and most gynecologists think they are not), then they progress to outright invasive cancer slowly, over many years, and the process is easy to interrupt. A thorough curettage may eliminate the more simple hyperplasias, and progesterone-like medications such as Provera or Megace are effective in preventing recurrences.

The precancerous tendencies of adenomatous hyperplasia are occasionally difficult to gauge precisely. The other hyperplasias (particularly atypical hyperplasia) are increasingly precancerous. Carcinoma *in situ* is the Latin name for the worst of these abnormalities short of invasive cancer. It is a localized cancer, almost ready to start its deadly invasion of surrounding tissues. Naturally, the more anxiety there is about cancer, the more pressure will be exerted toward undertaking hysterectomy. In truth, if the microscopic appearances are ominous, hysterectomy must be considered. However, it is not at all rare to come across women who were frightened into having a hysterectomy through insinuations that cancer was imminent, when the facts were much less ominous.

For years, the standard reaction to discovering *any* of the hyperplasias was to recommend hysterectomy. This was reasonable at a time when less was known about hyperplasias. The opinion in favor of hysterectomy was usually buttressed with a dictum attributed, among others, to Robert Meyer, the Austrian gynecologist whose ideas concerning endometriosis have been discussed in Chapter 7. Reacting to an instance of severe hyperplasia, Meyer reportedly said, "Nicht Karzinom, aber besser heraus." Loosely translated, this means, "Not cancer, but best removed." These days, for women whose endometrium shows no signs pathologists associate with cancerous tendencies, hysterectomy may be postponed safely.

The decision to operate (or not to operate) should come from a conference between your gynecologist and the pathologist, an expert in evaluating the microscopic appearance of tissues. Patients, either male or female, are almost never involved in such discussions, most likely because the language is likely to be incomprehensible to anyone lacking the necessary medical background. Occasionally, pathologists disagree among themselves about the exact significance of the changes observed. Further biopsies or a second curettage may be needed to obtain more tissue for analysis. Rarely, a second opinion should be obtained from a consultant pathologist; either your gynecologist or the pathologist will know how to arrange this consultation.

Treatment

For women in their thirties, the less ominous hyperplasias may be treated with a curettage, followed by efforts to reestablish ovulation by medical means. The drug usually used for this purpose is clomiphene citrate. Birth control pills may also be prescribed. If regular ovulation cannot be induced, and for women who are in their forties or older, endometrial cancer must be ruled out by means of biopsies, less often by curettage. Hormonal treatments must next be started. Most often drugs such as Provera, outlined in Chapter 8, are used. Other drugs with similar uses are megestrol acetate (Megace) and Norlutate. Depo-Provera is not approved by the FDA for this purpose, but it is a potentially useful injectable agent. There are serious medical and legal risks with using treatments not approved for specific purposes by the FDA, particularly the development of cancer during or shortly after treatment.

TABLE 12.3   Factors Increasing Your Risk of Endometrial Cancer

Obesity
Hypertension
Diabetes
Previous breast cancer
Use of estrogens without progesterone
Polycystic ovary disease
Previous heavy or irregular bleeding
Fibroids
Late menopause
Elevated lipid profile
Sonogram showing a thick and irregular endometrial lining

TABLE 12.4   Factors Decreasing Your Risk of Endometrial Cancer

Being underweight
Previous use of birth control pills
Use of progesterone with estrogen therapy
No abnormal bleeding in the past
Normal lipid profile
Sonograms showing a thin endometrial lining

After four to six months of medical treatment, it would not be unusual to rebiopsy the endometrial lining to check the effects of the medical treatment. If at any point the microscopic appearances of the endometrium are thought to be close to cancer, hysterectomy should not be discouraged.

Cancer of the endometrium, the lining of the uterus, is rare during pre-menopausal years, but there are exceptions to this rule: For instance, women who are overweight or have polycystic ovaries are at increased risk. Rarely and unaccountably, a premenopausal patient without an obvious risk factor is found to have endometrial cancer, one more instance of a woman (and her physician) receiving an inexplicable biological shock. Frequent use of endometrial biopsies after suspicious bleeding, particularly after the age of thirty-five or forty, is the only way to avoid this error. The occurrence of endometrial cancer is not entirely unpredictable. Table 12.3 shows the factors that increase your chances of developing this condition; Table 12.4 shows factors that diminish your chances of developing endometrial cancer.

Gynecologists usually believe that endometrial cancer is a disease of postmenopausal years only. The youngest woman I ever saw with this cancer was only twenty-six years old, and her diagnosis was delayed by months because her gynecologist was not aggressive enough to obtain an endometrial biopsy. The clues in her case were obesity and years of anovulatory bleeding. A tightly closed cervix did not simplify the procedure, but when the biopsy was taken, it gave the diagnosis almost immediately.

Bleeding during postmenopausal years calls for careful thinking, because cancer or precancerous conditions may be found. Rarely, an alert sonographer may notice, during an ultrasound examination, the thickened and irregular uterine lining characteristic of cancer. Less often, ovarian or tubal cancer may be diagnosed because of vaginal bleeding. The first clue to the existence of any of these conditions may be provided by an ultrasound

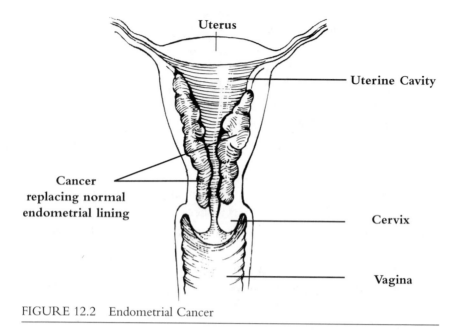

FIGURE 12.2   Endometrial Cancer

examination. If you are about to have hysteroscopy with curettage for post-menopausal bleeding, be sure that an ultrasound is taken first. You might also consider asking the technician to look at your endometrial lining carefully, and ask her (they are almost always women) to check this layer to note if it is thickened or irregular.

As noted, many postmenopausal patients bleed not because of cancer but in reaction to hormone therapy. Occasionally, nothing serious is ever found despite careful investigations. However, once cancer has been ruled out, meaning that all biopsies, sonograms, hysteroscopy, and curettage are negative, you should not be pressured into having a hysterectomy.

On occasion, unexpected disease is found. One woman I heard about had just turned seventy when she noted slight post-menopausal bleeding. She underwent all the investigations outlined above except the sonogram—she missed her appointment, which was never rescheduled. Everything was negative, yet she continued to bleed intermittently. When the sonogram was finally obtained, it showed a small mass surrounding an ovary. The mass was the body of a tubal cancer: a very rare disease, and one very difficult to diagnose at an early stage. Methodical adherence to details and to routines as well as careful thinking are required to avoid such dangerous surprises.

Other Reasons for Hysterectomy

Vaginal Bleeding

Fibroids and endometrial hyperplasias, which account for much of the abnormal bleeding experienced by women, have been discussed elsewhere in this book. Other causes include adenomyosis, polyps, cancer, breakthrough bleeding while using BCPs, and a host of other causes already discussed. However, there are several other reasons for excessive and unusual bleeding patterns you should know about. Some are related to stress. For instance, a young physician I knew told me that she usually began to spot the night before her examinations; before her final examinations, a time of exceptional stress, she bled more. Within hours of the 1987 stock market crash, a stockbroker had what she called a minor hemorrhage, although she had finished a normal period only the week before. A refugee from an East European country suddenly aborted her pregnancy of five months on hearing that her father had been arrested on trumped-up charges in her homeland. These episodes probably resulted from abrupt changes in uterine blood flow, but these ideas are speculative. It is usually impossible to investigate such events, and we can only guess at possible causes. A single bout of abnormal bleeding in a pre-menopausal woman who is not pregnant is rarely serious.

Occasionally, even a normal period might be misunderstood. Many years ago, during my residency in obstetrics and gynecology, a woman in her twenties came to the emergency room of a hospital in St. Louis, complaining of heavy vaginal bleeding. She was from the Ozarks and had recently come to St. Louis for her first job away from home. She first got pregnant at the age of twelve, before she had her first period. Subsequently, she was always either pregnant or had delivered and was nursing, thus she had never had any periods. She had also had a few miscarriages. She was familiar with these processes, but the unfamiliar bleeding and cramps took her by surprise: This was the first period she ever had. She left the hospital with much information about female physiology and a supply of BCPs, noticeably cheered by her newfound knowledge.

Sporadic abnormal bleeding is common in teenagers, in whom a normal menstrual pattern has yet to be established. It is rarely heavy; if it becomes problematic, it may be treated with low-dose BCPs. Excessive bleeding becomes more frequent again during the thirties and forties, when the womb begins to develop abnormalities. However, almost anything that goes wrong in the pelvis may involve bleeding, and textbooks cite lists of twenty or thirty less frequent but possible causes. For instance, if your gums bleed after brushing and you bleed for a long time after an accidental cut, you may have a rare bleeding tendency resembling hemophilia called von Willebrand's disease. Hemophilia itself is, for reasons involving genetics, exceptionally rare in women.

With abnormal bleeding, the first step is to determine the source of the bleeding. Your gynecologist can establish this fairly simply by inserting a speculum and identifying the cervix. Uterine and cervical bleeding may be seen flowing through the cervix, unless, of course, the bleeding has already stopped. Bleeding from the vaginal walls should be apparent immediately and should not be confused with uterine bleeding. Hemorrhoids or the bladder also may bleed, and this may confuse the picture occasionally, mostly when a language barrier prevents good communication. If you are not certain of the source of your bleeding, be sure to mention this to your gynecologist.

Bleeding originating from the vaginal walls may be due to infections, trauma, or lack of the hormone estrogen. Cancer of the vagina is rare, even in DES daughters—a topic discussed in the last chapter. These conditions may be identified through the careful use of a speculum. To survey the vaginal walls, the speculum must be turned sideways. Although this is not a comfortable experience, it is usually not too painful, either. Moreover, it is essential if there is any question about the source of the bleeding. I once examined a young woman whose syphilitic ulcer had gone unnoticed by her previous gynecologist. When he examined her, the metal blades of the speculum covered the posterior vaginal wall, the area involved. Plastic specula that are disposable have their disadvantages, too: They are cheaply made and may suddenly crack loudly or even break in mid-examination. If there is a choice, request the metal instrument. Appropriate cleansing procedures prevent the spread of communicable diseases by metal specula.

Cervical bleeding comes from polyps, cancer, infections, and erosions. If these are on the outside of the cervix, they are evident on speculum examination. Bleeding from inside the cervical canal resembles uterine bleeding flowing through the cervix, and it may take a minor operation called **hysteroscopy** to pinpoint the precise site and cause of the bleeding.

Uterine bleeding needs the most careful thinking. Pregnancy must be ruled out, because regardless of contraception, any sexually active woman may conceive without at first realizing it. If you are pregnant, bleeding maybe the first sign of a miscarriage, although most pregnancies continue despite the bleeding. Ectopic pregnancies usually cause pain before the bleeding starts, but this is not always the case.

A heavyset woman of about thirty, who had been on BCPs for years, began to bleed irregularly and consulted me some years ago. Her own gynecologist managed her problem by means of telephone discussions, increasing and then changing her pills. She found a new gynecologist, but he could only see her at the end of his evening session, which ended at 8 P.M. Because of her weight, she was not easy to examine; the gynecologist was probably too tired to think straight, and a pregnancy test was not ordered. When I examined her, I found nothing alarming either but arranged for a pregnancy test and a sonogram. A day later, to her surprise as well as to mine, I was called about a positive pregnancy test, but the sonogram showed no pregnancy in the womb. She had a tubal (or ectopic) pregnancy, an infrequent cause of painless bleeding, and one easy to miss in a woman using usually reliable contraception. In this instance, simple routine tests led to the correct diagnosis.

There are several other important causes of abnormal bleeding. In anovulatory bleeding, you may not ovulate for a month or two because of travel, stress, or abrupt gains or loss of weight. Thyroid disease, polycystic ovaries, obesity, and many other conditions such as diabetes may also upset the delicate and precise hormonal shifts needed for ovulation. A normal period is easily distinguishable from anovulatory flow. If cramps, breast fullness, PMS symptoms, weight gain, a bloated sensation, or any of your usual menstrual symptoms tells you that a period is about to begin, your period is ovulatory, and very likely normal. One of my patients regularly had a nightmare, or at least a very upsetting dream, a few days before her periods would begin. On the other hand, if your bleeding starts unexpectedly, with none of your usual symptoms, it is most likely anovulatory. Anovulatory bleeding is not always abnormal. In teenagers, it is common and usually corrects itself spontaneously. Much later, it may be the first sign that your menopause is approaching. If you have anovulatory cycles, you need gynecological advice if any of the following apply:

1.   You are trying to get pregnant;
2.   The bleeding is very heavy;
3.   You continue to bleed irregularly;
4.   The peculiar bleeding persists; or
5.   You are over thirty-five or forty years old.

The prolonged absence of periods due to anovulation may lead to high estrogen levels. Without progesterone, this may ultimately cause a condition called **endometrial hyperplasia**, which may in turn contribute, after many years, to the development of cancer. This scenario is not uncommon in women who are substantially overweight. Good gynecological care (or losing the excess weight) may prevent this outcome.

Uterine polyps are benign, fleshy, fingerlike growths, usually under an inch in length, that project into the uterine cavity and may cause heavy bleeding. Polyps are difficult to diagnose during curettage but easy to identify, and to remove, during hysteroscopy. If you have curettage after curettage without relief, you need hysteroscopy to identify polyps or perhaps small fibroids missed during previous investigations. Some years ago, one of my office nurses developed painful and excessive periods. She got her gynecological care elsewhere, but this consisted of curettages only. Simple office hysteroscopy revealed the source of her troubles: Tucked away, high in a corner, and missed at the time of the curettages, was a large polyp. This was removed without trouble, and she was cured of her symptoms.

Cancer may cause bleeding, a possibility that always needs careful consideration. Cervical cancer is rare these days, except in women who have neglected to have their annual examinations and Pap smears. A number of negative Pap smears in recent years is not a guarantee, but it is good evidence against cervical cancer. However, remember that Pap smears examine cervical cells only and cannot predict endometrial, tubal, or ovarian cancer. These topics have been discussed in the last chapter.

Abnormal bleeding may be caused by abnormalities of the arteries that feed blood to your womb. This is a rare condition, although it is possible that if gynecologists looked for it, they might find more cases. For this diagnosis to be made, you will need an **arteriogram**, an elaborate x-ray of the arteries leading to your womb. Treatment may be by hysterectomy. It is also possible to cut off the flow of blood to the womb by releasing tiny pellets of a material that coagulates (or clots) the blood in the uterine arteries, thereby blocking further bleeding. This procedure, called **uterine artery embolization**, is an advanced technique that should be performed only by expert radiologists in first-rate hospitals. Embolization starts with an arteriogram, followed by the injection of the pellets noted above; further details of this procedure are given in Chapter 9.

Intrauterine contraceptive devices (IUCDs) often cause some irregular cramping and bleeding. If the pain is not worse than a few cramps and the bleeding is tolerable, the IUCD may be left in place. An occasional blood count and the prescription of iron tablets usually prevent development of dangerous anemia. Rarely, the abnormal bleeding is caused by an IUCD that was thought to have been removed but is in fact still in the womb.

Uterine Prolapse and Procidentia

Prolapse, a condition that affects millions of American women, is the gradual descent of the womb into the vagina. In the worst cases, the body of the uterus ultimately emerges from the vagina and may be seen between the woman's thighs. Figure 13.1 shows an instance of complete prolapse of the womb; this is called **procidentia**. Prolapse is caused by numerous

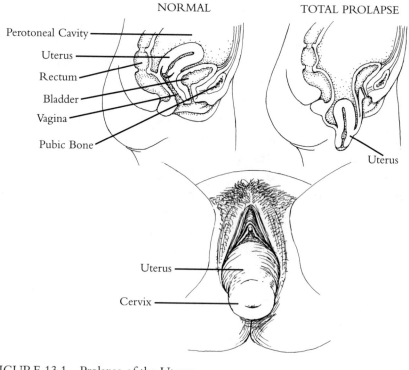

NORMAL   TOTAL PROLAPSE

Perotoneal Cavity

Uterus

Rectum

Bladder

Vagina

Pubic Bone

Uterus

Uterus

Cervix

FIGURE 13.1   Prolapse of the Uterus

pregnancies and by prolonged or difficult labors, which call for much pushing (bearing down) to deliver the baby. The birth of large babies is particularly damaging to the muscles and ligaments supporting the womb in its usual place, but modern research using ultrasound scans has shown that even a normal delivery disrupts pelvic supports. Women who have never delivered a baby vaginally rarely develop prolapse. Obesity, heavy physical labor, and the constant coughing and straining of chronic bronchitis or asthma may all contribute to causing this condition. Losing weight and avoiding strenuous work may help, but not if your womb is already hanging halfway out of your vagina.

Prolapse may cause a dragging feeling in the lower part of the pelvis and stress incontinence, or the involuntary loss of urine. A moderate degree of prolapse, with the womb descending into the upper vagina but without incontinence, is not unusual after two or three deliveries. Surgery is not warranted to correct such a minor abnormality but should be reserved for women with more marked prolapse and incontinence or procidentia. Hysterectomy used to be part and parcel of surgery for these major pelvic problems. While this view is somewhat obsolete, you must understand that surgery is a better solution for you than pessaries might be and that the success of your surgery, whatever is done, depends heavily on the skills of your surgeon. Experienced pelvic surgeons may not want to guarantee that they will be able to avoid hysterectomy: Much will depend on what is found forty minutes after the operation commences, particularly the strength of ligaments to be used for supporting pelvic structures. A relatively new procedure called sacro-spinous suspension is the best solution for many such problems; this operation is better performed after vaginal hysterectomy.

Urinary Stress Incontinence

Urinary stress incontinence (USI) is the involuntary loss of urine on exertion such as coughing, laughing, and exercising, which also affects millions of women. It may be caused by prolapse as well as other conditions. If not treated, it often worsens, with the woman wetting herself on getting up from a chair or even while walking. Women are often reticent about reporting this complaint, preferring to buy supplies of absorbent pads instead. The more carefully doctors inquire about stress incontinence and the older the women being questioned, the more USI is found.

Prolapse and incontinence often occur in the same woman, although either may be found without the other. Vaginal hysterectomy, usually combined with a procedure designed to tighten the vagina, used to be the standard surgical solution for these two problems. More recently, hysterectomy has been found to be inessential. It is crucial to find a surgeon highly competent at vaginal surgery, including the relatively simple repair that tightens vaginal tissues. The first operation to correct these abnormalities is critical. If it does not succeed, second, or third, and even fourth operations have progressively less chance of success.

As the size of the average family has decreased, prolapse, procidentia, and USI have become less frequent, as has the need for surgery tightening the vagina. Consequently, younger gynecologists are often not well trained in vaginal surgery and are familiar with only one or two basic operations. These considerations make finding the best surgeon for your first operation by far the most important of your choices.

In addition to prolapse, bladder infections and neurological conditions of the bladder may also cause the involuntary loss of urine. You should suspect that your problem is not simple USI if you recognize the following symptoms:

- You have to urinate very frequently (every half hour, perhaps hourly, during the day, or three or four times at night).
- There is much pain every time you have to pass urine.
- You get sudden, almost uncontrollable urges to pass urine, sometimes soon after emptying your bladder.
- You have no control at all over your bladder: Even at rest, unexpectedly and suddenly, you find urine is leaking out.

Interstitial cystitis and the urethral syndrome, and not USI, is the usual cause of the first three of these complaints. If these are your symptoms, it is essential not to have one of the standard gynecological operations because you may find that your symptoms worsen rather than improve. These symptoms are best investigated by a gynecologist or a urogynecologist, a specialist with additional training and skills in the management of urinary problems. If your problem is USI without prolapse, you may be better off in the hands of a urogynecologist or a competent urologist. Prolapse, however, is best handled by gynecologists. If you have both, you will have to search carefully to find an expert gynecologist. For the best results, and particularly if a previous operation has failed (meaning that the prolapse or incontinence have recurred), you need to research your options very carefully. Good departments of OB/GYN usually have a division of pelvic reconstructive surgery, with modern equipment including urodynamic tests. These test your bladder muscles to determine how they react to the bladder filling up, what happens when you cough or sneeze, and how your bladder empties. Some of the tests are simple; others need elaborate electronic equipment. The results of the tests may dictate that medications be tried instead of surgery. If you have already had surgery but have not been cured, be sure to get urodynamic testing before undergoing another operation.

The conditions just outlined may coexist with urinary tract infections, or the loss of urine due to prolapse may be compounded by neurological conditions. The most important of these goes by a variety of clumsy names: bladder dyssynergia, or the unstable bladder, or detrusor instability. In simple language, this means that bladder muscles involuntarily overreact to normal filling or to coughing, or straining, or even laughing or jumping and begin to expel urine when a normal bladder would not do so. Drugs and bladder retraining exercises are available to help with this condition. Unfortunately, the overactive bladder remains a difficult area for both women and their physicians: Neither may be happy with the results of treatment of complicated cases.

Nonsurgical Treatments for Urinary Stress Incontinence and Prolapse

Kegel's exercises and bladder retraining. You may be able to prevent prolapse and USI entirely by exercising after your deliveries or lessen these two ailments by exercising as soon as either condition is diagnosed. Kegel's exercises strengthen the pelvic floor muscles, known as the **levator muscles**, which include the PC (pubo-coccygeus) muscles some women know from books about sex. These muscles control three sphincters: the anal, urethral, and vaginal sphincters. To identify and strengthen them, sharply contract these muscles while you are passing urine, stopping and starting the flow by alternately squeezing and relaxing. The same may be done while you are sitting or standing, without anyone knowing that you are exercising. Five to ten minutes of Kegel's exercises five to ten times a day are usually recommended. The more you exercise, the better the results, although few women need to exercise an hour and forty minutes a day. You may also try the exercises during intercourse, contracting the muscles around your partner's penis, and this may enhance sexual pleasure.

Bladder drills and retraining exercises consist of teaching your bladder to empty frequently and on a rigid schedule: Every half-hour, then hourly, and so forth. With better control, the bladder learns not to empty itself unexpectedly. With improved bladder habits, the periods between voiding may be extended. These methods are becoming more available, usually through urogynecologists or urologists with an interest in the treatment of USI.

Estrogen replacement. The tissues of the postmenopausal woman may be low in estrogen. In addition to various other benefits, estrogen may restore strength and tone to pelvic and bladder muscles as well as all tissues involved in maintaining continence. Estrogen can be easily combined with Kegel's exercises, and the two, working in tandem, have produced excellent results for women after their menopause.

Pessaries and **cones.** The forerunners of the devices about to be described were mentioned in Egyptian papyri 3,000 or 4,000 years ago; other treatments were described by Hippocrates. Their modern descendants are not too different: rubber or plastic devices held in place by vaginal muscles. Some, like the cube pessary, a cube-shaped device with concave (hollowed-out) sides, are held in place by suction. A ball-shaped rubber device is inserted empty, then blown up to support the womb. The more common pessaries are doughnut or ring-shaped; these devices are supposed to keep the womb from prolapsing. If vaginal muscles are in poor shape to begin with, any device may pop out within minutes of being inserted. Anyone who is post-menopausal and is using a pessary should be on estrogens (unless for some reason these hormones cannot be used) to build up and maintain good vaginal tissues. Healthy tissues will also be less vulnerable to vaginal infections and ulceration, conditions likely to develop as the thin vaginal skin wears out from the prolonged use of a pessary.

Surgery may be postponed or avoided by using pessaries and cones, but these must be removed, cleaned, and reinserted: ideally once a week, but at least once a month. If this routine is forgotten, the device may become embedded in vaginal skin and cause ulcers, infections, or even a hemorrhage. This may happen to older women and those no longer sexually active. However, all forms of surgery may be avoided by using pessaries in a woman of seventy, only to become unavoidable because of a chronic, irreplaceable procidentia at eighty. The argument here is not for vaginal hysterectomy but for competent and well-timed surgery supporting the womb in its place.

Other medical treatments. An amazing variety of medications has been proposed to treat USI; such a profusion usually means that none is consistently useful. Antispasmodic agents, antiprostaglandins, anti–cholinergic drugs abound. Tricyclic antidepressants such as imipramine (Tofranil) and phenylpropolamine may be helpful, or calcium–channel blockers may work. Injections of tissuelike materials such as collagen into areas sur-rounding the urethra and electrical stimulation of the same area are still ex-perimental. Absorbent perineal pads are the last resort—perhaps more for the elderly woman than for her younger counterpart. If you need these treatments, you should be advised by expert urologists or urogynecologists, not by physicians with less extensive experience.

Surgical Treatments

Over 200 operations have been devised to correct stress incontinence, and over a dozen are still in common use. A large variety of operations may also be undertaken to cure prolapse. As said recently, such numbers mean that few of these operations have been accepted as superior to the others—in other words, most of these operations are problematic one way or another.

Surgery works best if there is a distinct anatomical abnormality that can be corrected. This abnormality usually consists of combinations of the fol-lowing: (1) a prolapsed uterus; (2) a cystocele, or cysto-urethrocele, which is a prolapse of your bladder or urethra into your vagina; or (3) a rectocele, or prolapse of your rectum into your vagina. After hysterectomy, the re-constructed vaginal vault, now containing bowel, may also prolapse. This is called an **enterocele**, and it may need surgical correction.

A review of operations for prolapse and USI would be well beyond the scope of a book about avoiding hysterectomy. An operation such as the Marshall-Marchetti operation, designed by gynecologists, competes with others such as those devised by urologists such as Drs. Burch, Pereyra, or Raz, all bearing their names. Some of the operations are performed ab-dominally, others laparoscopically, yet others vaginally combined with an abdominal component. More complex surgery, often after other operations have failed, involves supporting pelvic structures by means of slings: bury-ing bands of tissue, or artificial materials, deep in the pelvis. Gynecologists often prefer surgery designed by Marshall and Marchetti or by Burch; urol-ogists may prefer the Pereyra or Raz procedures. However, even in the hands of the most competent surgeons, success rates fall short of 100 per-cent. Even if successful for a few years, five or ten years after surgery, the leakage of urine may reappear. As has been emphasized, the selection of a surgeon to undertake your operation is the most important part of your care. Even an internist or other physician would have serious problems investigating who does the best Burch or Raz operation in a large city such as New York, Chicago, or Boston, let alone understand why a certain procedure might be ideal for a particular patient.

Every large city has one or two surgeons with a local reputation for vaginal surgery, and your gynecologist should know who they are. The least offensive way of asking a male gynecologist for the name of this surgeon is to ask him to whom he would refer *his* wife, mother, or sister for incontinence surgery. Female surgeons might be asked about the referral of female colleagues or family members. Perhaps the best and most reasonable approach would be to contact the chairperson or administrator of the department of OB/GYN at the nearest medical school or large hospital and ask for the name of the gynecologist best known for vaginal surgery skills. If you cannot find an expert locally, widen your search to the nearest university center. Finding an expert is well worth the expense incurred: Each successive operation has a gradually diminishing chance of success. There are complex reasons for this unsatisfactory situation. Surgery causes scarring, which makes the next operation more difficult. Also, if the cause of the leakage was not well understood before the first operation, simply resorting to a second (or third) round of surgery is unlikely to succeed.

Instead, before another operation, you should have a battery of tests usually called **urodynamics**, already discussed. The operations themselves are difficult to explain because the anatomy is complicated. The essence of the surgery is that the *bladder neck,* where the urethra enters the bladder, is pushed up to regain its original position higher in the pelvis. This can be achieved by pushing it up, working from the vagina, or by pulling it up from the abdominal cavity. Many modern operations are done laparoscopically, or at least without large incisions, usually employing two small cuts just above the pubic bone and one or two in the vagina.

Obstetric Emergencies

Very rarely, hysterectomy may become necessary because of an obstetrical emergency. A major hemorrhage or ruptured uterus—events that may be predictable—are usually involved. For instance, the current cesarean section rate, around 25 percent in most hospitals, poses dangers that became known only recently. In women who have had one or more cesarean sections, the obstetrician must check the location of the placenta (the after-birth) with great care, using sonograms. After a cesarean section, scar tissue may build up around the area where the womb was incised. If the woman conceives again, and the placenta (afterbirth) is located in this area, an abnormal attachment of the placenta to the womb may occur. This is called **placenta accreta**, and it may cause severe bleeding when efforts are made to detach the placenta after delivery. The more cesareans a woman has, the more likely this abnormally dense attachment will occur. Even if your gynecologist is well prepared, hysterectomy may be difficult or impossible to avoid when the bleeding starts. These are rare, lifesaving emergencies, and in these circumstances, there is no time to argue against hysterectomy.

On the other hand, be cautious about postpartum hysterectomy that may be urged on you for multiple reasons, none of which are particularly impressive or urgent. For instance, if you have fibroids, have chosen to have a tubal ligation, and had a prolapse before you became pregnant, hysterectomy may be recommended to you. The likelihood of complications is higher with immediate hysterectomy than with the simpler tubal ligation. Some time afterward, perhaps many years later, hysterectomy may become necessary after all. It is not an error or a failure to have a minor operation, possibly followed some years later by a necessary hysterectomy. Most women will never need the hysterectomy. Others may regret having it, for instance, if they want another child. Tubal ligations may be reversed; hysterectomy is final.

Salpingitis and Hysterectomy

Salpingitis, commonly abbreviated to PID (for pelvic inflammatory disease, another name for the same condition), or to chronic PID, is an infection of the fallopian tubes, sometimes called the oviducts. These two slender tendrils reach out from the top of the womb, one on each side, curving sideways and downward toward the ovaries, as shown in Figure 5.1. The infection is caused by bacteria that get to the tubes—most often by ascending from the vagina, through the uterus, possibly riding piggyback on sperm cells. Severe pelvic pain, chronic infections, infertility that is difficult (or impossible) to correct, and tubal (ectopic) pregnancies may all result

283

from a single sexual encounter, not to mention the HIV virus, and AIDS. These developments may be so unpredictable and devastating that special attention will be paid to their prevention.

There are over a dozen kinds of bacteria that may cause salpingitis. The most important of these are gonorrheal and chlamydial infections. Gonorrhea has been known since the last century when the German bacteriologist Albert Neisser described the bacteria. Chlamydial infections have been identified as a cause of tubal infections more recently. Syphilis, with which gonorrhea was confused for centuries, causes an entirely different and more serious illness. The famous eighteenth-century Scottish physician John Hunter experimentally inoculated himself with pus from a patient he thought had gonorrhea, but the doctor developed syphilis as well: His patient had both venereal diseases, not a rare event.

Venereal diseases caused by bacteria may be treated with antibiotics. Some women may not know that vaginal infections (vaginitis) have a tenuous connection only with PID. Douches are discouraged because they may wash vaginal bacteria, more or less innocent in the vagina, up into fallopian tubes, where they do not belong, causing PID. Viruses cause yet other kinds of infections. The human immunodeficiency virus (HIV) first races through the body and then disappears from view, only to resurface as AIDS many years later. The human papillomaviruses (HPVs) usually remain within the cervix and nearby skin surfaces, some ultimately causing warts or cancer of the cervix, also years later. Herpes, a serious acute illness at the start, often burns out gradually over the years. There are yet other venereal diseases, but the details are not appropriate for this book, nor are they frequent in the United States.

These infections present such a striking threat to women that their prevention, diagnosis, and treatment deserve further careful discussion. Avoiding venereal diseases may do more than save your womb: If you avoid HIV, it will save your life. Unfortunately, all these diseases may be inflicted on unsuspecting women by errant partners. A woman I saw a few years ago developed an unusually severe case of PID when she rejoined her husband, some time after he had relocated to New York from another continent. She had a complicated course that required two operations to drain large pelvic abscesses. From these, her cultures grew out gonococcal bacteria. She gave me a long, hard look when I mentioned the word "gonorrhea" and recommended that her husband also needed investigations and treatment.

Hysterectomy was avoided, but I doubt she'll ever conceive after the severe damage to her fallopian tubes.

How to Avoid Pelvic Infections

A single unprotected sexual encounter (or assault) can ruin or take away a woman's life, because venereal diseases now include AIDS. Avoiding venereal infections is essential for averting major disasters such as abscesses or contracting an infection with the HPV or HIV viruses. Precautions to help avoid PID follow:

- Use condoms. While not a guarantee, this may be the most effective precaution against venereal diseases and the transmission of HIV. Nevada prostitutes, who are regulated and use condoms, are reportedly rarely infected with this virus. New York prostitutes, who are not regulated, have unknown use of condoms, and possibly are more likely to use intravenous drugs, are often infected with HIV.
- BCPs protect against bacterial venereal disease, but not as much as condoms, and do not protect against AIDS or HPV. The cause of the protective effect of BCPs is uncertain. Most likely, it depends on a change in the small plug of mucus that seals the cervical canal, which becomes less permeable under the influence of the BCPs.
- You should avoid any sexual activity with a man who has a visible discharge, sores, or a wart anywhere on or near his penis. Condoms may offer some protection under these circumstances, but the price you may pay for not getting out of this difficult situation (or not dealing with it responsibly) may be very high.
- Get periodic checkups. Do not be embarrassed to ask for tests for gonorrhea, chlamydia, syphilis, and AIDS. If money is a problem, clinics run by larger hospitals or the department of health will perform these tests for you free of charge or for a "sliding fee" that depends on your income.
- If you have symptoms, get a checkup rapidly. If symptoms persist, return for another checkup.

- If you have PID, intravenous antibiotics in a hospital are preferable to outpatient care. Tell your partner that it is essential for him to be checked for infections. When dealing with any venereal disease, make sure that your partner receives appropriate treatments simultaneously with your treatments; otherwise, the infection may continue in both of you. Complete all courses of antibiotic treatments, and be sure to get vaginal medications to prevent the yeast (monilial) vaginitis that women on antibiotics often develop.
- Have your male partner get the occasional checkup. Venereal disease is rare among gay women, but there are, of course, no guarantees that it won't occur. An honest statement of facts—ideally including negative tests for gonorrhea, syphilis, chlamydia, and HIV—may be the most responsible way to deal with a new sexual partner of either gender.
- If you or your partner has had a bout of well-documented PID, double up on all the above precautions.
- If you or your partner choose to be sexually involved with more than one person, both of you must understand the responsibilities involved.
- If you are found to have one venereal disease, be sure to be checked for all other venereal diseases.

The Diagnosis of Pelvic Infections

Pelvic infections are diagnosed with great frequency by gynecologists, but as Chapter 10 showed, this diagnosis is often inaccurate. You may not have PID, but you may receive this diagnosis anyway. Even worse, you may have PID that is quietly destroying your fertility but be congratulated on your excellent health. How can you know for sure what is happening to your body?

If salpingitis (PID) causes symptoms, the major complaint is always pain, and there is much tenderness on bimanual examination. However, there are so many other gynecological diseases that also cause pain and tenderness that additional evidence of salpingitis must be sought. Further, to complicate this situation, salpingitis caused by chlamydia organisms may cause no symptoms at all. To simplify this complex situation, your gynecologist must get two or three blood tests and two cultures from you.

TABLE 13.1   Important Tests for Salpingitis

Name of Test	Results Normal	Abnormal
White blood cell count	4,000–11,000	Above 12,000
Sedimentation rate[a]	Less than 20	Above 20
C-reactive protein[a]	Negative	Positive
Gonococcus culture from cervix	Negative	Positive
Chlamydia culture from cervix	Negative	Positive
Ultrasound scan	Normal organs	Cysts, masses, fluid in the pelvis

[a] For complicated reasons, many gynecologists do not use these tests. I recommend them, but they are not as important as the others.

Without these, errors are possible. It happens frequently that salpingitis is misdiagnosed, thus you should know which tests your gynecologist must order to support this diagnosis, as well as the meaning of the results. You will find this information above in Table 13.1.

If all these tests are normal, it's unlikely that you have PID. If you are not in a monogamous relationship, you should also consider getting periodic cultures for gonorrhea and for chlamydial infections. These infections may remain silent for long spells of time and then flare up.

A detailed understanding of PID is important because too many of these diagnoses are casually made and are not as accurate as you may assume. Pain is a frequent complaint in women, as is tenderness on pelvic examination. However, these findings could point to a variety of diagnoses. If symptoms are unusual or severe, blood tests, cultures, and ultrasound scans should be taken. By far the best diagnostic measure to determine the exact diagnosis is laparoscopy, discussed in Chapters 5 and 10. Too many women believe that they have chronic infections when in fact they have endometriosis, ovulatory pains, a transient pain for which there is no reliable diagnosis, or the chronic pain state.

The Treatment of Pelvic Infections

Acute infections do not need hysterectomy; they need antibiotics. One of my patients went through a divorce, moved away from New York, developed severe PID, and was admitted to her local hospital. She was started on antibiotics, but three days later was still in severe pain, with fever spikes and abnormal blood tests. Hysterectomy was then proposed, and she was scheduled to have this operation the following day. She improved overnight, but (not surprisingly) did not recover entirely. Nevertheless, hysterectomy was performed on this young woman, who might have wanted to have more children. She sued her gynecologist and won. Another day or two of treatment with antibiotics would probably have avoided the heartache and legal turmoil that followed the surgery.

Milder infections remain in the fallopian tubes and usually respond well to modern antibiotics. More extensive infections spread into the pelvis and the abdomen, involving surrounding organs where they may cause much more serious illnesses, such as abscesses involving the tubes and the ovaries. The most common pelvic abscesses are called **TOAs (tubo-ovarian abscesses)**, but abscesses may occur in other sites as well. Abscesses inflict widespread damage to important tissues; because they tend to recur, they are regarded as chronic conditions. These, too, are treated with antibiotics, but the response is less certain. Like sinus infections, chronic tubal infections are difficult to eradicate. Recurrences need prolonged antibiotic treatment, sometimes surgery for draining abscesses, and often cause such misery that hysterectomy may be considered an acceptable alternative, simultaneously excising the tubes

The worst such infections were seen before the 1970s. Many appeared in the aftermath of criminal abortions, which frightened patients often denied undergoing. Then-current antibiotics were primitive, and little was understood about these infections. In those days, it was not unusual to have two or three frightened teenagers or young women in a large ward in a municipal hospital, all suffering from one of these infections; some died of complications rarely seen today.

One week in 1968, two such sisters were in my care. They had gone to the same abortionist, and both subsequently developed serious pelvic infections. The older sister came in two or three days before the younger. She was started on antibiotics, but her condition began to deteriorate. She survived after undergoing a hysterectomy. The younger sister was admitted already moribund, in shock from an overwhelming infection, and died within hours. Today, with fewer infected abortions and better antibiotics, such outcomes almost never occur.

Ruptured abscesses were fatal until gynecologists learned that releasing the pus and excising infected tissues could cure the illness. Performing a hysterectomy on a teenage patient was not undertaken without immense reluctance, and sometimes the decision was delayed until it was too late. Today, hysterectomy is avoidable: Releasing the pus and administering modern antibiotics usually get the infection under control. However, the damage to reproductive organs may be irreversible, causing infertility. Also, the infections tend to recur.

Hysterectomy may still be recommended to women with chronic salpingitis. Every time abscesses develop, the affected women must accept a prolonged hospital stay for intravenous antibiotics. The reason for the recurrence of abscesses is not known. These women have a number of other difficulties as well. For example, their fallopian tubes are damaged, causing ectopic (tubal) pregnancies and infertility. Chronic pain states are another common consequence of the recurring infections. Regardless of whether a woman accepts or declines hysterectomy under these circumstances, it may be too late to get her health back. Preventing these infections is not easy, but given the consequences, it is essential to try.

There are two important considerations to be noted here:

- As was the case with acute infections, it happens too often that the diagnosis of chronic salpingitis, or **chronic PID**, as this condition is often called, is an error. Women with chronic pelvic pain in particular are likely to be told that they have chronic PID without adequate investigation. If you have had to undergo surgery because of abscesses, the diagnosis is appropriate. Without a history of such surgery, and neither laparotomy nor laparoscopy that shows an ongoing or recent infection, the diagnosis is suspect. There is a third possibility—that adhesions are present; this is discussed in great detail in Chapter 10. These ideas may seem complicated, but they are, or should be, simple equations for any competent gynecologist. Table 13.3 applies almost as exactly to chronic infections as it applies to acute infections. If your tests show none of the abnormal findings in the column on the right, chronic tubal infections may not be the cause of your symptoms.
- If you do need hysterectomy—and I cannot say I am rigidly against this operation if you have had too much trouble from

properly diagnosed infections—you must sit down with your surgeon before your operation to discuss the fate of your ovaries. Ovaries retained in the course of surgery rarely get reinfected, but this is possible. My usual advice, or practice, has been to retain the healthier-looking ovary, and possibly excise the other ovary—but only if it looks damaged by repeated bouts of infection.

Backaches, retroversion, and chronic cervical infections are emphatically not adequate reasons to lose a womb, yet every few months I still hear of hysterectomies performed for such reasons. Backaches may be as bad as chronic pelvic pain, but hysterectomy is unlikely to provide relief for this condition. Retroversion is usually a harmless condition, at least in the absence of endometriosis or severe chronic PID. Chronic cervicitis is difficult to eliminate with antibiotics, but cryosurgery or the modern LEEP (or LLEETZ) procedures will cure it easily and safely. Laser excision will do the same at a higher cost. If neither is available to you, conization is even more expensive, but it will do the job.

··· 14 ···

Your Ovaries and Menopause

If you are interested in avoiding a hysterectomy but must undergo one, you will at least want to try to avoid losing your ovaries. However, you may now find that many gynecologists are uneasy about cooperating with your wish to keep your ovaries, regarding them as potential sources of trouble. Citing the risks of a dreaded disease, namely ovarian cancer, gynecologists often prefer to remove the ovaries from women older than forty or forty-five years of age once hysterectomy has been completed, even if the ovaries appear perfectly normal. The gravity with which urologists debate removing the testicles of older men with prostate cancer, thus castrating them, is generally missing from the briefer discussions that precede an equally castrating operation, the removal of ovaries from much younger women. This is inappropriate, because the biological consequences of castrating women are more extensive than the effects of castrating men.

Physicians know much less about the effects of castrating men than they know about parallel effects on women. **Orchiectomy**, the medical term for the surgical removal of the testicles, is so rarely performed in younger men that knowledge of the repercussions of the early loss of the testicles is very scanty. Nevertheless, orchiectomy is not thought to be followed by serious long-term disadvantages such as heart disease. Osteoporosis may occur but is not as severe as it is in women after castration. Contrary to popular thinking, sexually active men often remain interested in sex despite castration, and many continue to have normal erections, although without the hormone testosterone, which is made in the testicles, sexual drive begins to fail much earlier than it does among those not castrated. You may already know that testosterone is prescribed increasingly often for men as well as for women in an effort to recapture previous levels of sexual interest and drive. A few of my more skeptical colleagues think that at least some of the glowing testimonials are simply due to the placebo effect: If you believe that a drug (or surgery, or therapy of any kind) will have a certain beneficial effect, then you *will* notice this effect—even if the drug is inert or the intervention turns out to be innocuous, with no real influence.

As described earlier, even an uneventful hysterectomy, in which the ovaries are not removed, may, at least in some women, lead to the early onset of menopause. Much less often an incautious surgeon removes an ovary before realizing that the other ovary is already missing—removed by another surgeon, lost to torsion,[1] or damaged by previous surgery. If you are considering gynecological surgery, but particularly if you have a family history of ovarian cancer, the fate of your ovaries must be thought through very carefully.

Gynecological interest in removing ovaries is not new. In the nineteenth century, ovaries became the prime targets of so-called belly-rippers, surgeons who removed ovaries for reasons that were sexist as well as nonsensical. This attitude has persisted into at least the first half of the twentieth century. J. C. Doyle, a Beverly Hills gynecologist, reported on large numbers of unnecessary excisions in 1952. Reading about these operations is an embarrassing experience for modern gynecologists, who think that

---

[1] Rarely, a normal ovary may twist on its attachments, causing a transient bout of abdominal pain. It loses its blood supply, and unless the pedicle is untwisted (usually by means of surgery, possibly spontaneously), it begins to degenerate and is absorbed—in effect, it disappears slowly. There are no other consequences as long as the remaining ovary is normal—this ovary simply takes over the work of the lost ovary. A large cystic ovary may also twist, but this is usually detected because this event is more painful, and the ovary is often saved by surgery. Testicles may also undergo such spontaneous torsion, similarly requiring surgical care.

primitive ideas about removing ovaries did not survive into the twentieth century.

The reasons for the surgery may have changed, but the removal of ovaries has remained a fact of life. In 1965, 427,000 women had a hysterectomy performed, and 25 percent had their ovaries excised at the same time. By 1984, the number of hysterectomies grew to 675,000, with the proportion of women who had their ovaries removed increasing to 41 percent. The most recent figures are from 1993, and these show a further increase, to 52 percent. Increases have been most striking for women between the ages of 45 and 64: from 35 percent in 1965 to 66 percent in 1984. The reasons for the expansion in the use of bilateral salpingo-oophorectomy (or BSO, the initials gynecologists use to describe the removal of the ovaries and the fallopian tubes) are conjectural, by far the most prominent being concern about the development of ovarian cancer after hysterectomy. The growing proportion of women who undergo hysterectomy for endometriosis, a condition that often necessitates the excision of all ovarian tissue, may also explain, at least in part, the steep increases noted above. Unfortunately, the expansion comes at the time when the importance of the continued presence of ovarian hormones is receiving widespread publicity.

In certain states, laws have been enacted mandating that women about to undergo hysterectomy must sign not only the standard surgical consent but also an additional form intended for hysterectomy patients only. The form usually informs women that after the operation they will no longer be able to bear children. This statement must be signed even by incredulous sixty-five-year-old grandmothers who have cancer. Your ovaries have no such legal safeguards to protect them. The gynecologist who has obtained a consent for hysterectomy does not need to justify the removal of ovaries separately. Instead, "BSO" is added to the "hysterectomy" on the consent. The most frequent abbreviation is TAH-BSO, or total abdominal hysterectomy with bilateral salpingo-oophorectomy. In some areas of the United States, VH is the abbreviation for vaginal hysterectomy. The ovaries are difficult to reach during this operation; for this reason, they are excised during vaginal surgery less often than during abdominal surgery.

Recommending **oophorectomy**, the excision of the ovaries, rests on the premise that ovaries left in place after hysterectomy may later turn cystic or cancerous. About 3 to 5 percent of women will need surgery for the treatment of ovarian cysts that develop after the hysterectomy, and over 1 percent will develop ovarian cancer. These are rare events, but the development of ovarian cancer after hysterectomy is particularly devastating, with all involved sharply regretting the decision not to remove the ovaries well before cancer developed.

Competing with the fear of ovarian cancer is the fact that in premenopausal women, the abrupt loss of ovarian hormones causes the sudden onset of menopausal symptoms. These may be mild in some women but devastating in others, particularly in those under the age of forty. If the hormones are not replaced after such an operation, osteoporosis (and possibly heart disease) is likely to develop. These two illnesses are much more frequent than ovarian cancer. It makes no sense to remove organs to prevent cancer if women stand to develop more frequent and equally deadly conditions instead. However, I suspect that most women are more concerned with the specter of ovarian cancer occurring at any time, and perhaps soon, than with less clearly defined worries about the remote onset of bone and heart disease.

After menopause, the ovaries continue to function, secreting testosterone and similar "male" hormones such as androstenedione—not an unmixed blessing, since these hormones also cause an increased rate of growth of facial hair, and, in some, a so-called male-pattern loss of scalp hair: bald areas near the temples. The ovaries also continue to make prostaglandins, whose role in maintaining cardiovascular health remains to be investigated. Since either removing or retaining ovaries may cause serious complications, dogmatic insistence on either is inappropriate. Instead, women should understand the issues and their personal risks, and decide for themselves.

In the concluding sections of this book, we shall discuss ovarian cysts and cancer, the influence of your ovaries on your health, and hormone replacement therapy (HRT).

Ovarian Cysts

After menstruation, one of your ovaries begins to prepare for the next menstrual cycle by developing a small cyst. This is a grapelike structure, a sac of fluid with a thin wall that grows slowly for about two weeks, when it measures about 0.5 inches across and projects from the surface of the ovary. Next, it develops a small puncture, rupturing and collapsing pain-lessly, or perhaps with a twinge of pain, as you ovulate—this is called "mittelschmerz," German for "pain in the middle." A clump of cells, barely visible as a tiny speck of tissue, is now blown into the peritoneal cavity. In the middle of this cluster of cells is the ovum, ready to be fertilized. The cyst originally formed usually persists for an additional two weeks as the *corpus luteum* (Latin for a "yellow body"), a spongy collection of cells that makes estrogen and progesterone. Occasionally, the *corpus luteum* forms a cyst that persists as a *corpus luteum cyst,* a small and harmless structure that tends to disappear within a month or two. Other kinds of cysts may also appear. Most are innocuous, but a few are not. Unfortunately, without surgery it is generally not possible to be absolutely sure which kind you may have.

If you have an ovarian cyst, three factors determine how worrisome your situation may be: the size of your cyst, your age, and the sonographic appearance of the cyst. Small cysts, measuring less than an inch or two in size, are generally harmless. They are frequent, particularly in ovulating women. They come and go spontaneously and rarely cause difficulties. Every gynecologist has, in the course of a vaginal examination, inadvertently ruptured a small, thin-walled cyst; this is almost always a painless event. However, the larger the cyst, the more attention it requires. Gynecologists begin to worry about cysts when they are more than 2.5 inches in diameter, about as large as an apple or a peach.

Since ovarian cancer is rare before menopause, accelerating in frequency after the age of about fifty-five, your age is also important. A conscientious gynecologist will not want to dismiss the possibility of cancer just because the patient is young. As recently as ten years ago, gynecologists could not be sure what kind of cyst they were dealing with without waiting for it to go away, and removing it if it did not. This led to much surgery, some of which could be criticized as unnecessary—but only in retrospect, not a reasonable way to assess this situation.

Sonography has revolutionized gynecological thinking about ovarian cysts. High-resolution sonograms show details that distinguish harmless cysts, which need no surgery, from dangerous cysts, which may need urgent surgery. Sonography allows the exact measurement of cyst size and, most important, finds cysts not identified during gynecological examinations. However, such precise use needs sonography of high quality, including equipment for abdominal and vaginal sonograms. The latest device, called **transvaginal Doppler ultrasound**, estimates the flow of blood through ovarian arteries and veins. Cancer cells release chemicals that open up nearby arteries, thus increasing the flow of blood through nearby vessels. With modern ultrasound equipment, it may be possible to be reasonably sure what kind of cyst you have:

- A small cyst with thin walls, consisting of a single sac only and with normal blood flow through ovarian vessels, is usually harmless. If you are found to have this kind of cyst, it is reasonably safe to await the spontaneous disappearance of the cyst. This is probably true at any age, although if you want to be absolutely and 100-percent sure that the cyst is benign, only an examination of tissues surgically removed can give such a level of assurance.
- Thicker walls mean that the cyst is more solid and therefore less likely to vanish without surgery. The cyst might be deemed harmless, although there remains the possibility that it is cancerous or that it may twist, necessitating emergency surgery.
- A cyst that contains numerous smaller cysts, like a bunch of grapes in a plastic bag, suggests the possibility of cancer. A high rate of blood flow through ovarian vessels is another ominous finding. The presence of fluid within the pelvic or peritoneal cavities would further increase suspicion that cancer will be found. Careful evaluation and surgery, performed by a competent surgeon, is an urgent matter in this case. Ideally, the surgery should be performed by a gynecological oncologist (cancer specialist). Alternately, such a specialist should be rapidly available during surgery if cancer is found. Pathologists can usually identify cancer in tissues just excised using a rapid technique called "frozen section"; usually, again to be absolutely certain, they want to perform a more detailed examination that takes a day or two to complete.
- The presence of endometriosis may be suspected from the sonographic appearance of pelvic tissues and ovarian cysts, but this should be confirmed by laparoscopy.
- Specific types of cysts may also be recognized if sonography is combined with x-rays.
- A thick-walled cyst with solid contents may be x-rayed and found to have a calcium-containing, toothlike structure in its middle.

This is a **dermoid cyst,** which may also contain skin, hair, brain, bone or cartilage, or thyroid tissue, virtually any cellular matter found in the body. The thyroid tissue may become active, on rare occasions causing **hyperthyroidism**. Rarely, dermoid cysts develop cancerous elements. Dermoid cysts, which are fairly common in young women, warrant surgery: They will not disappear unless excised, and they may also twist, causing a surgical emergency.

- Another pattern of calcification, which shows up on x-rays as a flecked or mottled pattern, may suggest the presence of ovarian cancer.
- Many gynecologists suspect that only one common type of ovarian cyst, called "**serous**" because of its clear contents, may be precancerous. These cysts cause much anxiety to women and their gynecologists. Until recently, most ovarian cysts larger than a plum were regarded with great suspicion and required removal for diagnosis, to make sure they were not cancerous. Since they were usually excised, we may never find out exactly how often cancer might later develop in such cysts. However, there is evidence that some serous cysts, if left in place year after year, might turn cancerous.

Ovarian cysts have grown to monstrous sizes. One weighing 328 pounds was removed from a woman in Texas in 1905; the patient survived. The next largest cyst, reported from England in 1846, weighed 298 pounds. This tumor was managed by draining it, but the patient went into shock and died. Old engravings show women with these huge tumors lying on their side, immobilized by their vast, barrel-shaped bellies. The largest cyst I ever saw was so huge that with the woman sitting on a chair, the mass hung down between her legs, resting on the floor. Her skin was swollen and ulcerated by the friction of constant dragging. This cyst weighed a mere fifty pounds, so it is difficult to imagine what it may have felt like to have one six times larger.

The sudden appearance of severe lower abdominal pain may mean that the cyst has undergone torsion, a process in which it twists on its pedicle, or stalk. This represents an emergency, which requires surgery as soon as the diagnosis is confirmed, usually by means of an ultrasound examination.

Ovarian Cancer

The idea of cancer strikes fear into everyone. In women, only too often it starts in organs that are symbolically sacred. The female breasts are first on this list: By current estimates from the American Cancer Society, if she lives long enough, one woman in eight or nine will develop breast cancer, a gloomy frequency to contemplate. Ovarian cancer comes next, fresh in memory because of the well-publicized deaths of well-known people such as comedian Gilda Radner and Connecticut governor Ella Grasso. Women know how difficult it is to cure this most feared form of cancer, which strikes about one woman in sixty or seventy.

The ovaries are complex organs that can develop a prodigiously large variety of tumors. Ovarian cancer has been found in a fetus by the thirtieth week of pregnancy, causing premature labor and the delivery of a stillborn baby. One of my most upsetting gynecological memories dates back to the morning when I was called by a surgeon operating on a seven-year-old for presumed appendicitis. Instead of that disease, he found unmistakable and widespread ovarian cancer, involving both ovaries. I began to remove these, at which point the hospital's gynecological oncologist arrived and took over the operation. This relieved me of the task of performing hysterectomy on a mere child, something I regarded as inevitable but emotionally very difficult. Despite hysterectomy and chemotherapy, she died within the year.

Organs such as the bowel, breasts, or the lungs develop three or four basic types of cancer, but the ovaries can grow well over a dozen types of cancer. Most are cystic, containing many fluid-filled sacs; others are solid. Some appear so unusual under the microscope that they baffle the pathologists trying to classify them. Moreover, ovarian cancers are notoriously difficult to treat successfully. Again, it seems as if Nature had conspired against women, who die of breast, ovarian, and uterine cancers about twice as often, and often at an earlier age, than men die of genital cancers. Testicular cancer is about one-third as common as ovarian cancer, but with chemotherapy, the results of treatment have improved dramatically: 6,500 women die annually of ovarian cancer, but only 300 men die of testicular cancer. Prostatic cancer is easier to diagnose and to treat than ovarian cancer. If men had more rectal examinations, biochemical screening tests

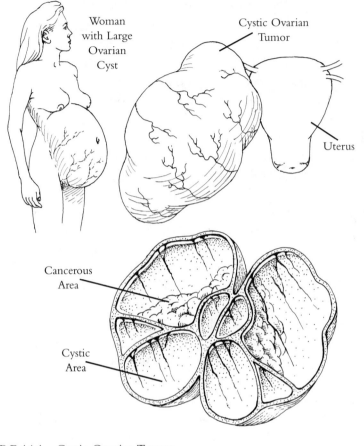

FIGURE 14.1   Cystic Ovarian Tumor

called PSA, biopsies of the prostate gland, and perhaps rectal sonograms, deaths from prostatic cancer would probably diminish. This is not true of ovarian cancer, which strikes silently and mercilessly, with most victims diagnosed at an advanced, difficult-to-treat stage. Recent data released by the American Cancer Society indicate that about 180,000 cases of breast cancer will occur annually in women, and much the same number of prostate cancer cases in men. However, nearly 41,000 women will die annually from breast cancer; about 32,000 men will die from prostate cancer.

The Growth and Detection of Ovarian Cancer

The appearance of ovarian cancer is an ominous event. By the time it is discovered, most often the cancer is so widely disseminated that surgery cannot be relied upon to remove all the cancerous tissues. This early spread usually occurs when cancer breaks through the thin capsule surrounding the ovary. Cancerous cells are now spilled into the peritoneal cavity and may reach and implant on distant organs such as the liver and the bowel within days, an almost explosively sudden occurrence. Cancer may also spread through the bloodstream and the lymphatics. Since there is little hope of removing all the cancerous areas by surgical means, chemotherapy (or radiation) is required. These slow the growth of malignant cells, but in the end, the cancerous nodules become resistant to chemotherapy, and no more radiation can be given. Only about 20–25 percent of women are alive and free of disease five years after treatment was started among the largest group of victims: those in whom the diagnosis was made with the cancer already disseminated. This dismal prognosis, and the difficult and painful course ovarian cancer often follows, has prompted a strong interest in the prophylactic removal of the ovaries.

In 1963, I attended a course at Harvard Medical School, where the insidious and rapid spread of ovarian cancer was illustrated with an example. A woman in her late forties was scheduled to have a hysterectomy for fibroids, but on opening the abdomen, the fibroids were found to be smaller than expected. This was not an unusual event in those days, before sonography became available (nor is such a story unusual, even today). There was no sign of any other disease, and the surgeon proceeded with the standard operation, removing her womb, ovaries, and tubes. The next day, the pathologist found a hazelnut-sized nodule of a virulent form of cancer deep in one of the ovaries. This cancer was detected at an exceptionally early stage, and hopes were high that her life would be saved. Nevertheless, the woman developed metastatic disease and died within two years.

The Causes of Ovarian Cancer

Discouragingly little is known about the causes of ovarian cancer. The strongest clues we have involve a genetic tendency toward genital and breast cancer, clues we'll discuss shortly. Earlier studies have indicated that talcum powder, used by some women as a hygienic measure, may be a culprit. The powder, which is chemically similar to asbestos, is known to migrate from perineal and vulval areas, surrounding vaginal lips, into the vagina and toward the peritoneal cavity and, therefore, the ovaries. Surgeons used to use talcum powder in and on their sterile gloves as a dry lubricant; this was another way for the powder to enter the abdomen and the pelvis. A study from Harvard Medical School some years ago suggested that women who used talcum powder to keep themselves dry more than 10,000 times during menstrual years increased their chances of developing ovarian cancer almost threefold. However, even if this theory were true, the use of talcum powder is unlikely to account for much ovarian cancer.

A typical Western diet, rich in milk and other animal fats, is another suspect. Japanese women residing in Japan have a low likelihood of developing ovarian cancer; once in the United States and consuming a Western diet, their incidence of ovarian cancer becomes similar to that of their American sisters. The levels of hormones that cause ovulation, and particularly FSH, increase sharply around menopause. This is also a time when the frequency of the disease increases; some researchers suspect that these hormones may have a role in causing ovarian cancer. This notion is reinforced by recent studies according to which fertility-enhancing drugs—prominently including FSH—also increase infertile women's chances of developing ovarian cancer. Uninterrupted ovulation (common in women who fail to conceive) is also slightly conducive to the development of ovarian cancer: Infertile women, those who postpone their first pregnancy, and those with fewer children are all at a slightly higher risk. Pregnancies afford some protection, as do BCPs, which inhibit ovulation; according to recent calculations, BCPs may prevent 1,700 cases of ovarian cancer a year in the United States.

The Role of Heredity

The most interesting speculations concern the role of heredity in the development of ovarian cancer. A strong family history of cancer is a powerful omen that the same illness might strike again. If a woman's mother *and* a sister have developed ovarian cancer, and particularly if these cancers were detected at an early age, her chances of the same fate may be close to 50 percent. With two second-degree relatives who had ovarian cancer, the corresponding figure is 25 percent. The prophylactic removal of the ovaries is an option that must be offered to women who have such a background. If there are distant relatives with ovarian cancer, the risk is much lower, but

still higher than the average, "baseline" rate. There is also a connection between breast and ovarian cancers: If your mother had one of these, you are
more likely to develop either. Some families have a strong background of
colonic, endometrial, ovarian, and possibly other cancers. A good case may
be made for recommending that every woman should construct a family
tree that shows the cause of death for everyone in the family—often a suggestive pattern emerges only when a trained geneticist assembles the entire
picture for an individual and her family.

The Gilda Radner Familial Ovarian Cancer Registry in Buffalo, New
York (800-OVARIAN), part of Roswell Park Cancer Institute, has seen
sharp increases in the numbers of families with such cancers reported to
them. Chromosomal abnormalities such as the BRCA genes and others
have been recognized in women with familial breast, ovarian, and colon
cancer. In such women, the disease often strikes at an early age: in their
thirties and forties. If you do not have a clear idea if the women in your
family might have had ovarian cancer, you should investigate this. (For instance, if your mother died of cancer when you were young, and the event
was so shocking that no one in your family ever discussed the details with
anyone, you should try to find out the cause of her death.) If there is a pattern of cancer in your family, you need careful surveillance of your ovaries,
a difficult project we'll discuss shortly. You should also discuss the prophylactic removal of your ovaries, possibly around the age of thirty-five, or
when you have had all the children you want, with a **gynecological oncologist**, a specialist whose main professional interest is the prevention and
treatment of gynecological cancer. The oncologist may in turn want to
send you to a **geneticist,** who specializes in identifying people who have
a chromosomal predisposition to the development of cancer. (Geneticists
have another important role: They advise pregnant women about genetic
and other risks to the fetus.)

The Frequency of Ovarian Cancer

The frequency with which ovarian cancer strikes has been studied with
great care, and the figures tell a discouraging story. Overall, about 1 woman
in 70, or 1.4 percent, will develop ovarian cancer. More recent figures suggest that one woman in 55, or 1.8 percent of women born in the United
States will face this problem. Swedish and Norwegian figures are slightly
higher. Rural Japanese women have a very low risk; but if they move to

America, they begin to develop ovarian cancer at the rate of their new compatriots. In the light of such pessimistic facts, the drive to remove the ovaries of women who are undergoing a hysterectomy is understandable, at least to gynecologists and women familiar with the ravages of ovarian cancer. The usual recommendation has been to perform the additional surgery on women older than 40, 45, or 50, a decade or two before the disease is the most likely to strike. More recently, the age at which the additional surgery is recommended has increased to 50 or over 50. The justifications for these recommendations must be considered very carefully.

Prophylactic Removal of the Ovaries

According to most experts, but contrary to elementary logic, removing one ovary has little effect on reducing the chances of developing ovarian cancer later in life. Unfortunately, a very small number of women have developed ovarian cancer despite the prophylactic removal of both ovaries, an astonishing development that shows how difficult it is to be absolutely sure of anything in medicine. Sometimes the surgery was performed too late, after microscopic areas of cancer from the ovaries had already metastasized (spread) to other organs. In other cases, ovaries were free of disease and were completely removed; yet some years later, an illness very similar to ovarian cancer developed. These rare but striking events have received widespread publicity among gynecologists, who have been left wondering where the cancer might have started. Peritoneal cells are the probable site of origin, because in the embryo, these cells and the surface cells of the ovaries develop from identical precursor cells. There may be cells capable of transformation into ovarian cancer scattered throughout the peritoneal layer. Whether this is an elegant explanation or an inaccurate guess disguised as an explanation remains to be seen.

Screening for Ovarian Cancer: Sonography

The early symptoms of ovarian cancer are entirely inconspicuous. A bloated feeling, vague abdominal discomfort, and dyspepsia (indigestion) are usually mentioned. These symptoms may appear in women who are healthy, and they may occur in victims of ovarian cancer when it is already too late for effective intervention. The usual sequence is that symptoms appear just before the abdomen begins to swell up. On examination, fluid and a tumor (or tumors) are found in the pelvis or the lower abdomen. At this point, to the consternation of all involved, it is often too late for successful treatment.

Screening is available to help with the early diagnosis of cancer in many organs. Unfortunately, screening for ovarian cancer has not been a success story, and after hysterectomy with conservation of the ovaries, you cannot rely on medical science to prevent ovarian cancer. For instance, regular and careful vaginal examinations are very unlikely to detect cancer in its earliest stages. The story from Harvard University, mentioned earlier, illustrates the difficulties accurately, although it was admittedly an extreme example of the potential deadliness of these tumors.

Periodic ultrasound examinations have been proposed for screening. At first these were done abdominally; then similar equipment became available for vaginal ultrasound examinations. The latest research uses ultrasound equipment that gives estimates of blood flow through ovarian vessels using color-enhanced television monitors, called Doppler ultrasound. The cost of equipment limited to simple vaginal ultrasound is currently in the $30,000 to $50,000 range. However, state-of-the-art Doppler ultrasound with color enhancement may cost closer to $75,000 and will be found in well-equipped hospitals only. Over 1,000 sonograms need to be taken to detect a single case of ovarian cancer. For this woman, a distinct advantage has been gained: Her cancer was found some months earlier, *possibly* (but not necessarily) with a better chance of a cure; discovering a so-called stage 4 cancer, already disseminated to distant sites, is not as much of a success as it may seem. Lives may be saved, but only if these cancers are discovered before they have spread widely, and this happens less often than hoped for.

Screening provides expensive care, with sonograms, gynecological consultations, and even surgery in search of an earlier diagnosis resulting in a slight gain by a few women. Women and gynecologists like the reassurance provided by this approach, although insurance companies likely do not. Costs are intruding in a major way into all aspects of medical care. If you own a business and pay for your own health insurance, you will be familiar with these conflicts. Screening for ovarian cancer is a good example of care that is very expensive and for which there is an increasing demand. However, and unfortunately, ovarian screening will save a woman's life on rare occasions only.

The strange new world of advanced ovarian cancer screening calls for much surgery that, to everyone's relief, has negative results. This, again, is not entirely a success story because occasionally a patient dies from an operation that, at least in retrospect, was avoidable. Screening may, paradoxically, lead to more unnecessary hysterectomies, too. The usual scenario is that a routine sonogram shows a small ovarian cyst in a menopausal woman, and her gynecologist recalls that the ovaries of such women should be small and inactive. Hugh Barber, an eminent cancer specialist at Lenox Hill Hospital in New York City, has long taught that the menopausal ovary should be so small that it could not be felt on bimanual examination. This observation was originally based on only three post-menopausal women, whose slightly enlarged, and therefore palpable, ovaries were found to be cancerous. These women were first reported in 1971, when they were said to have a case of the **post-menopausal palpable ovary syndrome (PMPO syndrome).** Subsequent studies confirmed the notion that any enlargement of a postmenopausal ovary must be investigated to ensure that it is not cancerous. The presence of a small cyst implies some activity, and it also causes a slight increase in size, hence anxieties about the situation are not misguided.

The medical malpractice situation, with large awards for failure to diagnose lethal forms of cancer, also encourages gynecologists to make every effort to avoid such lawsuits by operating whenever there is the least possibility of cancer. From the gynecologist's point of view, there is nothing much to gain and much to lose by not operating. Hysterectomy with removal of the ovaries and fallopian tubes is not rare under these circumstances: After all, the specimen removed has a cyst, although it is usually small. Most cancer specialists, working in academic hospitals, have no interest in operating on small ovarian cysts that are discovered by routine sonography but are benign by advanced sonographic techniques. Different rules often apply in peripheral hospitals where, as we have seen, there are fewer stringent and enforced guidelines against unnecessary surgery.

Another difficulty with screening is that the ideal frequency of screening is not known. If a disease goes from inconspicuous to widespread in a few months, annual screening may not help much.

Screening for Ovarian Cancer: The CA 125 Test

There are other tests in use for ovarian cancer screening. By far the best known is called CA 125, a substance usually described as a "tumor marker." CA 125 is a chemical normally present in your blood in small amounts, defined as less than 35 or 65 units per cubic centimeter. Levels are elevated if you have cancer and many other diseases, particularly endometriosis. The following are important facts about this test:

- Results are often inconclusive. Slight elevations of CA 125 may be a normal finding in a few women. Endometriosis, fibroids, pregnancy, inflammatory diseases such as salpingitis, and a host of cancerous and medical conditions may also cause slight elevations, usually well below 100 or 200 units. Levels are higher during menstruation and lower after menopause. If the CA 125 level is elevated, and there is no ovarian cancer, the breasts and the colon must also be checked out. Even if an ovarian cancer is found, the same investigations must be carried out. There may be breast or colon cancer spreading (metastasizing) to the ovaries, or *two* malignant conditions developing simultaneously. It would be a serious error to find and treat one cancer only, leaving the other to progress.
- Substantial elevations of CA 125 levels, from a few hundred to over 1,000 units per cubic centimeter, may be due to ovarian cancer. By this time, the cancer can probably be felt with examining fingers or detected by means of sonograms. Unfortunately, increases in CA 125 levels are found mostly in women with ovarian cancers arising from the capsule of the ovary, called "epithelial" cancers. Although these are the most common kind of ovarian cancer, other forms also occur, and CA 125 levels are not useful for detecting them, limiting the value of the test for screening purposes.
- The most useful role of the test is in monitoring progress after surgery for epithelial ovarian cancer. Recurrences may be detected earlier if rising CA 125 levels are found weeks or months, or years after surgery and chemotherapy.

Regular examinations, CA 125 levels, and expertly performed sonograms might give you a slight edge in the early detection of ovarian cancer, and the reassurance of negative tests is always welcome. However, do not be persuaded to have a hysterectomy solely because you have elevated CA 125 levels. Instead, get a second opinion from a competent gynecologist. Vaginal ultrasound examinations, mammograms, and tests for colon cancer may be all that you need. Laparoscopy may be warranted if the CA 125 levels are high; hysterectomy is not.

More recent, but so far unconfirmed, research from St. Bartholomew's Hospital in London indicates that elevated CA 125 levels may foretell the increased likelihood of ovarian cancer developing months or years later. One article claims that if CA 125 levels are elevated, ovarian cancer may be thirty-six times as likely to strike as in the absence of elevated levels. Such claims attract popular coverage but lack credibility until the work is replicated elsewhere with similar results.

Borderline Ovarian Tumors

You may have heard of a relatively new, and often remarkably benign, kind of ovarian cancer called **borderline ovarian cancer of low malignancy.** About 3,000 cases are diagnosed annually in the United States, more often in pre-menopausal women. These tumors are, as the name suggests, fairly benign. Often the cancer is confined to the inner lining of an ovarian cyst, and with no evidence of spread, long-term survival is close to 100 percent. Even if spread to surrounding structures, long-term survival is still remarkably good at about 70 percent. A frequent quandary with this diagnosis concerns the extent of the operation to be undertaken. If the pathologists are certain that their diagnosis is correct and there is no evidence of spread, only the ovary involved must be removed. Hysterectomy is not essential. The opposite ovary, if it looks benign, may also be left behind in an effort to preserve fertility. Unfortunately, the more tissue left behind, the higher the probability of a recurrence. Such a recurrence is still relatively benign—not as malignant as other, standard ovarian cancers—nevertheless, not removing the opposite ovary may later lead to serious problems.

Ovarian Cancer After Hysterectomy

On the surface, it would appear rare that cancer develops in ovaries that were "left behind" after hysterectomy. One instance was described decades ago in a letter to the editor of the *New England Journal of Medicine*. A female physician whose mother developed ovarian cancer wrote the letter, deploring the fact that when her mother had her hysterectomy, they were not told that this might happen. I do not remember a single such case from my personal experience, but this may be because my practice never performed large numbers of hysterectomies. However, any individual's experience is likely to be an inaccurate guide, and cancer experts tell a different story about hysterectomy with conservation of the ovaries.

Recent articles in gynecological journals claim that cancer in ovaries left behind after hysterectomy is a serious problem. A woman's lifetime chance of developing ovarian cancer is around 1.5 percent, and this figure remains unchanged for women who have had a hysterectomy with just one ovary left behind. Hervy Averette, a prominent gynecological cancer specialist from Miami, has reported that in a group of 755 women with ovarian cancer, 12.6 percent had undergone previous hysterectomy. Of these women, 7.9 percent had the operation after the age of 40. These cancers could have been prevented by a policy of routine removal of the ovaries if hysterectomy were performed after age 40. Other authors cited by Averette showed that 5 to 14 percent of women with ovarian cancer had a hysterectomy some years before the ovarian cancer appeared. Averette estimated that if hysterectomy with the routine removal of ovaries were performed past the age of 40, at least 1,000 cases of ovarian cancer, or about 5 percent of the 20,000 new cases in the United States, would be prevented each year. Unfortunately, such calculations depend on an unacceptably high rate of hysterectomies.

Most recent students of ovarian cancer have arrived at similar conclusions. Some gynecologists thought that an ovary that looks normal during surgery would not turn cancerous for at least a few years. Others have cited cases of ovarian cancer appearing within two or three years of hysterectomy, a particularly tragic event. The speed with which ovarian cancer develops and spreads, probably within months, makes it likely that finding a perfectly normal-looking ovary at surgery is no guarantee against ovarian cancer appearing later. One of my colleagues at Metropolitan Hospital, the Scottish oncologist Donald Clark, recalled one hysterectomy on a woman in her mid-forties. The ovaries appeared normal, and, in consonance with the patient's wishes, were left behind. Ovarian cancer was diagnosed three months later; in due course she died.

Such views are not unanimous. One study, published in 1986 by the epidemiologist N. S. Weiss, showed that the risk of ovarian cancer diminished substantially for the first five years after hysterectomy. However, after the sixth year, the frequency of cancer began to increase, even exceeding the levels found among women who did not have a hysterectomy. Brooks

Ranney, a gynecologist with a large private practice in Yankton, South Dakota, has reported his experiences, according to which ovarian cancer was a very rare event after hysterectomy. These opinions throw conflicting light on the problem: the likelihood of cancer developing in ovaries that were not removed at the time of hysterectomy.

Averette's work shows that at least 5 percent of women with ovarian cancer underwent hysterectomy at which the ovaries could have been removed. Avoiding ovarian cancer through an exceptionally high hysterectomy rate seems perverse and unfair. While fairness may not be the best principle to adhere to when dealing with a life-threatening disease, it must be the woman's prerogative to be given the facts, even if they are confusing, and to be allowed to decide for herself. If hysterectomy is inevitable, my practice has been to recommend the removal of ovaries after the age of forty-five, but only after discussing both sides of the question and making sure that hormone replacement would be accepted.

Since these issues are complicated, you should, if at all possible, not make rapid decisions or accept last-minute changes of plans just before surgery. If there is no emergency, you should have at least a week to consider the issues and make an informed decision. Knowing about these matters also means that in the unlikely event of an emergency, you will be able to participate in your care more effectively.

Another advantage of removing ovaries is that it prevents later complications, some of them requiring surgery. Ovarian cysts will not form if the ovaries are removed with hysterectomy. As already discussed, about 3 to 5 percent of women will develop ovarian cysts requiring repeat surgery after hysterectomy with retention of the ovaries. This shocking event happened to one of my patients.

I did the hysterectomy for this woman, a professional dancer, during the early 1980s, when she was in her mid-forties. Jackie had large fibroids, and the bleeding began to interfere with her career. The hormonal medications we tried did not produce much improvement. I gave her my usual presentation about ovarian cancer, heart disease, and osteoporosis before the operation. Jackie chose to keep her ovaries. Her surgery went well, and she continued without trouble for a few years afterward. I lost touch with her only when she moved out of New York City. Then she called me in a panic: She had developed lower abdominal pain, was found to have a pelvic mass, and an ultrasound scan showed an ominous picture. There was a larger ovarian cyst on one side, a smaller cyst on the opposite side, and much free-floating fluid in her pelvis surrounding the cysts. In short, she had a textbook case of ovarian cancer.

I rushed her through the standard workup expected before ovarian cancer surgery but, to my delight and astonishment, found the unexpected. She had two benign ovarian cysts, the larger with a twisted pedicle, or stalk, but no sign of cancer. The fluid was a consequence of the twisting. After this scare (by this time she was close to fifty), she finally decided to have her ovaries removed.

So far, it would appear that in the name of cancer prevention, ovaries may have to be removed prophylactically with abdominal or pelvic surgery from all women older than, say, forty, forty-five, or fifty. However, this is emphatically not the whole story, because there is a serious omission in our calculations. Here we must return to the loss of estrogen that follows the removal of pre-menopausal ovaries. This loss has serious adverse consequences for bones, and possibly for the heart. The gains from the removal of potentially cancer-bearing organs may not compare with losses accumulating from osteoporosis and heart disease if estrogen replacement therapy (ERT) is not instituted and continued.

Leon Speroff, a prominent gynecological endocrinologist from Portland, Oregon, addressed this issue in 1991 in the pages of the *American Journal of Obstetrics and Gynecology.* He came to the conclusion that for women who may not continue to take estrogen replacement therapy, it would be wiser not to remove ovaries unless there is a compelling reason to do so. You should note that with each choice, you are planning ahead for your next thirty or forty years, trying to assess what is better for the remainder of your life: removing your ovaries and replacing the hormones they produce or leaving them in your body and considering hormone treatment when you reach your natural menopause. To complete the picture, we must also address the thorny question of hormone replacement for women who become menopausal either spontaneously or because of gynecological surgery.

Menopause and Its Consequences

Record numbers of American women are now entering their late forties and early fifties; most will spend about one-third of their lives after menopause. Mentioning menopause no longer evokes an embarrassed silence. In fact, women's outspoken interest in this subject has recently produced a surge of articles, books, and fervent discussions about menopause. There have also been complaints that menopause has been "medicalized" and taken away from women. You may be relieved that you can no longer get pregnant, your PMS finally disappears, your fibroids shrink, or your endometriosis begins to fade. Unfortunately, the advantages come with a high price tag. Menopausal symptoms such as hot flashes and vaginal dryness appear in many women. Some find that their skin begins to look and feel thin and dry. Scalp and pubic hair may thin and fall out in handfuls; hair appears in new and unwanted places, including on the upper lips, the chin, and around the nipples. You may not be overly concerned with these purely cosmetic matters, but some years later more serious menopause-related conditions may appear, including heart disease and osteoporosis. Your ovaries have been protecting your health in the past by producing estrogen, and the appearance of many of these conditions is tied to reduced ovarian functions.

Menopause begins with ovaries aging and containing fewer egg cells capable of maturing and going on to ovulation. The hypothalamus and the pituitary try to resist this change by secreting more follicle stimulating hormone and luteinizing hormone (FSH and LH) to prod the ovaries back into activity. Increasing levels of these hormones begin to appear in the blood. Moderately high levels indicate that menopause is beginning. It may be months or years before the ovary finally stops responding to FSH and LH; meanwhile, the hormones are occasionally successful in producing ovulation. This so-called menopausal woman now ovulates, and she may even get pregnant. Such women have conceived in their late fifties and in their early sixties, although the majority of the pregnancies ended in miscarriages.

Yet higher values of FSH and LH prove that menopause is an established fact. Blood levels of FSH may increase tenfold after menopause. The hormone is excreted in the urine, an important source of hormones that was put to good use. Some of the earliest work on using these hormones to stimulate ovulation in infertile women was carried out in the 1950s and 1960s by extracting the hormones from barrelfuls of urine provided by menopausal nuns in Rome, Italy.

Pre-menopausal ovaries produce large amounts of estrogen, protecting your body and well-being in innumerable ways. As long as you ovulate, progesterone is also produced. This combination of hormones tends to prevent the development of endometrial (and possibly breast) cancer. With menopause, ovulation ceases, and progesterone all but disappears. The ovaries continue to produce, at least for a while, smaller amounts of estrogen. However, your body replaces the lost estrogen in a roundabout and ingenious way.

The ovaries and the adrenal glands, located just above the kidneys, have already been making two hormones, testosterone and androstenedione. These hormones are secreted, in much larger amounts, by men, but the ovaries, particularly after menopause, also produce them. Various tissues now convert these hormones to estrone, a hormone not as potent as estradiol. These processes are known as "peripheral conversion" because they take place away from your ovaries, in other organs and peripheral tissues, most notably in fat cells. The estrogens produced in this fashion mute the consequences of the loss of ovarian estradiol, but unconverted testosterone and androstenedione have adverse effects of their own. In addition to possibly causing baldness and the "male-distribution" hair loss noted earlier, the mix of lipids (fats such as cholesterol and others) appearing in the blood after menopause is not as good for your heart as the estradiol-induced mixture of lipids you had before. The net effect is an increased risk of coronary artery disease, possibly causing anginal pains and heart attacks.

Not all postmenopausal women are short of estrogen. Some women experience trouble because they have too many fat cells converting testosterone and androstenedione to estrone, developing excess amounts of estrogen. Without progesterone, estrogenic stimulation of the endometrium may produce endometrial hyperplasia. In some women, the hyperplasia continues long enough to turn into cancer. Fortunately, this sequence is preventable through the prolonged use of simple medical treatments with progesterone-like hormones.

You may not need elaborate hormone studies to understand what is happening in your body. If you are thin, sedentary, and a smoker, you probably need estrogen to protect you against osteoporosis and heart disease, but your chances of endometrial cancer are low. If you are substantially overweight and hirsute (hairy), and particularly if you also have diabetes or high blood pressure, you may have too much testosterone, androstenedione, and estrogens in your tissues, some of these changes increasing your chances of endometrial cancer. Your overall risks are smallest if you are fortunate enough to be of average weight, but ERT is probably beneficial for you even in the absence of the risk factors discussed.

Your ovaries and uterus may produce other substances that influence your state of health. Research conducted by Winnifred Cutler, Ph.D., some years ago, has shown that after menopause, regular intercourse, at least once a week, results in higher levels of estrogen. Prostaglandins, chemicals that appear ubiquitously in your tissues with a myriad of functions, are also produced in the uterus. However, their role in maintaining your health is not well understood.

It must be admitted that hormone replacement therapy has been a regular roller-coaster of advances and reversals trumpeted with immense publicity, and later reversed in quiet. Because of unarguable benefits to bones, I still recommend it, but this is not an easy decision.

The Signs of Menopause

The official definition of menopause is the absence of periods for a full year. In some women, menstrual periods may stop abruptly; in others they are phased out gradually, over a year or two. There may be much irregular bleeding before periods stop permanently. If you are not well informed about these processes, you may be persuaded to have an unnecessary hysterectomy. Irregular bleeding during the menopausal years should be investigated, ideally with endometrial biopsies and sonograms and possibly by means of hysteroscopy. A variety of treatments can be used to stop the excessive flow; hysterectomy should be reserved for cancer and certain precancerous changes, as discussed in Chapter 12.

The surgical loss of your ovaries before your spontaneous menopause (more bluntly described as castration) causes an immediate loss of estrogen. This is similar to menopausal losses; but because it is abrupt, its effects are usually more pronounced. The sudden onset of menopausal signs after surgery tells you that an essential substance has been lost. Hot flashes and other symptoms may appear within a day or two of the removal of the ovaries. Whether appearing spontaneously or in the wake of surgery, the signs are collectively referred to as the **menopausal syndrome** and consist of the following:

- Hot flashes are the most prominent sign of menopause. These consist of a feeling of warmth, often with profuse sweating, creeping over the face, the neck, the upper half of the body, and extending as far as the arms or the scalp. Some women have told me that their entire body throbs, sweating on the outside but chilled inside. These flashes appear without much warning, even during sleep, but more often under stressful circumstances. They may be short, lasting half a minute; other attacks are much longer. Many women find them uncomfortable; others call them disabling, particularly if they disturb work or sleep patterns.

Hot flashes (in England, they are called flushes) occur in over half of all women in Western societies. Anthropologists tell us that they are less frequent in more remote cultures. These women may have a different physiology, foods, and activity levels; cultural conditioning may also determine women's awareness or experience of these symptoms. Hot flashes usually last months or but may last years. They are thought to be due to diminished estrogen levels, but there is more to these annoying signs than we understand. Estrogen levels of women who have hot flashes are low, but not necessarily lower than the estrogen levels of women without them. More important, women can be short of estrogen without hot flashes. This seems good, except it also means that you may be short of estrogen without knowing it, your bones and heart gradually deteriorating without warning.

Testicles produce very little estrogen, but hot flashes may appear in men whose who have been castrated or who have certain hormonal diseases. GnRH analogs, discussed in Chapter 8, produce menopausal hot flashes in women and similar (but milder) sensations in men, who may get these or similar drugs as treatment for prostate or testicular cancer.

- Unwelcome changes in estrogen-dependent tissues are another consequence of menopause. The breasts and the womb shrink, the vaginal lining becomes dry, and sexual responses may be slower to appear and may not be as pronounced as before menopause.
- Nervousness, anxiety, depression, and irritability may occur. Poor sleep patterns or insomnia may cause a feeling of exhaustion. You may experience palpitations and joint pains. The exact role the loss of estrogen plays in producing these symptoms is difficult to delineate. As PMS sufferers know, the brain responds to hormones

profoundly, but in ways we cannot explain. Physicians and researchers have tried to correlate hormone levels with mood
changes and have pointed to a variety of experimental data to
support their ideas. Most experts are skeptical of such easy explanations. In an interview, Raphael Good, a Miami authority with
both OB/GYN and psychiatric training and a founding member
of the American Society for Psychosomatic Obstetrics and Gynecology, agreed with the view that the influence of hormones, of
giving or losing them, is exceedingly difficult to assess. It has been
observed that replacing estrogens usually produces an improved
mood, but it is difficult to account scientifically for this effect. The
most prevalent theory goes like this: Menopause causes hot
flashes, hot flashes cause insomnia, insomnia causes exhaustion and
irritability, hence the relief of hot flashes produces better moods.
It seems to me that this theory fails to tell us enough about the
mood changes women encounter while taking estrogen, but this
is the best "story" today.

• Heart disease is a rare condition before menopause but begins to
occur much more frequently several years after periods have
stopped, finally approaching male levels of heart disease.

• **Osteoporosis**, the loss of calcium and bone tissue, is one of the
most common conditions women develop decades after
menopause. If you have osteoporosis, you may be prone to fractures such as broken hips and forearm bones or a collapsed spine.
Fractured hips (the bone that breaks is actually the hip end of the
thighbone) are particularly lethal. Many women with these fractures die within a few months of the fracture. This may happen to
elderly women, whose poorly healed fractures render them
bedridden and who consequently develop complications such as
pneumonia.

To remedy these conditions, medical experts are almost unanimous in
recommending hormone replacement, particularly to women at high risk.
The earlier the age of menopause (see the next section), the higher the risk
of heart disease and osteoporosis. Ballet dancers and athletes often do not
ovulate, their ovaries producing little estrogen and no progesterone; these
women may develop osteoporosis at an unusually early age. Unfortunately,

unless hot flashes develop, osteoporosis is another silent disease: If you wait until a bone is fractured, the damage may be difficult or almost impossible to reverse. In fact, the first sign of osteoporosis is often an unexpected fracture: A bone is subjected to a stress it should be able to cope with—not a bone-crunching fall, just a slight fall that should do little more than jar your body. Nevertheless, a bone snaps. Plain x-rays cannot diagnose such a weakness; only more elaborate (and expensive) scans can do this.

Thin women need more protection than larger women. Exercise and calcium help, but not as much as estrogen. Smoking promotes osteoporosis, but it remains to be seen whether increasing the amount of estrogen customarily prescribed compensates for this effect. Complicated new treatments are now available for women with osteoporosis: drugs such as Fosamax, Raloxifene, and Calcitonin; a detailed discussion of these would be beyond the scope of this book.

Premature Menopause

In some women, menopause may appear prematurely, before the age of thirty-five or forty. Sometimes the cause is obvious: For example, pelvic radiation for cancer and chemotherapy for illnesses such as Hodgkin's disease may be responsible. Mumps may damage ovaries just as it may damage testicles. And as already discussed, hysterectomy may inadvertently result in the loss of ovarian function. More recent research has shown that immune diseases and chromosomal abnormalities may also be responsible.

You can tell if your menopause is approaching, even though you are still menstruating, by the following signs:

- You begin to have hot flashes and night sweats.
- Blood tests show higher-than-average levels of the two hormones mentioned earlier, FSH and LH.
- Your periods become less regular, less symptomatic, or completely pain-free. An impending menopause may also cause scanty periods. If you begin to bleed without any warning signs, such as cramps or breast swelling, the "period" is probably anovulatory, and this may be a sign of impending menopause.
- You feel hot all the time or begin to feel palpitations.
- Your breasts become less dense.

• You notice that vaginal lubrication diminishes and intercourse becomes painful.

Hormone Replacement Therapy

Hormone replacement therapy, abbreviated to HRT (or ERT for estrogen replacement therapy) is a complicated subject, which deserves its own book. There are several good books available, and some of these are listed among the references at the end of this book.

I have summarized the important issues you should understand but suggest that you read more about this subject. *The New Ourselves, Growing Older*, by Paula B. Doress-Worters and Diana L. Siegal (Peter Smith Publishers, 1996) is a valuable resource for menopause and a host of related subjects. The authors are wary of HRT, but they are honest and intelligent.

There are two ways of taking hormones. In the United States, the preferred way is called the sequential method, which is an imitation of the normal menstrual cycle. It consists of taking 0.625 or 1 mgm of estrogen a day from the first day of the month. The daily dose is continued for two weeks, when a progestational drug (also known as a progestin) is added for the next twelve to fourteen days: Now two hormones are taken daily. The dose of the second drug, usually medroxyprogesterone acetate (MPA, sold as Provera or Cycrin), used to be 10 mgm a day. Gynecologists then began to appreciate that MPA had adverse effects on serum lipids and possibly on moods, causing feelings of depression. With this in mind, the recommended dose of MPA was reduced to 5, or even 2.5, mgm daily. When the above course of medications has been completed, both drugs are stopped until the next cycle begins on the first day of the next month. There are other ways to take these hormones, but the variations are probably unimportant as long as a progestational drug is also consumed. Symptoms such as nausea, breast fullness, and slight spotting or bleeding may follow such a cycle, similar to the signs of a normal menstrual period or the symptoms that accompany and follow a course of BCPs.

In Europe, a different method is in use. No effort is made to imitate normal menstrual hormone activity. Instead, both hormones are taken every single day without interruption. The amounts of the hormones are similar to or identical with the amounts taken sequentially.

My preference is for the European method, which avoids the need for checking the calendar every day to find out which pills to take; many American gynecologists have switched to this approach that many women find less cumbersome. After a few months, the endometrium gets used to the monotonous levels of hormones, and breakthrough bleeding disappears or diminishes substantially. Nausea, breast complaints, and abdominal bloating are either absent or usually much less severe with this method, and there should be no mood swings.

Another European method deserves mention. Some experts recommend adding testosterone to the other hormones you may be prescribed. Testosterone is thought to improve libido and may help prevent osteoporosis. It is also likely to cause the growth of hair with a male pattern (that is, on the face, the upper lip, in the midline of the belly, and possibly between the breasts and on the nipples). Much depends on the dose taken; Canadian researchers Morrie Gelfand and Barbara Sherwin are convinced that the lower doses they recommend do not produce hairiness and are strong proponents of testosterone. With a few exceptions, American experts are less enthusiastic about this use of testosterone.

Before hormone replacement is started, you must get a complete physical examination. This should include your blood pressure, an examination of your breasts, mammograms, a pelvic examination with a Pap smear, blood tests for lipids, and at least a stool test for evidence of intestinal bleeding (or, even better, an elaborate test called sigmoidoscopy) to rule out colon cancer. Gynecologists do not usually take routine endometrial biopsies, reserving this test for women with abnormal bleeding. Follow-up visits must be scheduled, usually at intervals of six months.

There is only one serious objection to the data on which the recommendation to take estrogen is based. It is possible that the women who took hormone replacement were healthier to begin with and that their use of hormones was part of what they perceived was a healthy lifestyle. Two studies, supported by the National Institutes of Health, address these and similar issues. The first study, called Postmenopausal Estrogen/Progesterone Interventions, or PEPI, is already tracking a small number of women taking estrogen alone, or taking three combinations of estrogen with progesterone, or taking a placebo (an inert tablet) only. A much larger study, called the Women's Health Initiative (WHI) has been in progress for nearly ten years. WHI will collect data on over 100,000 menopausal women taking similar medications and is planned to last for fourteen years.

There are several problems with hormone replacement therapy, and we must not gloss over these. For example, many women given prescriptions for the hormones under discussion do not fill them or they take them for a few months only. Part of the reason for this may be that the media have emphasized headline-producing cancer-related disadvantages and down-played less attention-grabbing issues such as heart and bone disease. Also, women are probably more concerned with the apparently more immediate and dramatic threat of breast cancer than the more distant dangers of fractures and heart disease. The possibility that your chances of developing breast cancer may be increased by taking estrogen has received enormous publicity and is the focus of intense research. Some studies show no such effect, others show a minimal increase in breast cancer rates, and yet others show substantial increases among long-term users of high doses.

Also, hormone replacement, particularly if used in the cyclic pattern preferred by many American gynecologists, may cause some vaginal bleeding. This is a nuisance, but it should certainly not be used to convince you to undergo hysterectomy. Abnormal bleeding is easy to investigate with biopsies and sonograms. Women may be switched to the European regimen; if abnormalities are found, there are good surgical methods for dealing with them.

Many women are strongly opposed to the idea of decades of hormones for millions of women who are perfectly well. HRT may call for women to undergo potentially elaborate and expensive investigations and treatments, which are easy for them to misunderstand and for physicians to misuse. In addition to worrisome complications already discussed, such as vaginal bleeding and the links to endometrial and possibly breast cancer, there may be other difficulties if HRT is offered indiscriminately to most women as soon as they start their menopausal years. For instance, the medical community is uncertain whether the results of research based on predominantly white women are appropriate for recommending HRT to millions of women with a different ancestry. HRT may promote gallbladder disease and the formation of clots in veins. Its use is also contentious in women who are hypertensive or diabetic or who suffer from other medical conditions.

Medical research is habitually reported in articles that conclude by pleading for further research; HRT is complicated by the paucity of research on the use of progestational drugs such as Provera year after year. Estrogens have been under careful surveillance for well over twenty years. Whether the reassuring statistics developed during these years are reassuring enough and whether they can be extrapolated to forty or fifty years of continuous use remain open questions. Despite these drawbacks, I believe that there are sufficient benefits to the bones and the heart to justify the use of hormones.

Judging by the attention it has received in books and magazines and in sharp contrast to the silence of previous decades, menopause is one of the most interesting (and debated) health subjects for women. Along with exercise, calcium supplementation, and a healthy diet, HRT is, for many women, an important part of keeping well, fit, and in good shape.

Menopause-related research and the number of medical articles addressing menopausal issues have increased in a sharp crescendo. The North American Menopause Society (NAMS) is a well-established organization with excellent credentials. However, a measure of caution is essential. Some (perhaps much) menopause-related activity is commercial, driven by drug companies that manufacture the hormones and by physicians setting up "Women's Centers" and "Menopause Clinics." But it is not unreasonable to draw a parallel between the enormous attention arteriosclerotic heart disease began to receive in the 1960s and the recent upswing of interest in menopausal studies. The former led to men jogging and keeping fit, giving up smoking, watching their weight and cholesterol levels, and getting medical attention in the form of stress tests (cardiograms taken while exercising) and angiograms (x-rays of the vessels that supply the heart with blood). With all this attention, men now have fewer heart attacks and enjoy better health. It is women's turn now. Women are increasingly involved in cardiovascular and menopausal research, in finding out what is best for them. And we may reasonably expect that in time the net results will be equally good: better medical care, by doctors and by women themselves, and, ultimately, improved health for women.

APPENDIX

References, Resources, and Recommended Reading

References

This book provides you with information far more extensive and up-to-date than anything currently available apart from recent medical textbooks and articles in medical journals. The sources of many statements are identified in full in the text, thus many of these references are not repeated in this section. Readers may find it difficult to obtain texts and papers from, for example, the *New England Journal of Medicine*, or from a journal such as *Obstetrics and Gynecology*. To circumvent this, whenever possible, I have included references easily available to women in bookshops and libraries. However, if you are motivated enough to undertake some research, relatives or friends with access to a medical library (found in most hospitals and Departments of OB/GYN) may be willing to provide you with photocopies or printouts. Research librarians in public or medical libraries may also be able to help. Most important, popular services such as America Online (AOL) and Web sites such as Medline, Medscape, Grateful Med, and others are increasingly available to anyone with a computer and Internet connections to verify and expand the ideas presented in this book.

Another excellent Web site is <http://www.feminist.com>, with an exceptionally wide array of information.

If you need an excellent guide to gynecology in general, I recommend *The Complete Guide to Women's Health,* by Bruce D. Shepard, M.D., and Carroll A. Shepard, R.N., Ph.D. (Plume, New York, 1997). For an entirely different point of view, read *Our Bodies, Ourselves for the New Millennium,* by members of the Boston Women's Health Book Collective (Touchstone/Simon & Schuster, New York, 1998). *Our Bodies, Ourselves* is a classic; it presents a wealth of well-documented and thoroughly researched ideas, treating selected topics in an intelligent, humanitarian, distinctly political, and staunchly feminist point of view. However, and inevitably, it cannot cover all areas equitably. Sexuality, sexual health, and fertility-related topics are given about 240 pages; childbearing receives nearly 100 pages; gynecological and general medical topics are covered more cursorily in 90 pages. Hysterectomy and fibroids are discussed; pelvic pain is noted mostly in connection with intercourse; chronic pelvic pain is not mentioned. *The New Ourselves, Growing Older: Women Aging with Knowledge and Power,* by Diana Laskin Siegal, Paula Brown Doress-Worters, Wendy Sanford, and members of the Boston Women's Health Book Collective (Touchstone/Simon & Schuster, New York, 1994), treats menopause logically and thoughtfully.

Textbooks of gynecology written for medical students are not difficult to read and are less expensive than gynecological consultations. I recommend two: *Obstetrics and Gynecology,* by C. Beckmann and others (Williams & Wilkins, Baltimore, 1998); and *Essentials of Obstetrics and Gynecology,* by N. F. Hacker and J. G. Moore (W. B. Saunders, Philadelphia, 1998).

Te Linde's Operative Gynecology, edited by J. A. Thompson and J. D. Rock (Lippincott-Raven, Philadelphia, 1997), was written for gynecologists, but much of its over 1,600 pages should be comprehensible to intelligent women (or men). *Te Linde's* is an encyclopedic compendium of information; it is candid about unnecessary hysterectomies and about the complications, advantages, and disadvantages of gynecological surgery as well as some of its psychological aspects. Sections of the most recent (eighth) edition, published on the fiftieth anniversary of the first edition, are no longer up-to-date, but a new edition may be expected within a year or two.

Most medical terms are explained when first mentioned; they may also be traced through the index. You can also consult *Dorland's Illustrated Med-*

ical Dictionary (W. B. Saunders, Philadelphia, 2000) and *Stedman's Medical Dictionary* (Lippincott, Williams & Wilkins, Baltimore, 2000). If you have problems understanding medical texts, nurses or hospital-based social workers may be able to help you.

Many gynecological self-help books, including those dealing with alternatives to hysterectomy, are obsolete but continue to be sold. Any text published before the late 1990s, for example, will not discuss uterine artery embolization (UAE) for fibroids, a procedure that has attracted considerable public interest. Complete and impartial information about UAE is difficult to come by; it is provided in Chapter 9. Meanwhile, beware of spending time and money on information that may no longer be valid by checking the year of publication of any book or article, or the dates when updated or revised versions appeared.

If you are computer-savvy and connected to the Internet, you have a vast world of information at your fingertips and could spend many hours gathering and printing reams of materials. The immediate problem is that anyone who subscribes to a service such as AOL or has set up a Web site may post information available all over the world. Search engines cannot distinguish between impartial and expert advice, a gynecologist (or a radiologist) promoting his (or her) practice, and proponents of miscellaneous, possibly idiosyncratic views. Conversely, the Internet may be your most practical way to reach a so-called invasive radiologist who can perform uterine artery embolization (and is looking for patients) or a gynecologist hoping to increase his volume of laparoscopic myomectomies. Remember: dot.com is not about *communicating*, it is about *commerce;* many Web sites will prompt you with metronomic regularity to buy (or to subscribe to) something. The suffix .org stands for nonprofit (but not necessarily nonpartisan) organization; .edu originates from an educational institution; .gov from a governmental agency. For instance, cdc.gov tells you that the sponsoring organization is the Atlanta-based Centers for Disease Control.

Recommended Web sites are PubMed, previously sponsored by the National Library of Medicine but now allied with <http://www.all-heart.com>; Grateful Med; <http://www.NOAH.cuny.edu> from a consortium of New York City educational organizations. The Cochrane Collaboration, originally from Australia but now a worldwide consortium, provides excellent reviews of medical research and state-of-the-art practices, as does the Rand Corporation from California. Medscape, through which you can also log on to Medline, will help you obtain summaries of articles published in the medical literature. Internet addresses and search engines have undergone revolutionary changes in recent years; I expect that the above will remain accessible and useful in the years to come.

You will not find much information about chronic pelvic pain (CPP) in popular books, even in books about hysterectomy, or on the Internet. This may be because CPP is unusually complicated, because it has always been difficult to make sense of the profusion of dozens of possible causes and treatments, and perhaps because psychological factors are virtually impossible to write about without antagonizing readers. Treatments including hysterectomy for CPP remain controversial; it remains to be seen how effective the GnRH agonists will prove in the long term.

You may wish to read two excellent books about CPP written for medical professionals that contain many chapters easily accessible to nonprofessional readers: *Chronic Pelvic Pain: An Integrated Approach*, edited by J. F. Steege, D. A. Metzger, and B. S. Levy (W. B. Saunders, Philadelphia, 1998); and *Chronic Pelvic Pain: Evaluation and Management*, edited by R. E. Blackwell and D. L. Olive (Springer-Verlag, New York, 1998).

Detailed information about fibroids and endometriosis, beyond the four chapters in this book, is not easy to obtain. Sites such as <http:www.amazon.com> and <http:www.barnesandnoble.com> (or a visit to a good bookstore) will yield many books about these problems—perfectly adequate volumes containing a collection of simple, basic facts, but not as complete as the materials in this book. Books published before about 1998 rarely contain information about uterine artery embolization (UAE), a procedure that caught major public interest during the late 1990s. However, see two books and other materials by Mary Lou Ballweg and the Endometriosis Association, listed in the Recommended Reading section below.

Resources

American Association of Acupuncture and Oriental Medicine
4101 Lake Boone Trail, Suite 201
Raleigh, NC 27607
(919) 787-5181

American Association of Gynecological Laparoscopists
13021 East Florence Avenue
Santa Fe Springs, CA 90670
(800) 554-AAGL

American Association of Sex Educators,
    Counselors, and Therapists
435 North Michigan Avenue, Suite 1717
Chicago, IL
(312) 644-0828

American Cancer Society
1559 Clifton Road, NE
Atlanta, GA
(800) 952-7664 or (404) 320-3333

American College of Obstetricians and
    Gynecologists
409 Twelfth Street SW
Washington, DC
(202) 638-5577

American Medical Women's Association
801 North Fairfax Street, Suite 400
Alexandria, VA 22314
(703) 838-0500

American Society for Psychosomatic OB/GYN
409 Twelfth Street SW
Washington, DC
(202) 863-2414 or 863-2516

American Society for Reproductive Medicine
1209 Montgomery Highway
Birmingham, AL 35216
(205) 978-5000

Boston Women's Health Book Collective
240-A Elm Street
Somerville, MA 02144
(617) 625-0271

Breast Cancer Action
55 New Montgomery Street, Suite 323
San Francisco, CA 94105
(415) 243-9301

Endometriosis Association
8585 North 76th Place
Milwaukee, WI 53225
(800) 992-3636 or (414) 355-2200

Gilda Radner Familial Ovarian Cancer Registry
Department of Gynecologic Oncology, Roswell Park Cancer Institute
Elm and Carlton Streets
Buffalo, NY 14263
(800) OVARIAN

Help for Incontinent People
P.O. Box 544
Union, SC
(800) 252-3337

Interstitial Cystitis Association of America
51 Monroe Street, Suite 1402
Rockville, MD 20850
(800) HELP-ICA

National Cancer Institute Office of Cancer Communications
National Cancer Institute
NIH Building 31, Room 10A24
Bethesda, MD 20892
(800) 4-CANCER

National Osteoporosis Foundation
P.O. Box 96616
Department N1
Washington, DC 20077
(800) 223-9994

North American Menopause Society
P.O. Box 94527
Cleveland, OH 44101
(440) 442-7550

Sex Information and Education Council
130 West 42nd Street
New York, NY 10036
(212) 819-9770

Women's Cancer Resource Center
3023 Shattuck Street
Berkeley, CA 94705
(510) 548-9286

Recommended Reading

The following additional sources may prove useful if you wish to read more about the subjects covered in this book:

American Cancer Society. *Cancer Facts and Figures, 2000.*

Angier, N. *Woman: An Intimate Geography.* Doubleday and Co., New York, 2000. A kaleidoscopic and astonishingly colorful and detailed account of the way women think and how their bodies work. Written by the prize-winning reporter for the *New York Times;* highly recommended.

Bachmann, G. "Hysterectomy: A Critical Review." *Journal of Reproductive Medicine,* 1990, 35:839. An excellent review with an extensive list of references, some too dated to be useful. Gloria Bachmann is an expert who has had a lifelong interest in various aspects of hysterectomy; her writings are an essential resource for women.

Ballweg, M. J., and the Endometriosis Association (EA). The EA was established nearly twenty-five years ago; it provides support for women with "endo" and is also active in education and research. EA headquarters are in Milwaukee, WI; they can be reached at (800) 992-3636 or at (414) 355-2200. In addition to numerous other resources, Mary Lou Ballweg, EA's president, and the Endometriosis Association have produced two books: *The Endometriosis Sourcebook* (Contemporary Books, Chicago, 1995) and *Overcoming Endometriosis* (Congdon & Weed, 1987).

Barbieri, R. L., and A. J. Friedman. *Gonadotropin Releasing Hormone Analogs: Applications in Gynecology.* Elsevier, New York, 1991.

Beard, R. W., and others. "Bilateral Oophorectomy and Hysterectomy in the Treatment of Intractable Pelvic Pain Associated with Pelvic Congestion." *British Journal of Obstetrics and Gynaecology,* 1991, 98:988. Beard, the most respected gynecologist and researcher of CPP in the United Kingdom, has for many years advocated the excision of the womb and the ovaries for women with severe CPP.

Bonica, J. *The Management of Pain.* 2 vols. Lea and Febiger, 1990. A two-volume text by one of the pioneers of chronic pain studies. Bonica, who died recently, coined and popularized a new concept: chronic pain states. Also see the two books by P. Wall listed below.

Bradley, L. D., and J. S. Newman. "Uterine Artery Embolization for the Treatment of Fibroids." *The Female Patient* (Chatham, NJ), 2000, 25, 2:71.

Broder, M. S., and others. "The Appropriateness of Recommendations for Hysterectomy." *Obstetrics and Gynecology,* 2000, 95:199.

Carlson, K. J., and others. "The Maine Women's Health Study: I. Outcomes of Hysterectomy." *Obstetrics and Gynecology,* 1994 83:556. Based on a relatively small number of operations (418), Karen J. Carlson reports that hysterectomy was highly effective in relieving chronic pelvic pain, with few new problems encountered after surgery.

Carlson, K. J., D. H. Nichols, and I. Schiff. "Indications for Hysterectomy." *New England Journal of Medicine,* March 25, 1993, 328:856.

Chalker, R., and K. E. Whitmore. *Overcoming Bladder Disorders.* Harper and Row, New York, 1990.

Damasio, A. *Descartes' Error: Emotion, Reason, and the Human Brain.* Grosset-Putnam, New York, 1994.

––––––. *The Feeling of What Happens.* Harcourt, New York, 2000.

Dennerstein, L., and others. "Sexual Response Following Hysterectomy and Oophorectomy." *Obstetrics and Gynecology*, 1977, 49:92.

Dexeus, S., and others. "Preservation of the Ovaries: A Controversial Subject." *European Journal of Obstetrics, Gynecology and Reproductive Biology*, 1988, 28:146.

Fedele, L., and others. "The Risk of Recurrence After Myomectomy." *British Journal of Obstetrics and Gynaecology*, 1991, 98:385. A well-known gynecologist and researcher from Milan, Italy, reports a recurrence rate of 27 percent during the first ten years after myomectomy.

Goldstein, S. R., and L. Ashner. *The Estrogen Alternative.* Berkley Publishing, New York, 1999. Covers estrogen and newer drugs such as Raloxifene, effective in preventing osteoporosis, and possibly preventing breast cancer.

Hardman, J. *Goodman and Gilman's* The Pharmacological Basis of Therapeutics. McGraw-Hill Publishers, New York, 1996. An academic tome, not for those afraid of detail, but containing encyclopedic information about drugs.

Harrison, K. *The Kiss.* William Morrow & Co., New York, 1998. The celebrated account of a young woman's affair with her father.

Herman, J. L. *Father-Daughter Incest.* Reprint, Harvard University Press, Boston, 2000.

———. *Trauma and Recovery.* Basic Books, New York, 1997.

Hillis, S. D., and others. "The Effectiveness of Hysterectomy for Chronic Pelvic Pain." *Obstetrics and Gynecology*, 1995, 86:941. Susan Hillis reports that most women with CPP have long-term improvement, but some continue to experience long-term pain.

Kjerulff, K. H., and others. "The Effectiveness of Hysterectomy." *Obstetrics and Gynecology*, 2000, 95, 3:319. Reports on the effect of surgery on the various symptoms of nearly 1,300 women from Maryland. To reduce a long and detailed paper to one sentence: 92 percent improved; 8 percent did not improve.

Leonardo, R. A. *History of Gynecology.* Froben Press, New York, 1944.

Lerner, J., and R. Jaffe. "Scholarly Debate: Should Women Undergo Routine Ovarian Cancer Screening?" *The Female Patient* (Chatham, NJ), 2000, 25, 6:20. Two experts agree to disagree.

Longo, D. "The Rise and Fall of Battey's Operation: A Fashion in Surgery." *Bulletins of the History of Medicine*, 1979, 53:244.

Love, S., with K. Lindsey. *Dr. Susan Love's Hormone Book: Making Informed Choices About Menopause.* Random House, New York, 1997. Dr. Susan Love and Karen Lindsey of *Breast Book* fame have written another intelligent, down-to-earth yet sophisticated book. Highly recommended.

Love, S. with K. Lindsey. *Dr. Susan Love's Breast Book.* Perseus Books, Boston, 2000.

Miller, N. F. "Hysterectomy: Therapeutic Necessity or Surgical Racket?" *American Journal of Obstetrics and Gynecology,* 1946, 51:804. The first major attack on unnecessary hysterectomy.

Nachtigall, L., and J. R. Heilman. *Estrogen.* Harperinformation, New York, 2000. An excellent introduction from Lila Nachtigall, an expert on hormone replacement therapy.

National Cancer Institute. "Low Malignant Potential Tumor of the Ovary." NCI, Bethesda, MD. Call (800) 4 CANCER.

_____. Twenty-four-hour information service with prerecorded messages: (800) 4 CANCER.

_____. "What Are Clinical Trials All About?" NCI, Bethesda, MD. Call (800) 4 CANCER.

_____. "What You Need to Know About Cancer of the Cervix." NCI, Bethesda, MD. Call (800) 4 CANCER.

Netter, F. H. *The CIBA Collection of Medical Illustrations, Vol. 2: The Reproductive System.* CIBA Pharmaceutical Company, New Jersey, 1977.

Piver, M. S., and G. Wilder. *Gilda's Disease.* Prometheus Books, New York, 1996. Piver is a senior GYN oncologist at Roswell Park, a prominent cancer center in Buffalo, New York; Gene Wilder was comedian Gilda Radner's husband at the time of her death from ovarian cancer.

Rapkin, A. J., and L. D. Kames. "The Pain Management Approach to Chronic Pelvic Pain." *Journal of Reproductive Medicine,* 1987, 32:323. Andrea Rapkin is one of the best-known American experts on CPP. This paper outlines the treatments she advocates. However, due to its vintage, this article does not mention recent advances such as treatment with the GnRH agonists.

Reiter, R. C., ed. "Chronic Pelvic Pain." In *Clinical Obstetrics and Gynecology,* Vol. 33, p. 117 (Lippincott, New York, 1990). An excellent overall review; however, because it was published in 1990, this book does not contain any information about the treatment of CPP with GnRH agonists.

Schofield, M. J., and others. "Self-Reported Long-term Outcomes of Hysterectomy." *British Journal of Obstetrics and Gynaecology,* 1991, 98:1129. Reports good overall satisfaction with surgery in New Zealand.

Shorter, E. *From Paralysis to Fatigue: A History of Psychosomatic Illness in the Modern Era.* The Free Press/Macmillan, New York, 1992.

Showalter, E. *The Female Malady: Women, Madness, and English Culture.* Viking Penguin, New York, 1989.

"Special Surveillance for Reproductive Health." *MMWR: Morbidity and Mortality Weekly Review,* August 8, 1997, Vol. 46, No. SS-4. Provides a variety of hysterectomy-related statistics from 1980 through 1993 and gives references for earlier years as well as other relevant information.

Speert, H. *Obstetrics and Gynecology in America: A History.* Waverly Press, Baltimore, 1980.

Stovall, T. G., and others. "Hysterectomy for Chronic Pelvic Pain of Presumed Uterine Etiology." *Obstetrics and Gynecology,* 1990, 75:676. Despite serious statistical problems, this paper shows that at least some women with CPP are helped by hysterectomy. However, and mysteriously, a few remain unchanged, or their problems increase.

Stringer, N. H. "Pirfenidone and Tibolone." *The Female Patient* (Chatham, NJ), 2000, 25, 5:28.

Verkauf, B. "Myomectomy for Fertility Enhancement and Preservation." *Fertility and Sterility,* 1992, 58:1.

Wall, P. *Textbook of Pain.* 2 vols. W. B. Saunders, Philadelphia, 1999. An extensive encyclopedia. Two-volume books such as Wall's and Bonica's are extraordinarily expensive, about $250 each per set—more appropriate for professionals in pain management, an established specialty, or for medical libraries. More suitable for nonmedical readers is the next entry, a shorter, popular account by Wall, another pioneer.

_____. *Pain: The Science of Suffering.* Columbia University Press, New York, 2000.

Wangensteen, O. H., and S. D. Wangensteen. *The Rise of Surgery.* University of Minnesota Press, Minneapolis, 1978.

Wright, R. C. "Hysterectomy: Past, Present, and Future." Editorial, *Obstetrics and Gynecology,* 1969, 33:560. Of historical interest only.

INDEX